BIOMEDICAL DEVICE TECHNOLOGY

ABOUT THE AUTHOR

Anthony Y. K. Chan graduated in Electrical Engineering (B.Sc. Hon.) from the University of Hong Kong in 1979, completed a M.Sc. degree in Engineering from the same university, and worked for a number of years as a project engineer in electrical instrumentations, control, and systems. In 1987, he completed a Master of Engineering Degree (M.Eng.) in Clinical Engineering from the University of British Columbia in Canada. He also holds a Certificate in Hospital Services Management from the Canadian Healthcare Association. Anthony was the director and manager of biomedical engineering in a number of Canadian acute care hospitals. He is currently the Program Head of the Biomedical Engineering Technology Program at the British Columbia Institute of Technology and Adjunct Professor of the Biological and Chemical Engineering Department of the University of British Columbia. He is a Professional Engineer, a Chartered Engineer, and a Certified Clinical Engineer.

BIOMEDICAL DEVICE TECHNOLOGY

Principles and Design

By

ANTHONY Y. K. CHAN, MSc, MEng, PEng, CCE

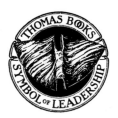

CHARLES C THOMAS • PUBLISHER, LTD.
Springfield • Illinois • U.S.A.

Published and Distributed Throughout the World by

CHARLES C THOMAS • PUBLISHER, LTD.
2600 South First Street
Springfield, Illinois 62704

© 2008 by CHARLES C THOMAS • PUBLISHER, LTD.

ISBN 978-0-398-07699-3 (hard)
ISBN 978-0-398-07700-6 (paper)

Library of Congress Catalog Card Number: 2006050066

With THOMAS BOOKS *careful attention is given to all details of manufacturing
and design. It is the Publisher's desire to present books that are satisfactory as to their
physical qualities and artistic possibilities and appropriate for their particular use.*
THOMAS BOOKS *will be true to those laws of quality that assure a good name
and good will.*

Printed in the United States of America
SM-R-3

Library of Congress Cataloging-in-Publication Data

Chan, Anthony Y. K.
    Biomedical device technology : principles and design / by Anthony Y. K.
Chan.
        p. cm.
    Includes bibliographical references and index.
    ISBN 978-0-398-07699-3 -- ISBN 978-0-398-07700-6 (pbk.)
    1. Medical instruments and apparatus. 2. Medical technology. 3.
Biomedical engineering. I. Title.

R856.C43 2007
610.28--dc22

                                                            2006050066

To my wife, Elaine
and
my daughters, Victoria and Tiffany

PREFACE

For many years, the tools available to physicians were limited to a few simple handpieces such as stethoscopes, thermometers, and syringes; medical professionals primarily relied on their senses and skills to perform diagnosis and disease mitigation. Today, diagnosis of medical problems is heavily dependent on the analysis of information made available by sophisticated medical machineries such as electrocardiographs, ultrasound scanners, and laboratory analyzers. Patient treatments often involve specialized equipment such as cardiac pacemakers and electrosurgical units. Such biomedical instrumentations play a critical and indispensable role in modern medicine.

In order to design, build, maintain, and effectively deploy medical devices, one must understand not only their design and construction but also how they interact with the human body. This book provides a comprehensive approach studying the principles and design of biomedical devices as well as their applications in medicine. It is written for engineers and technologists who are interested in understanding the principles, design, and applications of medical device technology. The book is also intended to be used as a textbook or reference for biomedical device technology courses in universities and colleges.

The most common reason of medical device obsolescence is changes in technology. For example, vacuum tubes in the 1960s, discrete semiconductors in the 1970s, integrated circuits in the 1980s, microprocessors in the 1990s, and networked multiprocessor software-driven systems in today's devices. The average life span of medical devices has been diminishing; current medical devices have a life span of about 5 to 7 years. It is unrealistic to write a book on medical devices and expect that the technology described will remain current and valid for years. On the other hand, the principles of medical device applications, the origins of physiological signals and their methods of acquisition, and the concepts of signal analysis and processing will remain largely unchanged. This book focuses on the functions and principles of medical devices (which are the invariant components) and uses specific designs and constructions to illustrate the concepts where appropriate.

The first part of this book discusses the fundamental building blocks of biomedical instrumentations. Starting from an introduction of the origins of biological signals, the essential functional building blocks of a typical medical device are studied. These functional blocks include electrodes and transducers, biopotential amplifiers, signal conditioners and processors, electrical safety and isolation, output devices, and visual display systems. The next section of the book covers a number of biomedical devices. Their clinical applications, principles of operations, functional building blocks, special features, performance specifications, as well as common problems and safety precautions are discussed. Architectural and schematic diagrams are used where appropriate to illustrate how specific device functions are being implemented.

Due to the vast variety of biomedical devices available in health care, it is impractical to include all of them in a single book. This book selectively covers diagnostic and therapeutic devices that are either commonly used or whose principles and design represent typical applications of the technology. To limit the scope, medical imaging equipment and laboratory instrumentations are excluded from this book.

Three Appendices are included at the end of the book. These are appended for those who are not familiar with these concepts yet an understanding in these areas will enhance the comprehension of the subject matters in the book. They are: A–1. A Primer on Fourier Analysis; A–2. Overview of Medical Telemetry Development; and A–3. Medical Gas Supply Systems.

I would like to take the opportunity to acknowledge Euclid Seeram, who encouraged and inspired me to embark in writing, and Michael Thomas for agreeing to publish and giving me the extra time to finish this book.

Anthony Y. K. Chan

CONTENTS

APPENDICES

BIOMEDICAL DEVICE TECHNOLOGY

Chapter 1

OVERVIEW OF BIOMEDICAL
INSTRUMENTATION

OBJECTIVES

- Define "medical device."
- Analyze biomedical instrumentation using a systems approach.
- Explain the origin and characteristics of biopotentials and common physiological signals.
- Explain the importance and approaches of human factor engineering in medical device design.
- List common input, output, and control signals of medical devices.
- Identify the special constraints encountered in the design of biomedical devices.
- Define biocompatibility and list common biomaterials used in medical devices.
- Explain the tissue responses and approaches to achieve biocompatibility.
- Identify the basic functional building blocks of medical instrumentation.

CHAPTER CONTENTS

1. Introduction
2. Classification of Medical Devices
3. Systems Approach
4. Origins of Biopotentials
5. Physiological Signals

3

6. Human Machine Interface
7. Input, Output, and Control Signals
8. Constraints in Biomedical Signal Measurements
9. Concepts on Biocompatibility
10. Functional Building Blocks of Medical Instrumentation

INTRODUCTION

Medical devices come with different designs and complexity. They can be as simple as a tongue depressor, as compact as a rate-responsive demand pacemaker, or as sophisticated as a surgical robot. Although most medical devices use similar technology as their commercial counterparts, there are many fundamental differences between devices used in medicine and devices used in other applications. This chapter will look at the definition of medical devices and the characteristics that differentiate a medical device from other household or commercial products.

According to the United States Food and Drug Administration (FDA), a "medical device" is defined as:

> "an instrument, apparatus, implement, machine, contrivance, implant, in vitro reagent, or other similar or related article, including a component part, or accessory which is:
>
> - recognized in the official National Formulary, or the United States Pharmacopoeia, or any supplement to them,
> - intended for use in the diagnosis of disease or other conditions, or in the cure, mitigation, treatment, or prevention of disease, in man or other animals, or
> - intended to affect the structure or any function of the body of man or other animals, and which does not achieve any of its primary intended purposes through chemical action within or on the body of man or other animals and which is not dependent upon being metabolized for the achievement of any of its primary intended purposes."

A "medical device" is similarly defined in the Canadian Food and Drugs Act, as:

> "Any article, instrument, apparatus or contrivance, including any component, part or accessory thereof, manufactured, sold or represented for use in:
>
> (a) the diagnosis, treatment, mitigation or prevention of a disease, disorder or abnormal physical state, or the symptoms thereof, in humans or animals;
> (b) restoring, correcting or modifying a body function, or the body structure of humans or animals;

(c) the diagnosis of pregnancy in humans or animals; or

(d) the care of humans or animals during pregnancy, and at, and after, birth of the offspring, including care of the offspring, and includes a contraceptive device but does not include a drug."

Apart from the obvious, it is clear from these definitions that in vitro diagnostic products such as medical laboratory instruments are medical devices. Furthermore, accessories, reagents, or spare parts associated with a medical device are also considered to be medical devices. An obvious example of this is the electrodes of a heart monitor. Another example, which may not be as obvious, is the power adapter to a medical device such as a laryngoscope. Both of these accessories are considered as medical devices and are therefore regulated by the premarketing and postmarketing regulatory controls.

CLASSIFICATION OF MEDICAL DEVICES

There are many different approaches to classify or group medical devices. Devices can be grouped by their functions, their technologies, or their applications. A description of some common classification methods follows.

Classified by Functions

Grouping medical devices by their functions is by far the most common way to classify medical devices. Devices can be separated into two main categories: diagnostic and therapeutic.

Diagnostic devices are used to determine physical signs and diseases and/or injury without alteration of the structure and function of the biological system. However, some diagnostic devices may alter the biological system to a certain extent due to their applications. For example, a real-time blood gas analyzer may require invasive catheters (which puncture the skin into a blood vessel) to take PCO_2 measurement. A computer tomography scanner will impose ionization radiation (transfer energy) on the human body in order to obtain the medical images.

Diagnostic devices whose functions are to determine the changes of certain physiological parameters over a period of time are often referred to as monitoring devices. As the main purpose of this class of devices is trending, absolute accuracy may not be as important as their repeatability. Examples of monitoring devices are heart rate monitors used to detect variation of heart rates during a course of drug therapy, and noninvasive blood pressure monitors to watch arterial blood pressure immediately after surgery.

Therapeutic devices are designed to effect structural or functional changes that lead to improved overall function of the patient. Examples of such devices are electrosurgical units in surgery, linear accelerators in cancer treatment, and infusion devices in fluid management therapy. Assistive devices are a group of devices used to restore an existing function of the human body. They may be considered a subset of therapeutic devices. Examples are demand pacemakers to restore normal heart rhythm, hearing aids to assist hearing, and wheelchairs to enhance mobility of the disabled.

Based on the methods of application, these device classes can be further subdivided into invasive or noninvasive, automatic or manual.

Classified by Physical Parameters

Medical devices can also be grouped by the physical parameters that they are measuring. For example, a blood pressure monitor is a pressure monitoring device, an airway spirometer is a flow measurement device, and a tympanic thermometer is a temperature-sensing device.

Classified by Principles of Transduction

Some medical devices are grouped according to the types of transducers used at the patient-machine interface such as resistive, inductive, or ultrasonic.

Classified by Physiological Systems

Medical devices may also be grouped by their related human physiological systems. Examples of such grouping are blood pressure monitors and electrocardiographs as cardiovascular devices, and respirators and mechanical ventilators as pulmonary devices.

Classified by Clinical Medical Specialties

In another model, devices are grouped according to the medical specialties (such as pediatrics, obstetrics, etc.) in which they are being used. For example, a fetal monitor is considered as an obstetric device, an x-ray machine as a radiological device.

Classified by Risk Classes

For biomedical engineers and regulatory personnel, medical devices are often referred to by their risk class. Risk classes are created to differentiate devices by rating their risk level on patients. A device risk classification determines the degree of scrutiny and regulatory control imposed on the manufacturers and users by regulatory bodies to ensure their safety and efficacy in clinical use. Table 1–1 shows examples of medical devices in each risk class under the Canadian Medical Device Regulations. Similar risk classifications are used in the United States and Europe.

Table 1–1.
Risk Classification

Four risk classes–from Class I (lowest risk) to Class IV (highest risk)	
Class I	conductive electrode gel, band-aids
Class II	latex gloves, contact lenses
Class III	IV bags, indwelling catheters
Class IV	heart valve implants, defibrillators

SYSTEMS APPROACH

In simple terms, a system is defined as a group of things or parts or processes working together under certain relationships. A system transforms a set of input entities to a set of output entities. Within a system there are aspects, variables, or parameters that mutually act on each other. A closed system is self-contained on a specific level and is separated from and not influenced by the environment, whereas an open system is influenced by the environmental conditions by which it is surrounded. Figure 1–1 shows an example of a system. The elements within a system and their relationships as well as the environment can affect the performance of the system. A more complicated system may contain multiple numbers of subsystems or simple systems.

In analyzing a large complex system, one can divide the system into several smaller subsystems with the output from one subsystem connected to the input of another. The simplest subsystem consists of an input, an output, and a process as shown in Figure 1–2. The process that takes the output and feeds it back to the input in order to modify the output is called a feedback process. A system with feedback is called a closed-loop system, whereas a system without any feedback is called an open-loop system. Most systems that we encounter contain feedback paths and hence are closed-loop systems.

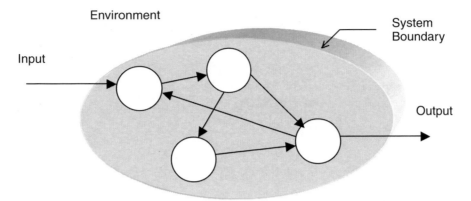

Figure 1–1. Typical System.

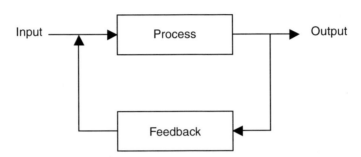

Figure 1–2. Basic Subsystem.

Listening to radio is an example of a simple closed-loop system. The input to the system is the radio broadcast in the form of an electromagnetic wave that is received by the radio. The radio processes the received signal and produces the audible sound such as music. If the music (output) is not loud enough, you turn up the volume to increase the sound level. In doing this, you become the feedback process that analyzes the loudness of the music and produces the action to turn up the volume.

The systems approach is basically a generalized technique to understand organized complexity. It provides a unified framework or a way of thinking about the systems and can be developed to handle specific problems. In order to solve a problem, one must look at all components within the system and analyze the input and output of each subsystem in view to isolate the problem and establish the relationships of the problem with respect to each component in the system.

Using block diagrams to analyze complex devices is an application of the systems approach. Figure 1–3 shows a compact disc (CD) music player system. The input to the CD player is the musical CD, the output is sound (or music), and the feedback is the listener who will replace the CD when it has finished playing or turn down the volume if it is too loud. If the CD player is not working properly, one may buy a new one and discard the malfunctioning unit.

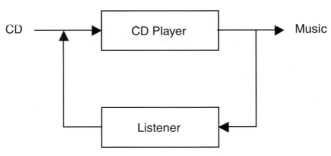

Figure 1–3. CD System.

The CD player can be divided into its functional blocks as shown in Figure 1–4. One may be able to troubleshoot and isolate the problem to one of the functional blocks. In this case, it will be cheaper just to replace the malfunctioning block. For example, if the speakers are not working, it may be more economical to get a pair of replacement speakers than to replace the entire CD player.

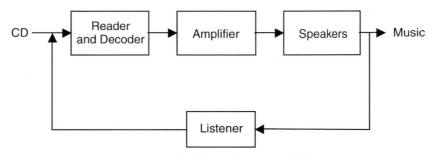

Figure 1–4. CD Player Functional Block.

Similarly, a complex biomedical device can be broken down into its functional building blocks. Figure 1–5 shows a block diagram of an electrocardiogram (ECG) system. The input to the device is the biopotential from the heart activities. The electrodes pick up this tiny electrical signal from the patient and send it to the amplifier block to increase the signal amplitude. The amplified ECG signal is then sent to the signal analysis block to extract information such as the heart rate. Finally, the ECG signal is sent to the output block such as a paper chart recorded to produce a hard copy of the ECG tracing. These blocks can be further subdivided, eventually down to the individual component level. Note that the cardiology technologist is also considered a part of the system. He or she serves as the feedback loop by monitoring the output and modifying the input.

When analyzing or troubleshooting a medical device, it is important to understand the functions of each building block, and what to expect from the output when a known input is applied to the block. Furthermore, medical devices are, in most cases, conceptualized, designed, and built from a combination of functional building blocks or modules.

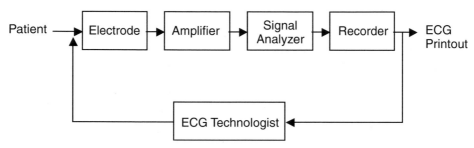

Figure 1–5. ECG Block Diagram.

ORIGINS OF BIOPOTENTIALS

The source of electrical events in biological tissue is the ions in the electrolyte solution, as opposed to the electrons in electrical circuits. Biopotential is an electrical voltage caused by a flow of ions through biological tissues. It was first studied by Luigi Galvani, an Italian physiologist and physicist, in 1786. In living cells, there is an ongoing flow of ions (predominantly sodium-Na^+, potassium-K^+ and chloride-Cl^-) across the cell membrane. The cell membrane allows some ions to go through readily but resists others. Hence it is called a semipermeable membrane.

There are two fundamental causes of ion flow in the body: diffusion and drift. Fick's law states that if there is a high concentration of particles in one region and they are free to move, they will flow in a direction that equalizes the concentration; the force that results in the movement of charges is called diffusion force. The movement of charged particles (such as ions) that is due to the force of an electric field (static forces of attraction and repulsion) constitutes particle drift. Each cell in the body has a potential voltage across the cell membrane known as the single-cell membrane potential.

Under equilibrium, the net flow of charges across the cell membrane is zero. However, due to an imbalance of positive and negative ions internal and external to the cell, the potential inside a living cell is about –50 mV to –100 mV with respect to the potential outside it (Figure 1–6). This membrane potential is the result of the diffusion and drift of ions across the high resistance but semipermeable cell membrane, predominantly sodium [Na^+] and potassium [K^+] ions moving in and out of the cell. Because of the semipermeable nature of the membrane, Na^+ is partially restricted from passing into the cell. In addition, a process called the sodium-potassium pump moves sodium ions at two to five times the rate out of the cell than potassium ions into the cell. However, in the presence of diffusion and drift, an equilibrium point is established when the net flow of ions across the cell's membrane becomes zero. As there are more positive ions (Na^+) moved outside the cells than positive ions (K^+) moved into the cell, under equilibrium, the inside of the cell is more negative than the outside. Therefore, the inside of the cell is negative with respect to the outside. This is called the cell's resting potential, which is typically about –70 mV.

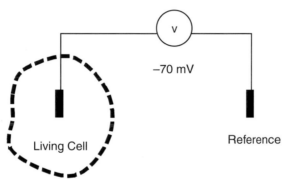

Figure 1–6. Cell Membrane Potential.

If the potential across the cell membrane is raised, for example by an external stimulation, to a level that exceeds the threshold, the permeability of the cell membrane will change, causing a flow of Na^+ ions into the cell. This inrush of positive ions will create a positive change in the cell's membrane potential to about 20 mV to 40 mV more positive than the potential outside the cell. This action potential lasts for about 1 to 2 milliseconds. As long as the action potential exists, the cell is said to be depolarized. The membrane potential will drop eventually as the sodium-potassium pump repolarizes the cell to its resting state (–70 mV). This process is called repolarization and the time period is called the refractory period. During the refractory period, the cell is not responsive to any stimulation.

The events of depolarization and repolarization are shown in Figure 1–7.

The rise in the membrane potential from its resting stage (when stimulated) and return to the resting state is called the action potential. Cell potentials form the basis of all electrical activities in the body, including such activities as the electrocardiogram (ECG), electroencephalogram (EEG), electrooculogram (EOG), electroretinogram (ERG), and electromyogram (EMG).

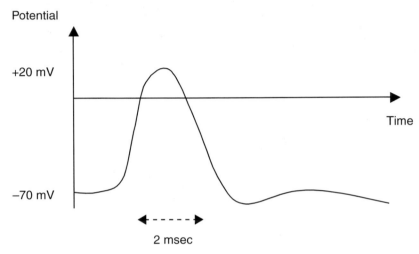

Figure 1–7. Action Potential.

When a cell is depolarized (during which the membrane potential changes from negative to positive), the cells next to it may be triggered into depolarization. This disturbance is propagated either to adjacent cells, resulting in the entire tissue becoming depolarized (in an entire motor group), or along the length of the cell from one cell to the next (in a single motor unit or a nerve fiber).

In most biopotential signal measurements, unless one is using a needle electrode to measure the action potential of a single cell, the measured signal is the result of multiple action potentials from a group of cells or tissue. The amplitude and shape of the biopotential are largely dependent on the location of the measurement site and the signal sources. Furthermore, the biopotential signal will be altered as it propagates along the body tissue to the sensors. A typical example of biopotential measurement is measuring electrical heart activities using skin electrodes (electrocardiogram or ECG). Figure 1–8 shows a typical ECG waveform showing the electrical heart potential when a pair of electrodes is placed on the chest of the patient. This biopotential, which is the result of all action potentials from the heart tissue transmitted to the skin surface, is very different in amplitude and shape from the action potential from a single cell shown in Figure 1–7. In addition, placing the skin electrodes at different locations on the patient will produce very different looking ECG waveforms.

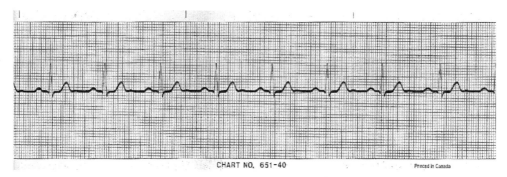

Figure 1–8. Typical ECG Obtained from Skin Electrodes.

PHYSIOLOGICAL SIGNALS

Biopotentials represent a substantial proportion of human physiological signals. In addition, there are other forms of physiological signals, such as pressure and temperature, all of which contain information that reflects the well-being of an individual. Monitoring and analyzing such parameters is of interest to medical professionals. Different physiological signals have different characteristics. Some physiological signals are very small compared with other background signals and noise; some change rapidly during the course of their measurement. Therefore, different transducers with matching characteristics are necessary in medical devices to accurately measure these signals. Table 1–2 shows some examples of common physiological signals; their characteristics and examples of the transduction techniques used to capture these signals are also listed. The range and bandwidth quoted in the list are nominal values, which may not include some extreme cases. An example is severe hypothermia, in which the body temperature can become many degrees below 32°C.

An example of a physiological signal measurement is the electrocardiogram. When skin electrodes are placed on the surface of a patient's chest, they pick up a small electrical potential at the skin surface from the activities of the heart. If one plots this potential against time, this is called an electrocardiogram. An example of an electrocardiogram is shown in Figure 1–8. The spike is called the R-wave, which coincides with the contraction phase of the ventricles. The time interval between two adjacent R-waves represents one heart cycle. The amplitude and the shape of the ECG signal depend on the physiological state of the patient as well as the locations and the types of electrodes used. From Table 1–2, the amplitude of the R-wave may vary from 0.5 to 4 mV, and the ECG waveform has a frequency range or bandwidth from 0.01 to 150Hz.

There are many more physiological signals than those listed in the table. While some are common parameters in clinical settings (e.g., body temperature), others are used sparingly (e.g., electroretinogram).

Table 1–2.
Characteristics of Common Physiological Parameters

Physiological Parameters	*Physical Units and Range of Measurement*	*Signal Frequency Range of Bandwidth*	*Measurement Method or Transducer Used*
Blood Flow	1 to 300 mL/s	0 to 20 Hz	Ultrasound Doppler flowmeter
Blood Pressure–Arterial	20 to 400 mmHg	0 to 50 Hz	Sphygmomanometer
Blood Pressure–Venous	0 to 50 mmHg	0 to 50 Hz	Semiconductor strain gauge
Blood pH	6.8 to 7.8	0 to 2 Hz	pH electrode
Cardiac Output	3 to 25 L/min	0 to 20 Hz	Thermistor (thermodilution)
Electrocardiography (ECG)	0.5 to 4 mV	0.01 to 150 Hz	Skin electrodes
Electroencephalography (EEG)–scalp	5 to 300 μV	0 to 150 Hz	Scalp electrodes
EEG–brain surface or depth	10 to 5,000 μV	0 to 150 Hz	Cortical or depth electrodes
Electromyography (EMG)	0.1 to 5 mV	0 to 10,000 Hz	Needle electrodes
Nerve Potentials	0.01 to 3 mV	0 to 10,000 Hz	Needle electrodes
Oxygen Saturation– Arterial (noninvasive)	85 to 100%	0 to 50 Hz	Differential light absorption
Respiratory Rate	5 to 25 breath/min	0.1 to 10 Hz	Skin electrodes (impedance pneumography)
Tidal Volume	50 to 1,000 ml	0.1 to 10 Hz	Spirometer
Temperature–Body	32 to 40°C	0 to 0.1 Hz	Thermistor

HUMAN-MACHINE INTERFACE

A medical device is designed to assist clinicians to perform certain diagnostic or therapeutic functions. In fulfilling these functions, a device interfaces with the patients as well as the clinical users. Figure 1–9 shows the interfaces between a medical device, the patient, and the clinical staff. For a diagnostic device, the physiological signal from the patient is picked up and processed by the device; the processed information such as the heart rhythm from an ECG monitor or blood pressure waveform from an arterial blood line is displayed by the device and reviewed by the clinical staff. For a therapeutic device, the clinical staff will, using the device, apply certain actions on the patient. For example, a surgeon may activate the electrosurgical hand piece during a procedure to coagulate a blood vessel. In another case, a nurse may set up an intravenous infusion line to deliver medication to a patient.

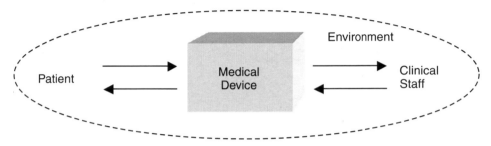

Figure 1–9. Human-Machine Interface.

These interfaces are important and often critical in the design of biomedical devices. An effective patient-machine interface is achieved through carefully choosing a transducer suitable for the application. For example, an implanted pH sensor must pick up the small changes in the hydrogen ion concentration in the blood; at the same time it also must withstand the corrosive body environment, maintain its sensitivity, and be nontoxic to the patient.

Other than safety and efficacy, human factor is another important consideration in designing medical devices. Despite the fact that human error is a major contributing factor toward clinical incidents involving medical devices, human factor is often overlooked in medical device design and in device acquisitions. The goal to achieve in user-interface design is to improve efficiency, reduce error, and prevent injury. Human factor engineering is a systematic, interactive design process that is critical to achieve an effective user-interface. It involves the use of various methods and tools throughout the design life cycle. Classical human factor engineering involves analysis of sensory limitations, perceptual and cognitive limitations, and effector limitations of the device users as well as the patients. Sensory limitation analysis evaluates the responses of the human visual, auditory, tactile, and olfactory systems. Perceptual and cognitive limitation analysis studies the nervous system's response to the sensory information. Perception refers to how people identify and organize sensory input; cognition refers to higher-level mental phenomena such as abstract reasoning, formulating strategies, formation of hypothesis, et cetera. Effector limitation analysis evaluates the outputs or responses of the operators (e.g., the reaction time, force-exerting capability, etc.).

There are three subjects to be focused on in human factor design in medical devices: the user, the patient, and the support staff. The three areas of limitations described above must be considered in each case (Figure 1–10).

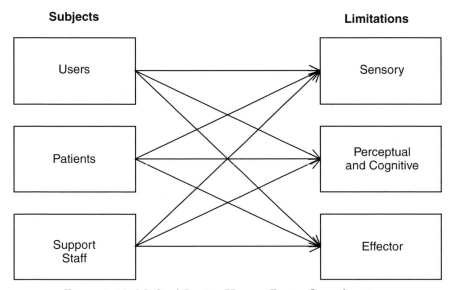

Figure 1–10. Medical Device Human Factor Considerations.

User Focus

For diagnostic devices, users rely on the information from the medical device to perform diagnosis. The display of information should be clear and unambiguous. It is especially important in clinical settings, where errors are often intolerable. In a situation in which visual alarms might be overlooked, loud audible alarms to alert one to critical events should be available. For therapeutic devices, ergonomic studies should be carried out in the design stage to ensure that the procedures could be performed in an effective and efficient manner. Critical devices should be intuitive and easy to set up. For example, a paramedic should be able to correctly perform a cardiac defibrillation without going through complicated initialization procedures since every second counts when a patient is in cardiac arrest.

A systems approach to analyze human interface related to users should consider the following:

- User characteristics
- Operating environment
- Human mental status
- Task priority
- Work flow

Human interface outputs may involve hand, finger, foot, head, eye, voice, et cetera. Each should be studied to identify the most appropriate choice for the application. A device should be ergonomically designed to minimize the strain and potential risk to the users, including long-term health hazards. For example, a heavy X-ray tube can create shoulder problems for radiology technologists who spend most of their working days maneuvering X-ray tubes over patients. Studies show that user fatigue is a major contributor to user errors. User fatigues include motor, visual, cognitive, and memory.

Traditionally, human factor engineering is task-oriented. It examines and optimizes tasks to improve output quality, reduce time spent, and minimize the rate of error. Proactive human interface designers tend to be user-centered, who integrate the physical and mental states of the user into the design, including the level of fatigue and stress, as well as recruit emotional feedback. Ideally, a good human interface design will produce a device that is both user-intuitive and efficient. However, in most cases, there is a balance and trade-off between the two. An intuitive design is easy to use, that is, a user can learn to operate the device in a short time. However, the operation of such a device may not be efficient. An example of such a device is a PACS (picture archiving and communication system) using a standard computer mouse as the human machine interface between the user and the PACS. The mouse is intuitive to most users. However, a radiologist may require going through a large number of moves and clicks to complete a single task. On the other hand, a specially designed, multibutton, task-oriented controller may be difficult to learn initially but will become more efficient once the radiologist has gotten used to it. Figure 1–11 shows the efficiency-time learning curve of a device by a new user. The learning time for an intuitive device is shorter than a specially designed device, but the efficiency is much lower once the user becomes proficient with the specially designed device.

Patient Focus

Traditionally, in designing a medical device, much attention is given to the safety and efficacy of the system. However, it is also important to look at

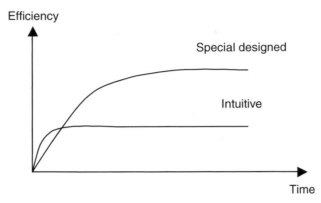

Figure 1–11. Learning Curve.

the design from the patient's perspectives. A good medical device design should be aesthetically pleasing to the eye and will not interfere with the normal routines of the patient. Some examples to illustrate the importance of human factor design related to patients are:

- A model of an infrared ear thermometer looks like a pistol with a trigger. The patient may feel threatened when the clinician points it into his or her ear and pulls the trigger.
- A motorized fan in an infant incubator is too noisy. It disturbs the sleep of the baby and may even inflict hearing damage.
- For a person who requires 24-hour mechanical ventilation, a tracheostomy tube that cannot be concealed properly may affect his (or her) social life.

Support Staff Focus

In designing a medical device, the ergonomics of maintenance tasks such as cleaning and servicing are often overlooked. Apart from its desired application, a medical device will be handled by many parties during its life cycle. A device that has difficult-to-assess hollow cavities will have problems in cleaning and sterilization and hence is not suitable for some medical procedures. Some devices are not service-friendly; many poorly designed devices require extensive dismantling in order to get access to replacement parts such as lightbulbs and batteries. Other devices may not have taken into consideration the operating environment, which in most cases will result in expensive and labor-intensive maintenance. An example is a fan-cooled device used in a dusty environment. In addition, poor design of accessories may increase the chance of incorrect assembly, which can impose unnecessary risk on the patients.

INPUT, OUTPUT, AND CONTROL SIGNALS

A simple system has a single input and a single output. When we study a medical device using the systems approach, the first step is to analyze the input to the device. In most cases, input signal to biomedical devices are physiological signals. In order to study the characteristics of the output, one must understand the nature of the processes that the device applies to the input. In addition to the main input and output signals, most medical devices have one or more control inputs (Figure 1–12). These control inputs are used by the operator to select the functions and control the device. Table 1–3 lists some examples of input, output, and control signals in biomedical devices.

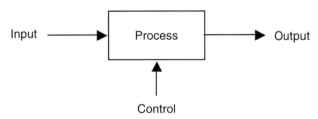

Figure 1–12. Medical Device System.

Table 1–3.
Examples of Medical Device Input/Output

Signal Input
       Electrical potential in ECG
       Pressure signal in blood pressure monitoring
       Heat in body temperature measurement
       Carbon dioxide partial pressure in end-tidal CO_2 monitoring

Device Output
       Printout in paper chart recorder
       Signal waveform in CRT display
       Alarm signal in audible tone
       Heat energy from a thermal blanket
       Grayscale image on an X-ray film
       Fluid flow from an infusion pump

Control Input
       Exposure technique settings on an X-ray machine
       Sensitivity setting on a medical display
       Total infusion volume setting on an infusion pump
       Alarm settings on an ECG monitor

CONSTRAINTS IN BIOMEDICAL SIGNAL MEASUREMENTS

Medical devices in many respects are similar to devices we use in everyday life. In fact, most technologies used in health care were adapted from the same technologies used in the military, industrial, and commercial applications. Since medical devices are used on humans, their reliability and safety requirements are usually more stringent than other devices. In addition, medical devices are often used in situations in which patients are vulnerable to even minor errors; therefore, special consideration in minimizing risk is necessary in designing medical devices. Listed next are some of the factors and constraints in designing medical devices.

Low Signal Level

The level of biological signal can be very small, for example, on the order of microvolts (μV) in EEG measurements. Therefore, very sensitive transducers as well as good noise rejection methods are required.

Inaccessible Measurement Site

Many signal sources are inside the human body and hidden by other anatomy. Biomedical measurements and procedures often require invasive means to obtain access to specific anatomy. For example, to access a nerve fiber for electrical activity measurement, the electrode must go through the skin, muscle, and other tissues.

Small Physical Size

Some measurement sites are very small. In order to measure the signal coming from these tiny sites while at the same time to avoid picking up the surrounding activities, special sensors that allow isolated measurement at the source are required. For example, in EMG measurement, needle electrodes with insulated stems are used to measure the electrical signal produced at a specific group of muscle fibers.

Difficult to Isolate Signal from Interfering Sources

As we cannot voluntarily turn ON or OFF, or remove tissue or organ to take a measurement, the measurand is subjected to much interference. As an example, in fetal monitoring, fetal heart activities are often masked by the stronger maternal heartbeats. It requires special techniques to extract information from these interfering signals.

Signal Varies with Time

Human physiological signals are seldom deterministic; they always change with time and with the activities of the body. It is therefore not an easy task to establish the norm of such signals. An example of such is in arterial blood pressure measurement; the blood pressure of a person is usually higher in the morning than at other times of day.

Signal Varies Among Healthy Individuals

Since every human being is different, the same physiological signal from one person is different from that of another. It is not a straightforward task to establish what is normal or abnormal and what is healthy or unhealthy when looking at some of these physiological parameters. For example, there is a huge difference in normal resting heart rate between an athlete and a couch potato. Nevertheless, there are generally recognized normal ranges. For example, systolic arterial pressure between 90 and 120 mmHg is considered acceptable.

Origin and Propagation of Signal Is Not Fully Understood

The human body is very complicated and nonhomogeneous. There are many signal paths within the body, and interrelationships between physiological events are often not fully understood. For example, the ECG obtained by surface electrodes looks very different from that obtained by invasive electrodes placed inside the heart chamber.

Difficult to Establish Safe Level of Applied Energy to the Tissue

Very often, electrical current from a medical device, whether by intention or by accident, will flow through the patient's body. Although such energy will impose risk on the patient, it is often difficult to establish the minimum safety limits of such signals.

Biocompatibility

The parts of a medical device that are in contact with patients must be nontoxic and must not trigger adverse reaction. In addition, they must be able to withstand the chemical corrosive environment of the human body.

CONCEPTS ON BIOCOMPATIBILITY

Definitions

Biocompatibility refers to the compatibility of nonliving materials with living tissues and organisms, whereas histocompatibility refers to the compatibility of different tissues in connection with immunological response. Histocompatibility is associated primarily with the human lymphocyte antigen system. Rejection of transplants may be prevented by matching tissues according to histocompatibility and by the use of immunosuppressive drugs. Biocompatibility entails mechanical, chemical, pharmacological, and surface compatibility. It is about the interactions that take place between the materials and the body fluid, tissues, and the physiological responses to these reactions.

Biocompatibility of metallic materials is controlled by the electrochemical interaction that results in the release of metal ions or insoluble particles into the tissues and the toxicity of these released substances. Biocompatibility of polymers is, to a large extent, dependent on how the surrounding fluids extract residual monomers, additives, and degradation products. Other than the chemistry, biocompatibility is also influenced by other factors such as mechanical stress imposed on the material.

Mechanism of Reaction

The adverse results of incompatibility include the production of toxic chemicals, as well as the corrosion and degradation of the biomaterials, which may affect the function or create failure of the device or implant. Protein absorption of the implant and tissue infection may lead to premature failure, resulting in removal and other complications. Compatibility between medical devices and the human body falls under the heading of biocompatibility.

Biocompatibility is especially important for implants or devices that for a considerable length of time are in contact with or inside the human body. Common implant materials include metal, polymers, ceramics, and products from other tissues or organisms.

Tissue Response to Implants

During an implant procedure, the process often requires injuring the tissue. Such injury will invoke reaction such as vasodilation, leakage of fluid into the extravascular space, and plugging of lymphatics. These reactions produce classic inflammatory signs such as redness, swelling, and heat, which often lead to local pain. Soon after injury of the soft tissues, the mesenchymal cells evolve into migratory fibroblasts that move into the injured site; together with the scaffolding formed from fibrinogen in the inflammatory exudates, collagen is deposited onto the wound. The collagen will dissolve and redeposit during the next 2 to 4 weeks for its molecules to polymerize in order to align and create cross-links to return the wound closer to that of normal tissue. This restructuring process can take more than 6 months.

The body always tries to remove foreign materials. Foreign material may be extruded from the body (as in the case of a wood splinter), walled off if it cannot be moved, or ingested by macrophages if it is in particulate or fluid form. These tissue responses are additional reactions to the healing processes described above.

A typical tissue response involves polymorphonuclear leukocytes appearing near the implant site followed by macrophages (foreign body giant cells). However, if the implant is chemically and physically inert to the tissue, only a thin layer of collagenous tissue is developed to encapsulate the implant. If the implant is either a chemical or a physical irritant to the surrounding tissue, then inflammation occurs at the implant site. The inflammation will delay normal healing and may cause necrosis of tissues by chemical, mechanical, and thermal trauma.

The degree of the tissue response varies according to both the physical and chemical nature of the implants. Pure metals (except the noble metals) tend to evoke a severe tissue reaction. Titanium has minimum tissue reaction of all the common metals used in implants as long as its oxide layer remains intact to prevent diffusion of metal ions and oxygen. Corrosion-resistant alloys such as cobalt-chromium and stainless steel have a similar effect on tissue once they are passivated. Most ceramic materials are oxides such as TiO_2 and Al_2O_3. These materials show minimal tissue reactions with only a thin layer of encapsulation. Polymers are quite inert toward tissue if there are no additives such as antioxidants, plasticizers, antidiscoloring agents, et cetera. On the other hand, monomers can evoke an adverse reaction since they are very reactive. Therefore, the degree of polymerization is related to the extent of tissue reaction. As 100% polymerization is not achievable, different sizes of polymer can leach out and cause severe tissue reaction.

A very important requirement for implant or materials in contact with blood is blood compatibility. Blood compatibility includes creating blood clot and damaging protein, enzymes, and blood elements. Damage to blood elements includes hemolysis (rupture of red blood cells) and triggering of platelet release. Factors affecting blood compatibility include surface roughness and surface wettability. A nonthrombogenic surface can be created by coating the surface with heparin, negatively charging the surface, or coating the surface with nonthrombogenic materials.

Systemic effect can be linked to some biodegradable sutures and surgical adhesives, as well as particles released from wear and corrosion of metals and other implants. In addition, there are some concerns about the possible carcinogenicity of some materials used in implantation.

Characteristics of Materials Affecting Biocompatibility

The following material characteristics should be analyzed to determine biocompatibility:

- Stress–the force exerted per unit area on the material; stress can be tensile, compressive, or shear.
- Strain–the percentage dimensional deformation of the material.
- Viscoelesticity–the time-dependent response between stress and strain.
- Thermal properties–include melting point, boiling point, specific heat capacity, heat capacity, thermal conductivity, and thermal expansion coefficient.
- Surface property–measure of surface tension and contact angle between liquid and solid surface.
- Heat treatment–for example, quenching of metal or surface compression of glass and ceramics to improve material strength.
- Electrical properties–determination of resistivity and piezoelectric properties.
- Optical properties–measurement of refractive index and spectral absorptivity.
- Density and porosity–include measurement of solid volume fraction.
- Acoustic properties–include acoustic impedance and attenuation coefficient.
- Diffusion properties–determination of permeability coefficients.

Each of these characteristics should be analyzed for its intended applications. It should be noted that the same material may have different degrees of biocompatibility under different environments and different applications.

In Vitro and In Vivo Tests for Biocompatibility

Tests for biocompatibility should include both material and host responses. The usual approach in testing a new product is to perform an in vitro screening test for quick rejection of incompatible materials. In vitro tests can be divided into two general classes: (1) tissue culture methods, and (2) blood contact methods.

Tissue culture refers collectively to the practice of maintaining portions of living tissues in a viable state, including cell culture, tissue culture, and organ culture. Blood contact methods are performed only for blood contact applications such as cardiovascular devices. Both static and dynamic (flow) tests should be performed.

After screening by in vitro techniques, the product is moved to in vivo testing. It is the practice to test new implant materials or existing materials in significantly different applications. In vivo tests are often done in extended-time whole animal tests before human clinical trials. In vivo tests in general are divided into two types: (1) nonfunctional, and (2) functional.

In nonfunctional tests, the product material can be of any shape and is embedded passively in the tissue site for a period of time (e.g., a few weeks to 24 months). Nonfunctional tests focus on the direct interactions between the material of the product and the chemical and biological species of the implant environment. In addition to being implanted, functional tests require that the product be placed in the functional mode as close as possible to the conditions of its intended applications. The purpose of functional tests is to study both the host and material responses such as tissue in growth into porous materials, material fatigue, and production of wear particles in load-bearing devices. Functional tests are obviously more involved and costly than nonfunctional tests.

FUNCTIONAL BUILDING BLOCKS
OF MEDICAL INSTRUMENTATION

A typical diagnostic medical device acquires information from the patient, analyzes and processes the data, and presents the information to the clinician. In a therapeutic device, it processes the input from the clinician and applies the therapeutic energy to the patient. Figure 1–13 shows the functional building blocks of a typical medical device. It includes the following functional building blocks:

- Patient interface
- Analog processing

- Analog to digital conversion and digital to analog conversion
- Signal isolation
- Digital processing
- Memory
- User interface

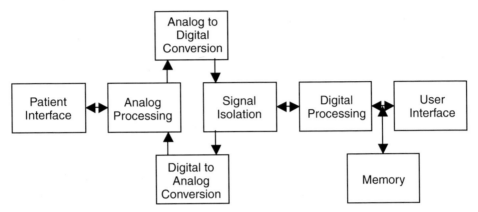

Figure 1–13. Functional Block Diagram of a Medical Instrument.

Patient Interface

In diagnostic devices, the patient interface includes transducers or sensors to pick up and convert the physiological signal (e.g., blood pressure) to an electrical signal. In therapeutic devices, the patient interface contains transducers that generate and apply energy to the patient (e.g., ultrasound physiotherapy unit).

Analog Processing

The analog processing contains electrical circuits such as amplifiers (to increase signal level) and filters (to remove any unwanted frequency components such as high-frequency noise from the signal). The signal until this point is still in its analog format.

Analog to Digital Conversion

The function of the analog to digital converter (ADC) is to convert the analog signal to its digital format. The signal coming from the ADC is a string of binary numbers (1's and 0's).

Digital to Analog Conversion

If an analog output is necessary, a digital to analog converter (DAC) will be required to convert the digital signal from its "1" and "0" states back to its analog format. A DAC reverses the process of an ADC.

Signal Isolation

The primary function of signal isolation is for microshock prevention in patient electrical safety. The isolation barrier, usually an optocoupler, provides a very high electrical impedance between the patient's applied parts and the power supply circuit to limit the amount of risk current flowing to or from the patient.

Digital Processing

After being digitized by the ADC, the signal is sent to the digital processing circuit. In a modern medical instrument, digital processing is done by one or more computers built into the system. The center of a digital computer is the central processing unit (CPU). Depending on the needs, the CPU may perform functions such as calculations, signal conditioning, pattern recognition, information extraction, et cetera.

Memory

Information such as waveforms or computed data is stored in its binary format in the memory module of the device. Signal stored in the memory can later be retrieved for display, analysis, or used to control other outputs.

User Interface

User interfaces can be output or input devices. Examples of output user interfaces are video displays for physiological waveforms and audio alarms. Examples of input devices are touch screen and trackballs.

Chapter 2

CONCEPTS IN SIGNAL MEASUREMENT, PROCESSING, AND ANALYSIS

OBJECTIVES

- List the typical elements in medical device specifications.
- Define common parameters found in device specifications, including accuracy, error, precision, resolution, reproducibility, sensitivity, linearity, hysteresis, and zero offset.
- Describe common steady state nonlinear input-output characteristics.
- Define transfer functions in time and frequency domains.
- Explain and analyze the effect of filters on biomedical signals.

CHAPTER CONTENTS

1. Introduction
2. Device Specifications
3. Steady State Versus Transient Characteristics
4. Linear Versus Nonlinear Steady State Characteristics
5. Time and Frequency Domains
6. Signal Processing and Analysis

INTRODUCTION

Most medical devices involve measurement or sensing one or more physiological signals, enhancing the signals of interest, and extracting useful information from the signals. The concepts of signal measurement, processing, and analysis are fundamental in understanding scientific instrumentations, including medical devices. This chapter provides an introductory overview of these concepts.

DEVICE SPECIFICATIONS

To understand the functions and performance of a medical device, one should start from reading the specifications of the device. Specifications of an instrument are the claims from the manufacturer on the performance of the instrument. The specification document of a medical device should contain at least the following information:

- List of device functions
- Input and output characteristics
- Performance statements
- Physical characteristics
- Environmental requirements
- Codes and regulations

Below is an example of a specification document of an electrocardiograph:

Instrument type: 12-channel, microcomputer-augmented, automatic electrocardiograph
Input channels: simultaneous acquisition of up to 12 channels
Frequency response: −3 dB @ 0.01 to 105 Hz
Sensitivities: 2.5, 5, 10, and 20 mm/mV, ±2%
Input impedance: > 50 MΩ
Common mode rejection ratio: > 106 dB
Recorder type: thermal digital dot array, 200 dots/in vertical resolution
Recorder speed: 1, 5, 25, and 50 mm/sec, ±3%
Digital sampling rate: 2,000 samples/sec/channel
ECG analysis frequency: 250 samples/sec
Display formats: user-selectable channel and lead configurations: 3, 4, 5, 6, and 12 channels
Dimensions: H × W × D = 90 cm × 42 cm × 75 cm
Weight: 30 kg
Power requirements: 90 VAC to 260 VAC, 50 or 60 Hz
Certification: UL 544 listed, meets ANSI/AAMI standards, complies with IEC 601 standards

---

Some common parameters found in medical device specifications are explained next.

The **error** (ε) of a single measured quantity is the measured value ($\mathbf{Q_m}$) minus the true value ($\mathbf{Q_t}$), or

$$\varepsilon = Q_m - Q_t.$$

There are three types of errors: gross error, systematic error, and random error.

- Gross error arises from incorrect use of the instrument (e.g., human error).
- Systematic error is due to a shortcoming of the instrument (e.g., defective or worn parts, adverse effect of the environment on the equipment).
- Random error is fluctuations that cannot be directly established or corrected (e.g., noise in photographic process).

Error may be expressed as absolute or relative.

- Absolute error is expressed in the specific units of measurement, e.g., 15 Ω $\pm$ 1 Ω. The graphical representation is shown in Figure 2–1a.
- Relative error is expressed as a ratio of the measured quantity, e.g., output reading $\pm$ 5%. (Figure 2–1b)
- An alternative way to express absolute error is percentage of full scale, e.g., 5% of full scale output. (Figure 2–1c).
- Or it can be a combination of the above, e.g., ± 1 Ω or 5% of output, whichever is greater. (Figure 2–1d)

Accuracy (**A**) is the error divided by the true value and is often expressed as a percentage.

$$A = \left[\frac{Q_m - Q_t}{Q_t} \right] \times 100\%$$

Accuracy usually varies over the normal range of the quantity measured. It can be expressed as a percentage of the reading or a percentage of full scale. For example, for a speedometer with $\pm 5.0\%$ accuracy, when it is reading 50 km/hr, the maximum error is ± 2.5 km/hr. If the speedometer is rated at $\pm 5.0\%$ full scale accuracy and the full scale reading is 200 km/hr, the maximum error of the measurement is ± 10 km/hr, irrespective of the reading.

The **precision** of a measurement expresses the number of distinguishable alternatives from which a given result is selected. For example, a meter that can measure a reading of three decimal places (e.g., 4.123 V) is more precise than one than can measure only two decimal places (e.g., 4.12 V).

Resolution is the smallest incremental quantity than can be measured with certainty. If the readout of a digital thermometer jumped from 20°C to 22°C and then to 24°C when it is used to measure the temperature of a bath

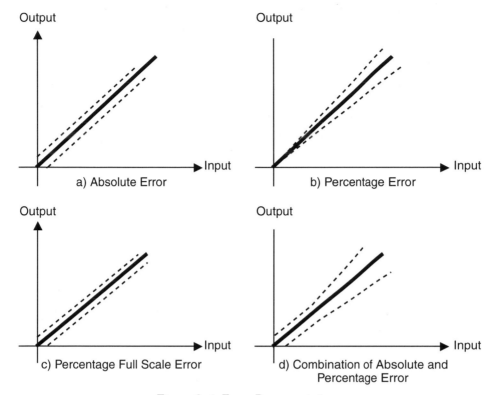

Figure 2–1. Error Representation.

of water slowly being heated by an electric water heater, the resolution of the thermometer is 2°C.

Reproducibility is the ability of an instrument to give the same output for equal inputs applied over some period of time.

Sensitivity is the ratio of the incremental output quantity to the incremental input quantity $(S = \frac{dy}{dx})$. It is the slope or tangent of the output versus input curve. Note that the sensitivity of an instrument is a constant only if the output-input relationship is linear. For a nonlinear transfer function (as shown in Figure 2–2), the sensitivity is different at different points on the curve $(S_1 \neq S_2)$.

Zero offset is the output quantity measured when the input is zero. Input zero offset is the input value applied to obtain a zero output reading. Zero offsets can be positive or negative.

Zero drift has occurred when all output values increase or decrease by the same amount.

A **sensitivity drift** has occurred when the slope (sensitivity) of the input-output curve has changed over a period of time.

Perfect **linearity** of an instrument requires that the calibration curve be

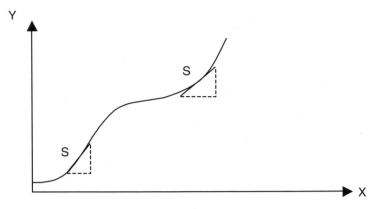

Figure 2–2. Sensitivity.

a straight line. That is, a linear instrument has the characteristics

$$y = mx + c,$$

where x is the input, y is the output, and m and c are both constants.

Independent **nonlinearity** expresses the maximum deviation of points from the least-squares fitted line as either $\pm$ P% of the reading or $\pm$ Q% of full scale, whichever is greater. Percentage nonlinearity (Figure 2–3) is defined as the maximum deviation of the input (D_{max}) from the curve to the least square fit straight line divided by the full scale input range (I_{fs}). It is sometimes referred to as % input nonlinearity (versus % output nonlinearity).

$$\% \text{ nonlinearity} = \frac{D_{max}}{I_{fs}} \times 100\%.$$

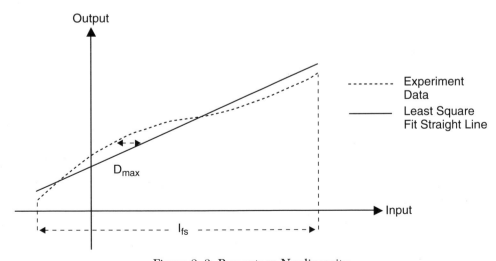

Figure 2–3. Percentage Nonlinearity.

An instrument complies with the listed specifications (such as accuracy, % nonlinearity) only within the specified **input ranges**. In other words, when the input of the instrument is beyond the specified input range, its characteristics may not be according to the labeled specifications.

Since biomedical transducers and instruments usually convert nonelectrical quantities to electrical quantities (voltage or current), its **input impedance** must be specified to evaluate the degree to which the instrument disturbs the quantity being measured.

Hysteresis measures the capability of the output to follow the change of the input in either direction. Hysteresis often occurs when the process is lossy.

Response time is the time required for the output to change from its previous state to a final settled value given the tolerance. (e.g., time to change to 90% of the steady state).

Calibration is the process of determining and recording the relationships between the values indicated by a measuring instrument and the true value of the measured quantity. Since the true value is usually difficult to obtain, the instrument is usually calibrated against a device that is traceable to a national standard.

Statistical control ensures that random variations in measured quantities (result from all factors that influence the measurement process) are tolerable. If random variables make the outputs nonreproducible, **statistical analysis** must be used to determine the error variation. In fact, many medical devices rely on statistical means to determine their calibration accuracy.

STEADY STATE VERSUS TRANSIENT CHARACTERISTICS

For a typical instrument, the output will change following a change in the input. Figure 2–4 shows a typical output response when a step input is applied to the system. Depending on the system characteristics, the output may experience a delay before it settles down (dotted line in Figure 2–4) or may get into oscillation right after the change of the input (solid line in Figure 2–4). However, in most instruments, this transient will eventually settle down to a steady state until the input is changed again.

The input-output characteristics when one ignores the initial transient period is called the steady state characteristics or static response of the system. When the input is a time-varying signal, one must take into account the transient characteristics of the system. For example, when the input is a fast-changing signal, the output may not be able to follow the input, that is, the output may not have enough time to reach its steady state before the input is changed again. In this case, the signal will suffer from distortion.

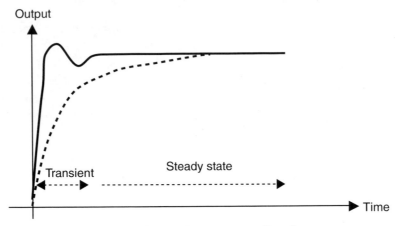

Figure 2–4. Output Response to a Step Input.

LINEAR VERSUS NONLINEAR STEADY STATE CHARACTERISTICS

A linear calibration curve is one that obeys the relationship

$$y = mx + c,$$

where x is the input,
y is the output, and
m and c are both constants.
Figure 2–5a shows a linear characteristics with $c = 0$.

Some common nonlinear characteristics are shown in Figure 2–5.
- **Saturation** occurs when the input is increased to a point where the output cannot be increased further. A linear operational amplifier will become saturated when the input is close to the power supply voltage.
- **Breakdown** is the phenomenon when the output abruptly starts to increase when the input changes slightly following a linear relationship. Some devices such as zener diodes have this type of nonlinear behavior.
- **Dead zone** is a range of the input where the output remains constant. A worn-out gear system usually has some dead space (dead zone).
- **Bang-bang** occurs when a minor reversal of the input creates an abrupt change in the output. This phenomenon can be observed in some thin metal diaphragm transducers. The diaphragm may flip from one side to another when the force applied to the center of the diaphragm changes direction.
- **Hysteresis** is the phenomenon that the input-output characteristic fol-

lows different pathways depending on whether the input is increasing or decreasing. Hysteresis results when some of the energy applied during an increasing input is not recovered when the input is reversed. The magnetization characteristic of a transformer is a perfect example where some applied energy is loss in the eddy current in the iron core.

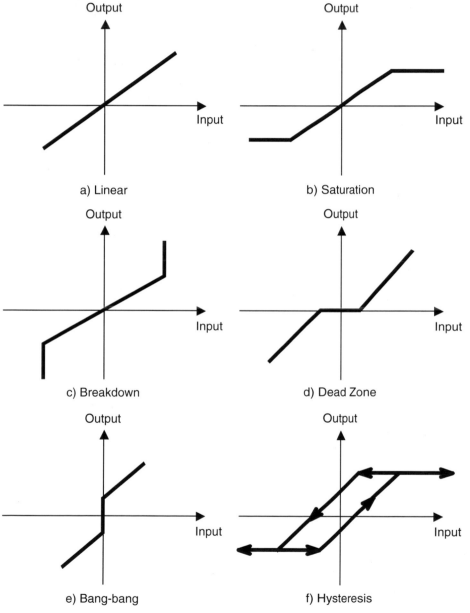

Figure 2–5 a) to f). Common Nonlinear Characteristics.

TIME AND FREQUENCY DOMAINS

A **time-varying signal** is a signal the amplitude of which changes with time. A **periodical signal** is a time-varying signal the waveshape of which repeats at regular time intervals. Mathematically, a periodical signal is given by:

$$G(t) = G(t + nT),$$

where n = any positive or negative integer,
and T = fundamental period.

A sinusoidal signal is an example of a periodical signal. The mathematical expression of a sinusoidal signal is

$$G(t) = A \sin(\omega t = \phi),$$

where A = a constant,
ω = angular velocity, and
ϕ = phase angle.

Any periodical signal can be represented (through **Fourier-series** expansion) by a combination of sinusoidal signals

$$G(t) = a_o + \sum_{n=1}^{\infty} [a_n \cos(n\,\omega_0 t) + b_n \sin(n\,\omega_0 t)],$$

where a_o, a_n, and b_n are time-invariant values depending on the shape of $G(t)$, and $\omega_o = 2\pi f_o = 2\pi/T$.

Using the preceding equation, the Fourier series of a symmetrical square waveform (Figure 2–6a) with amplitude of ± 1 V and a period of 1 sec is:

$$V(t) = 4V/\pi \,(\sin 2\pi t + 0.33\sin 6\pi t + 0.20\sin 10\pi t + 0.14\sin 14\pi t + \ldots).$$

The frequency domain plot or frequency spectrum of the same signal is shown in Figure 2–6b. A brief description of Fourier analysis can be found in Appendix A.1.

For a nonperiodical signal, the frequency spectrum is continuous instead of discrete. An example of an arterial blood pressure waveform is shown in Figure 2–7.

All biomedical signals are time-varying. Some signals may change very slowly with time (e.g., body temperature), while others may change more rapidly (e.g., an ECG). Although some appear to be periodical, in fact, each cycle of the signal differs from the others due to many factors. Physiological signals that appear to be periodical are considered pseudoperiodical. For example, each cycle of the invasive blood pressure waveform of a resting healthy person may look the same within a short period of time; however, the waveform and

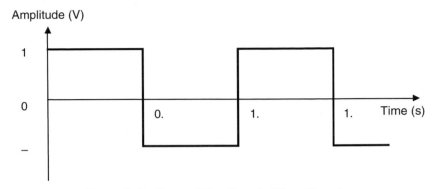

Figure 2–6a. Square Waveform in Time-Domain.

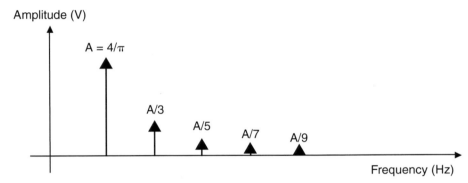

Figure 2–6b. Frequency Spectrum of the Square Wave in a.

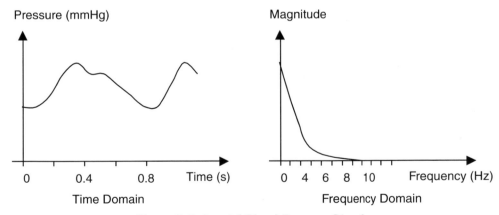

Figure 2–7. Arterial Blood Pressure Signal.

amplitude will be quite different when the person is engaged in different physical activities such as running. Furthermore, the waveform may be very different from cycle to cycle when the person has cardiovascular problems.

SIGNAL PROCESSING AND ANALYSIS

The purpose of signal processing and analysis in medical instrumentation is to extract useful information from the "raw" biological signals. For example, an ECG monitor can derive the rate of the heartbeats from the biopotential waveform of the heart activities. It also can generate an alarm signal to alert the clinician should the heart rate fall outside a predetermined range (e.g., greater than 120 bpm or less than 50 bpm).

Transfer Function

Mathematically, an operation or process (Figure 2–8) can be represented by a transfer function *f(t)*. When a signal *x(t)* is processed by the transfer function, the output *y(t)* is equals to the time convolution between the input signal and the transfer function. That is,

$$y(t) = \int_0^t f(t - \lambda)x(\lambda)d\lambda$$

or simply denoted by $y(t) = f(t)^* \ x(t)$.

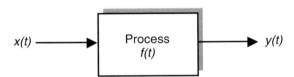

Figure 2–8. Time Domain Transfer Function.

In the frequency domain, the mathematical relationship between the output and input signals when the input is processed by the transfer function F (Figure 2–9) is given by:

$$Y(\omega) = F(\omega) \ X(\omega),$$

where $X(\omega)$ is the input signal,
$Y(\omega)$ is the output signal,
$F(\omega)$ is the transfer function of the process, and
ω = angular velocity = $2\pi f$.

Note that the output is simply equal to the input multiplied by the transfer function in the frequency domain. This is why signal analysis is often performed in the frequency domain.

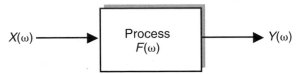

Figure 2–9. Frequency Domain Transfer Function.

Signal Filtering

A filter separates signals according to their frequencies. Most filters accomplish this by attenuating the part of the signal that is in one or more frequency regions. The transfer function of a filter is frequency-dependent. A filter can be represented by a transfer function $F(\omega)$. Filters can be low pass, high pass, band pass, or band reject. The four types of filters are shown in Figure 2–10. The cutoff frequency (corner frequency) of a filter is usually measured at –3dB from the midband amplitude (70.7% of the amplitude).

A low pass filter attenuates high frequencies above its cutoff frequency. An example of such is the filter used to remove baseline wandering signal in ECG monitoring; a 0.5Hz high pass filter is switched into the signal path to remove the low-frequency component caused by the movement of the patient. High pass filters attenuate low frequencies and allow high-frequency signals to pass through. Many biomedical devices have low pass filters with upper cutoff frequencies to remove unwanted high-frequency noise. A band pass filter is a combination of a high pass filter and a low pass filter, it eliminates unwanted low- and high-frequency signals while allowing the mid-frequency signals to go through. A band reject filter removes only a small bandwidth of frequency signal. A 60 Hz notch filter designed to remove 60 Hz power-induced noise is an example of a band reject filter. Filters can be inserted at any point in the signal pathway. Filters can be inherent (characteristics of the intrinsic or parasitic circuit components) or inserted to achieve a specific effect. For example, a low pass filter is inserted in the signal pathway to remove high-frequency noise from the signal, which results in a "cleaner" waveform.

Figure 2–11 shows the effect of filters on an ECG waveform. Figure 2–11a is acquired using a bandwidth from 0.05 to 125 Hz. In Figure 2–11b, the upper cutoff frequency is reduced from 125 Hz to 25 Hz. The effect of eliminating the high-frequency components in the waveform is the attenuation of the fast-changing events (i.e., reduction of the amplitude of the R-wave). Figure 2–11c shows the effect of increasing the lower cutoff frequency from 0.05 to 1.0 Hz. In this case, the low-frequency component of the signal is removed. Therefore, the waveform becomes more oscillatory.

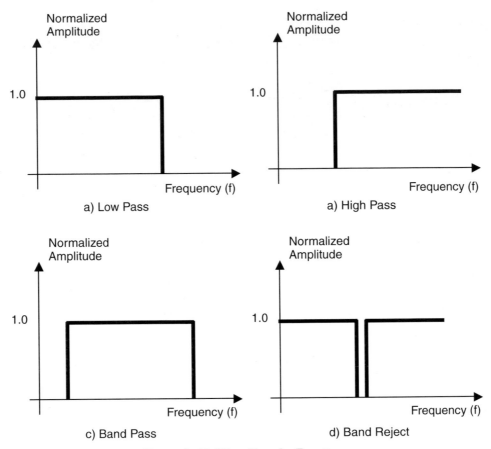

Figure 2–10. Filter Transfer Functions.

Signal Amplification and Attenuation

An amplifier increases (amplifies) the signal amplitude, while an attenuator decreases (attenuates) the signal amplitude. The transfer function of an amplifier is also called the amplification factor *(A)*. *A* is expressed as the ratio of the output *(Y)* to the input quantity *(X)*. That is:

$$A(\omega) = \frac{Y(\omega)}{X(\omega)}.$$

The amplification factor can be frequency-dependent (i.e., the value of *A* is different at different frequencies). The transfer function of an ideal amplifier or attenuator is independent of time and frequency (i.e., it has a constant magnitude at all frequencies).

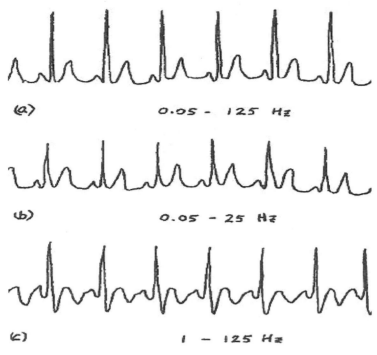

(a)   0.05 - 125 Hz

(b)   0.05 - 25 Hz

(c)   1 - 125 Hz

Figure 2–11. Effect of Filters on ECG Waveform.

Other Signal Processing Circuits

Other than filters and amplifiers, there are many other signal processors with different transfer function characteristics. Examples are integrators, differentiators, multipliers, adders, inverters, comparators, logarithm amplifiers, et cetera. Readers who want to learn more about these signal processing circuits should refer to an integrated electronic textbook. Although many medical devices still use analog signal processing circuits, more and more of these signal processing functions are performed digitally by software in modern computer-based devices.

Chapter 3

FUNDAMENTALS OF BIOMEDICAL TRANSDUCERS

OBJECTIVES

- Define the terms transducer, sensor, electrode, and actuator.
- Distinguish between the following modes of biological signal measurements: direct and indirect, intermittent and continuous, desired and interfering, invasive and noninvasive.
- Specify the three criteria for the faithful reproduction of an event.
- Evaluate the effect on physiological signal measurements due to amplitude nonlinearity, phase distortion, and bandwidth limitation.
- Analyze Wheatstone bridge circuits in medical instrumentation applications.

CHAPTER CONTENTS

1. Introduction
2. Definitions
3. Types of Transducers
4. Transducer Characteristics
5. Signal Conditioning
6. Transducer Excitation
7. Common Physiological Signal Transducers

INTRODUCTION

Medical devices are designed either to measure physiological parameters from the patient or to apply certain energy to the patient. To achieve that, a medical device must use a transducer to interface between the device and the patient. The transducer is usually the most critical component in a medical device as it must reliably and faithfully reproduce the signal to or from the patient. In addition, transducers are often in contact with or even implanted inside a human. Transducers in such applications must be stable and non-toxic to the human body. Ideally, a transducer should respond only to the energy that is desired to be measured and exclude the others. Most of the medical device constraints discussed in Chapter 1 are also applicable to bio-medical transducers.

DEFINITIONS

A **sensor** is a device that can sense changes of one physical quantity and transpose them systematically into a different physical quantity. Generally speaking, a **transducer** is defined as a device to convert energy from one form to another. For example, the heating element on the kitchen stove is a transducer that converts electrical energy to heat energy for cooking. In instrumentation, a transducer is a device whose main function is to convert the measurand to a signal that is compatible with a measurement or control system. The compatible signal is often an electrical signal. For example, an optical transducer may convert light intensity to an electrical voltage. In instrumentation or measurement applications, sensors and transducers are often use synonymously. An **electrode** is a transducer that directly acquires the electrical signal without the need to convert it to another form; that is, both input and output are electrical signals. On the other hand, an **actuator** is a transducer that produces a force or motion. An electrical motor is an example of an actuator that converts electricity to mechanical motion.

In many biomedical applications, the transducer or sensor converts a physiological event to an electrical signal. With the event available as an electrical signal, it is easier to use modern computer technology to process the physiological event and display the output in a user-friendly format. Figure 3–1 shows a simple block diagram of a physiological monitor.

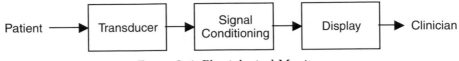

Figure 3–1. Physiological Monitor.

TYPES OF TRANSDUCERS

Passive Versus Active Transducers

Transducers can be passive or active. For a passive transducer, the input to the transducer produces change in a passive network parameter such as resistance, capacitance, or inductance. On the other hand, an active transducer, such as a piezoelectric crystal or a thermocouple, acts as a generator, producing force, current, or voltage in response to the input.

Direct Versus Indirect Mode of Transducers

For a direct transducer, the measurand is interfaced to and measured directly by the transducer. Blood pressure may be measured directly by placing a pressure transducer inside a blood vessel. The electrical cardiac signal is directly picked up by a set of electrodes placed on the chest of a patient. Both are examples of direct mode of transduction. In indirect mode, the transducer measures another measurand that bears a known relationship to the desired measurand. Indirect transducers are often used when the desired measurands are not readily accessible. An example of such indirect mode of transduction approach is in noninvasive blood pressure measurements, where the systolic, mean, and diastolic pressures are estimated from the oscillatory characteristics of the pressure in a pneumatic cuff applied over the upper arm of the subject.

Intermittent Versus Continuous Measurement

In some cases, it is important to monitor physiological parameters in a continuous manner. Continuously monitoring the heart rate and blood oxygen level of a patient during general anesthesia is an example. In other circumstances, a single measurement is sufficient to obtain a snapshot of the patient's condition. Measurement of oral temperature using a liquid-in-glass thermometer is an example of intermittent temperature measurement. In another application, periodical measurement to track changes is more appropriate. Charting the arterial blood pressure of a patient in the recovery room every 5 minutes is an example of periodical measurement.

Desired Versus Interfering Input

Desired input to a transducer is the signal that the transducer is designed to pick up. Interfering input is an unwanted signal that affects or corrupts the output of the transducer. For example, maternal heart rate is the interfering input in fetal heart rate monitoring. Interfering input is sometimes referred to as noise in the system. In medical applications, interfering input is usually compensated for by adjusting the sensor location, or through signal processing such as filtering.

Invasive Versus Noninvasive Method

A procedure that requires bypassing the skin of the patient is called an invasive procedure. Entering the body cavity such as through the mouth into the trachea is also considered to be invasive. In biomedical applications, measurement of a physiological signal often requires placing a transducer inside the patient's body. Using a needle electrode to measure myoelectric potential is an example of an invasive method of measurement. On the other hand, myoelectric measurements using skin (or surface) electrodes are noninvasive procedures.

TRANSDUCER CHARACTERISTICS

A transducer is often specified by the following:

- The quantity to be measured, or the measurand
- The principle of the conversion process
- The performance characteristics
- The physical characteristics

In biomedical measurements, common measurands are position, motion, velocity, acceleration, force, pressure, volume, flow, heat, temperature, humidity, light intensity, sound level, chemical composition, electric current, electric voltage, et cetera. Examples of their characteristics and method of measurements of some of these physiological parameters are tabulated in Table 1–2 in Chapter 1.

Many methods can be used to convert a physiological event to an electrical signal. The event can be made to modify, directly or indirectly, the electrical properties of the transducer, such as its resistance or inductance values. The primary functional component of a transducer or sensor is the transduction element. Many different transduction elements are suitable for health care applications. Table 3–1 lists some common transducer categories and their operating principles. Examples of transducers in each category are also listed in the table.

Table 3–1.
Transducers and Their Operating Principles

Transduction Elements	Correlating Properties	Examples
Resistive	Resistance–temperature	Thermistor to measure temperature
	Resistance–displacement due to pressure	Resistive strain gauge to measure pressure
Capacitive	Capacitance–motion	Capacitive blanket in neonatal apnea detection
Inductive	Inductance–displacement due to pressure	Linear variable differential transformer in pressure measurement
Photoelectric	Electric current– light energy	Photomultiplier in scintillation counter, red and infrared LEDs and detectors in pulse oximeter
Piezoelectric	Electric potential–force	Ultrasound transducer in blood flow detector
Thermoelectric	Electric potential– thermal energy	Thermocouple junctions in temperature measurement
Chemical	Electric current–chemical concentration	Polarographic cell in oxygen analyzer

Transducers should adhere to the following three criteria for the faithful reproduction of an event:

1. Amplitude linearity–ability to produce an output signal such that its amplitude is directly proportional to the input amplitude.
2. Adequate frequency response–ability to follow both rapid and slow changes.
3. Free from phase distortion–ability to maintain the time differences in the sinusoidal frequencies.

Amplitude Linearity

The output and input should follow a linear relationship within its operating range. The output will not resemble the input if the above is not true. A common example of a nonlinear input-output relationship is saturation of operational amplifier when the input becomes too large. In Figure 3–2, when the input is within the linear region of the operational amplifier, any change of the input will produce a change of output proportional to the change of input. When the input becomes too large, it drives the amplifier into saturation with the effect that the output will not increase further with the input; the waveform is "clipped."

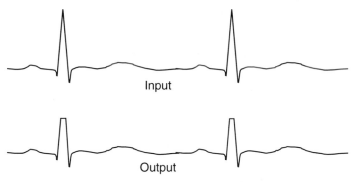

Figure 3–2. Effect of Nonlinearity (Saturation).

Adequate Frequency Response

In physiological signal measurements, the signals often change with time; body temperature changes slowly, whereas the heart potential (ECG) changes more rapidly. In order to accurately measure a changing signal, the transducer should be able to follow the changes of the input; that is, it must have a wide enough frequency response. Figure 3–3 shows the effect of inadequate frequency response. In this case, the high frequency of the ECG signal is attenuated or removed by the low pass filtering effect of the system. Note that in the output waveform, the amplitude of the R-wave is substantially reduced.

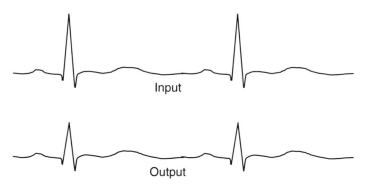

Figure 3–3. Effect of Inadequate High Frequency.

Free from Phase Distortion

A system that creates different time delay at different signal frequency will create phase distortion. As we know, any time-varying signal can be represented by a number of sinusoidal signals of different frequencies and amplitudes, and recombining or adding these signals will reproduce the original signal (Fourier analysis). However, if the transducer in the measurement process creates different time delays on the sinusoidal signal components, recombining these signals at the output of the transducer will produce a distorted signal (Figure 3–4). Phase distortion will prevent the faithful reproduction of an event.

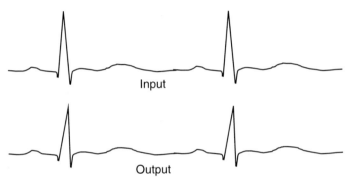

Figure 3–4. Effect of Phase Delay.

Any deviations from these three criteria will produce distorted output signals. Therefore, transducers must be carefully chosen to minimize distortion within the range of measurement. If signal distortion cannot be avoided due to nonideal transducers, additional electronic circuits may be used to compensate for such distortions.

SIGNAL CONDITIONING

A transducer output may be directly coupled to a display device to be viewed by the user. Very often, the output of a transducer is coupled to a signal conditioning circuit. A signal conditioning circuit can be as simple as a passive filter or as complicated as a digital signal processor. A very common signal conditioning circuit for passive transducers is a Wheatstone bridge. Many functional elements for signal conditioning commonly used in industrial electrical instrumentations are used in medical devices. These functional elements can be implemented using analog components or performed by software. In the latter case, the signal must be digitized and processed by a digital computer. Some common signal conditioning functions are amplifiers, filters, rectifiers, peak detectors, differentiators, integrators, et cetera.

TRANSDUCER EXCITATION

Transducers that vary their electrical values according to changes in their inputs are often used in biomedical applications. These transducers are usually coupled to operational amplifiers to increase their sensitivities and to reject noise. When the output of a transducer is a passive electrical parameter (e.g., resistance, capacitance, or inductance), it often requires an excitation to convert the passive output variable to a voltage signal. The excitation can be a constant voltage or a constant current source; it may be a DC or an AC signal of any frequencies. A common excitation method in biomedical transducers is the Wheatstone bridge.

A Wheatstone bridge is commonly used to couple a transducer to the other electronic circuits. Figure 3–5 shows a typical Wheatstone bridge with excitation voltage V_E and impedances Z_1, Z_2, Z_3, and Z_4 at each arm of the bridge.

The output of the bridge V_0 in the figure is:

$$V_0 = V_a - V_b = V_E \left(\frac{Z_3}{Z_3 + Z_4} - \frac{Z_2}{Z_2 + Z_1} \right) \qquad (1)$$

From the equation, when $\left(\dfrac{Z_3}{Z_3 + Z_4} - \dfrac{Z_2}{Z_2 + Z_1} \right) = 0$, the bridge output

voltage is zero $(V_0 = 0)$.

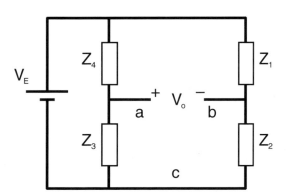

Figure 3–5. Wheatstone Bridge Circuit.

In most transducer applications, one of the bridge arm impedances is replaced by a transducer whose impedance changes with the parameter being measured. Figure 3–6 shows an example of such an arrangement. The transducer impedance can be written as $Z + \Delta Z$, where ΔZ is the impedance that changes with the quantity being measured and Z is the invariable part of the transducer impedance. In this example, the impedances in the remaining arms are all equal to Z.

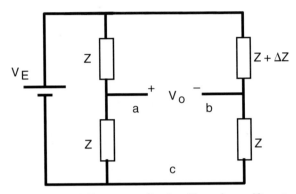

Figure 3–6. Wheatstone Bridge Transducer Circuit.

Substituting $Z_1 = Z + \Delta Z$, and $Z_2 = Z_3 = Z_4 = Z$ in equation (1) gives:

$$V_0 = V_E \frac{\Delta Z}{2(2Z + \Delta Z)} \tag{2}$$

Equation (2) shows that V_0 and ΔZ has a nonlinear relationship. However, if ΔZ is much smaller than Z $(\Delta Z << Z)$, equation (2) can be approximated by:

$$V_0 \quad \frac{V_E}{4} \Delta Z \tag{3}$$

Now consider the half bridge circuit in Figure 3–7, where there are two transducers $Z + \Delta Z$ and $Z - \Delta Z$, each on one arm of the bridge.

Substituting the $Z_1 = Z + \Delta Z$, $Z_2 = Z - \Delta Z$, $Z_3 = Z_4 = Z$ in equation (1) gives:

$$V_0 = \frac{V_E}{2Z} \Delta Z \tag{4}$$

Note that the bridge output V_0 is proportional to the change in transducer impedance ΔZ with a proportionality constant (or sensitivity) equals to $\frac{V_E}{2Z}$.

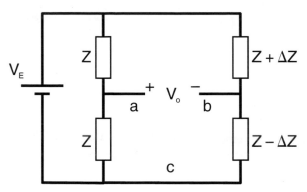

Figure 3–7. Half Bridge Transducer Circuit.

If we replace all the fixed impedances on the bridge arms with transducers as shown in Figure 3–8, the bridge circuit is called a full bridge.

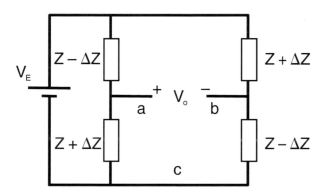

Figure 3–8. Full Bridge Transducer Circuit.

Substituting the $Z_1 = Z_3 == Z + \Delta Z$, $Z_2 = Z_4 = Z - \Delta Z$ in equation (1) gives:

$$V_0 = \frac{V_E}{Z} \Delta Z \qquad (5)$$

Similar to the half bridge, the full bridge output V_0 is proportional to the change in transducer impedance ΔZ. However, the proportionality constant for a full bridge circuit is $\frac{V_E}{Z}$, which is two times the value of a half bridge circuit.

Among the three bridge circuits discussed, a full bridge transducer circuit produces a linear output voltage with respect to changes in the transducer impedance and it has the highest sensitivity. However, it requires four matching transducers compared to two for the half bridge and only one for the typical bridge circuit.

COMMON PHYSIOLOGICAL SIGNAL TRANSDUCERS

In biomedical measurement, the transducer is a component of the medical device that picks up the physiological signal from the patient. It is also the interface between the device and the human body. The transducer with its excitation circuit and its associated analog signal processing components is sometimes referred to as the frontend of the medical device. There are many types of transducers in biomedical applications. Their characteristics, principles of operation, and design can be very different. The following major categories of biomedical transducers are covered in the next six chapters:

1. Pressure transducers
2. Temperature transducers
3. Motion transducers
4. Flow transducers
5. Optical transducers
6. Electrochemical transducers

Chapter 4

PRESSURE AND FORCE TRANSDUCERS

OBJECTIVES

- Understand different units of pressure measurement and perform unit conversion.
- Define absolute and gauge pressure.
- Explain the function of barometers and manometers.
- State the principles of bourdon tube, bellow, and diaphragm pressure meters.
- Define gauge factor for a resistive stain gauge and derive its dependent variables.
- Describe bonded and unbonded strain gauges, metal strain wire, and diaphragm strain gauges.
- Analyze the principles of piezoelectric pressure gauges.

CHAPTER CONTENTS

INTRODUCTION

If a force F is acting uniformly on and perpendicular to a surface of area A, the pressure P on the surface is defined as:

$$P = \frac{F}{A}$$

From this definition, a force transducer may be used for pressure measurement and vice versa. Pressure transducers have many applications in biomedical instrumentation. Blood pressure measurement is one of the routine procedures performed in medicine. Several types of pressure-sensing elements are discussed in this chapter.

BAROMETERS AND MANOMETERS

One of the earliest transducers used in measuring atmospheric pressure is the barometer. A simple mercury barometer is constructed from inverting a mercury-filled glass tube in a bath of mercury (Figure 4–1). When the tube is tall enough, a vacuum is created on top of the mercury column. The atmospheric pressure P_{atm} is calculated from the height of the mercury column h by the equation:

$$P_{atm} = \rho g h \qquad (1)$$

where ρ is the density of mercury (equal to 13.6×10^3 kg/m^3),
g is the acceleration due to gravity (equal to 9.8 m/s^2), and
h is the height of the mercury column measured in meters.

The S.I. unit of pressure is Pascal (Pa). At standard atmospheric pressure (STP), one atmosphere is equal to 101 kPa at temperature 273 K (0°C); the mercury column height h calculated from equation (1) is 760 mm. Therefore, at STP, one atmospheric pressure corresponds to a mercury column height of 760 mm, or simply 760 mmHg. If one uses water instead of mercury in the column, using 1,000 Kg/m^3 as the density of water, the height of the water column is calculated to be 10.3 m using the same equation. In addition to the S.I. unit, the two most commonly used pressure units in biomedical measurement are mmHg (e.g., for blood pressure measurement) and cmH$_2$O (e.g., for respiration pressure measurement). The conversion factors of some frequently used units in pressure measurement are tabulated in Table 4–1.

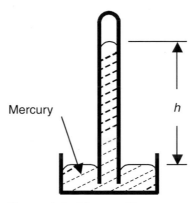

Figure 4–1. Mercury Barometer.

Table 4–1.
Pressure Unit Conversion

	Pa	mmHg	cmH₂O	psi	milli Bar
Pa	1	7.50×10^{-4}	1.02×10^{-2}	1.45×10^{-4}	1.00×10^{-2}
mmHg	133	1	1.36	1.93×10^{-2}	1.33
cmH₂O	98.1	0.735	1	1.42×10^{-2}	0.981
psi	6.89 3 103	51.7	70.3	1	
milli Bar	100	0.750	1.02	1.45×10^{-2}	1

Example 1

i) What is 760 mmHg in kPa?
ii) What is 2 cmH₂O in psi?

Solution:

i) In the first column of Table 4–1, the multiplication factor to convert mmHg to Pa is 133. Therefore, 760 mmHg = 133 × 760 Pa = 101,080 Pa = 101.08 kPa.
ii) In the fourth column of Table 4–1, the multiplication factor to convert cmH₂O to psi is 1.42×10^{-2}. Therefore, 2 cmH₂O = 2 × 1.42 × 10^{-2} = 2.84×10^{-2} psi.

In physiological pressure measurement, as the human body is constantly under one atmospheric pressure, the pressure measured is expressed as the pressure above atmospheric pressure instead of the absolute pressure P_{abs}. The pressure above atmospheric pressure is called gauge pressure P_{gauge}. The relationship between absolute, atmospheric, and gauge pressures is given by the equation:

$$P_{abs} = P_{gauge} + P_{atm} \qquad (2)$$

Whereas a barometer is used to measure the atmospheric pressure, a manometer can be used to measure the pressure from any source. Figure 4–2 shows a manometer constructed from a liquid-filled U-shaped glass tube with one end connected to a known constant pressure source P_b and the other end connected to the source to be measured. If the source pressure is P_a, using the Pascal principle, the relationship between P_a, P_b, the difference in liquid column height h, and the liquid density ρ is given by:

$$P_a = P_b + \rho gh \qquad (3)$$

In measuring gas pressure, one must remember that the pressure in a closed container changes with its temperature. The relationship between the gas pressure P, its volume V, and the temperature T is governed by the gas law, which states that:

$$PV = nRT$$

where nR is a constant.

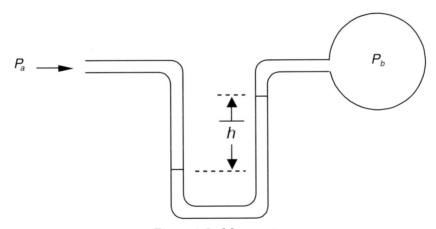

Figure 4–2. Manometer.

MECHANICAL PRESSURE GAUGES

Three types of mechanical pressure-sensing elements are often used in gas pressure measurement: bourdon tube, diaphragm, and bellow. A bourdon tube pressure transducer is shown in Figure 4–3; a bourdon tube is a hol-

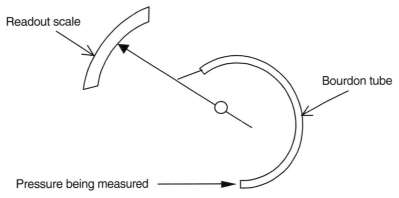

Figure 4–3. Bourdon Tube Pressure Gauge.

low metal coil with an oval-shaped cross section. When the pressure inside the coil increases, the pressure creates a force to unwrap the coiled tube. A mechanical linkage translates this movement into a pressure readout scale. The scale is calibrated against known pressure sources.

Figure 4–4 shows a diaphragm pressure transducer. When the pressure in the measurement chamber increases, the higher pressure on the measurement side pushes the diaphragm outward. The movement of the diaphragm is then converted to movement of a pointer needle to indicate the pressure to be measured.

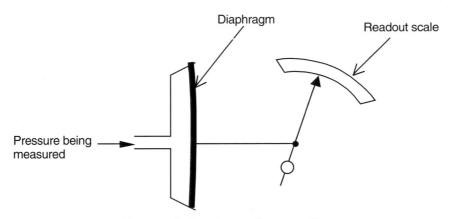

Figure 4–4. Diaphragm Pressure Gauge.

In Figure 4–5, a bellow is used as the sensing element. Similar to the diaphragm transducer, the bellow extends (or shortens) when the pressure inside the bellow becomes higher (or lower). Through a mechanical linkage, the bellow extension creates a motion on the pointer to indicate the pressure exerted on the bellow.

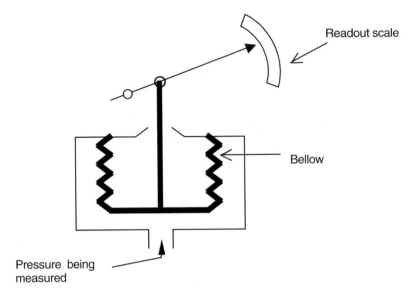

Figure 4–5. Bellow Gauge.

STRAIN GAUGES

Passive resistive sensors are commonly used in physiological measurement. The resistance of a resistor wire is given by the equation:

$$R = \rho\frac{L}{A} \tag{4}$$

where L is the length of the resistive wire, A is the cross-sectional area of the wire, and ρ is the resistivity.

A passive transducer can use one of the three parameters in equation (4) (length, area, and resistivity) to change its resistance, and thereby transduct the physiological event. The two most important examples are the transduction of pressure and the transduction of temperature. For example, a device known as a strain gauge can be used to measure force or pressure. A strain gauge is either a length of a thin conductor or a piece of semiconductor that is stressed or compressed in proportion to an applied force or pressure. The extension or contraction of the strain gauge element results in a change of the resistance.

Consider a piece of conductor wire, the resistance of which is given by equation (4). As the material is stretched, its length will increase and its cross-sectional area will decrease. Both of these changes will cause an increase in the resistance of the conductor. Alternatively, if the material is compressed, the length will decrease and the area will increase and therefore will cause a reduction in the conductor's resistance. In fact, for most materials, the unit increase in length is proportional to the unit decrease in diameter. This proportional constant is called Poisson's ratio v and is material-dependent. Poisson's ratio is defined as:

$$v = \frac{\Delta D/D}{\Delta L/L} \tag{5}$$

where $\Delta D/D$ is called the lateral strain, and $\Delta L/L$ is the axial strain.

Both the lateral and axial strains have no unit as the numerator and denominator in equation (5) have the same unit. However, the axial strain is often given a unit ε, and due to its small value, it is often expressed in $\mu\varepsilon$.

If one takes a partial derivative of R in equation (4), it becomes

$$\Delta R = \rho \frac{\Delta L}{A} - \rho L \frac{\Delta A}{A^2} + L \frac{\Delta \rho}{A} \tag{6}$$

Dividing both sides of the equation by R (the right-hand side by R and the left-hand side by $\rho \frac{L}{A}$) gives

$$\frac{\Delta R}{R} = \frac{\Delta L}{L} - \frac{\Delta A}{A} + \frac{\Delta \rho}{\rho} \tag{7}$$

For a cylindrical resistant wire, $A = \frac{\pi D^2}{4}$, where D is the diameter of the wire. Taking the partial derivative of this equation and dividing both side by A gives

$$\frac{\Delta A}{A} = 2 \frac{\Delta D}{D} \tag{8}$$

Substituting equation (8) into equation (7) gives

$$\frac{\Delta R}{R} = \frac{\Delta L}{L} - 2 \frac{\Delta D}{D} + \frac{\Delta \rho}{\rho} \tag{9}$$

Substituting equation (5) into equation (9) gives

$$\frac{\Delta R}{R} = \frac{\Delta L}{L} + 2v \frac{\Delta L}{L} + \frac{\Delta \rho}{\rho} = \frac{\Delta L}{L}(1 + 2v) + \frac{\Delta \rho}{\rho} \tag{10}$$

Equation (10) shows that both the change in resistivity and the change in length of the wire affect the resistance. The unit change of resistance per unit change in length of a strain gauge is called the gauge factor (G.F.).

$$G.F. = \frac{\Delta R/R}{\Delta L/L} \qquad (11)$$

From equations (10) and (11), the gauge factor G.F. is equal to

$$G.F. = \frac{\Delta R/R}{\Delta L/L} = (1 + 2v) + \frac{\Delta \rho/\rho}{\Delta L/L} \qquad (12)$$

The G.F. value is different from one material to another. For a metal strain gauge, $\frac{\Delta \rho}{\rho}$ is zero and the G.F. is between 2 and 4. For a semiconductor or piezoelectric strain gauge, $\frac{\Delta \rho}{\rho}$ is nonzero. The G.F. of a piezoelectric stain gauge can be several hundreds.

Example 2

For a metal wire resistive strain gauge with nominal resistance $Ro = 120.0\ \Omega$ and G.F. = 2.045, find the change in resistance if an axial strain of 7,320 $\mu\varepsilon$ is applied to the strain gauge.

Solution:

From equation 11

$$G.F. = \frac{\Delta R/R}{\Delta L/L}$$

$$\Rightarrow \qquad \Delta R = R \times G.F. \times \Delta L/L$$

$$\Rightarrow \qquad \Delta R = 120.0\ \Omega \times 2.045 \times 7320 \times 10^{-6} = 1.796\ \Omega$$

A strain gauge may be either bonded or unbonded. A bonded strain gauge means that the wire or semiconductor material is attached to a flexible bonding material, such as paper or plastic. It is then cemented to the surface of the structure to measure the strain. Unbonded strain gauges use posts to hold the ends of the gauge. The posts are attached to the structure to be measured. Figure 4–6 shows bonded and unbonded metal wired strain gauges.

Other than metal wire strain gauges, a common transducer element in pressure measurement is the diaphragm piezoresistive strain gauge. It is fabricated using semiconductor technology in which a layer of piezoresistive material is deposited on a flexible diaphragm and lead wires are bonded to

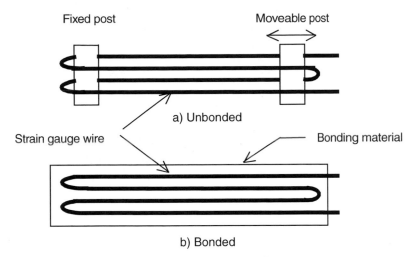

a) Unbonded

Strain gauge wire

Bonding material

b) Bonded

Figure 4–6. Wired Strain Gauges.

the strain gauge (Figure 4–7). The gauge resistance changes as the strain element on the diaphragm is deformed by the applied pressure. As the gauge factor of piezoresistive material is much higher than that of metal, it creates a much more sensitive pressure transducer than metal wire stain gauges. Furthermore, by controlling the position of the piezoresistive deposit on the diaphragm and its shape, it can produce a linear output response to the applied pressure.

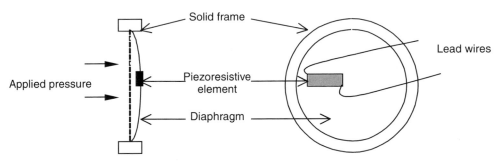

Figure 4–7. Diaphragm Piezoresistive Strain Gauge.

While the focus has been on the use of the strain gauge for the transduction of pressure, it does have many other biomedical applications. An interesting application in cardiology technology is the use of strain gauges to measure cardiac contractility. In this application, which is used for research purposes, a bonded strain gauge is sutured directly to the ventricular wall of the heart. The contractile force of the muscle fibers causes a change in the strain gauge resistance, which is then measured, processed, and displayed. Another example is a load cell to measure the body weight of a patient undergoing renal dialysis. A load cell is a transducer that converts a load (or force) acting on it to an analog electrical signal. An example of a load cell is shown in Figure 4–8, where the deformation of the bonded strain gauge on the beam is converted to a change in resistance.

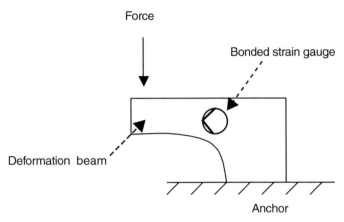

Figure 4–8. A Load Cell.

PIEZOELECTRIC PRESSURE TRANSDUCERS

Some materials such as quartz crystal and certain ceramic materials generate opposite electric charges at their surfaces when subjected to mechanical strain. Also, these materials produce physical deformation when an electric potential is applied. The charge Q produced is proportional to the applied force F (which created the strain on the material). The proportionality constant is called the piezoelectric constant K. Consider the circular disc piezoelectric transducer in Figure 4–9 with thickness d and cross-sectional area A. The charge Q created on the surface of the transducer is:

$$Q = k \times F$$

Assuming the transducer is a thin circular disc, with charge residing on the surface, the disc can be considered as a parallel plate capacitor with capacitance $C = \dfrac{\varepsilon A}{d}$. The voltage across the capacitor

$$V = \frac{Q}{C} = \frac{kF}{C} = \frac{kFd}{\varepsilon A} = \frac{Kd}{\varepsilon}\frac{F}{A} = \frac{kd}{\varepsilon}P \qquad (13)$$

It shows that the voltage measured across the surface of the transducer is proportional to the applied pressure.

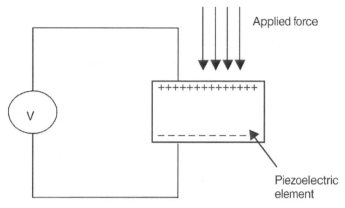

Figure 4–9. Circular Disc Piezoelectric Element.

A biomedical application of such a transducer is the ultrasound transmitter and receiver. In an ultrasound receiver, the sound pressure to be detected produces some mechanical strain on the piezoelectric element, which generates a potential difference whose amplitude varies according to the sound pressure. In an ultrasound transmitter, the electric signal imposes on the transducer produces deformation according to the amplitude and frequency of the signal. This physical deformation creates mechanical pressure waves in the medium in which the transducer element is submerged.

Example 3

A pressure transducer with nominal resistance $R_0 = 100 \ \Omega$ (at zero pressure) and sensitivity $S = 3.00 \ \Omega$ per 100 mmHg is placed on one arm of a Wheatstone bridge as shown in the figure below. If the resistors R_1, R_2, and R_3 are all 100 Ω and the excitation voltage $V_E = 5.00$ V, find the change in output voltage V_0 when the pressure is increased from 0 to 60.0 mmHg.

Solution:

When $P = 0$ mmHg, $R_x = R_1 = R_2 = R_3 = 100 \ \Omega$, the bridge output $V_0 = 0.0$ V (balanced bridge).

When the applied pressure $P = 60.0$ mmHg, the change in resistance of the transducer $\Delta R_x = S \times \Delta P = 3.00 \ \Omega/100$ mmHg $\times 60.0$ mmHg $= 1.80 \ \Omega$.

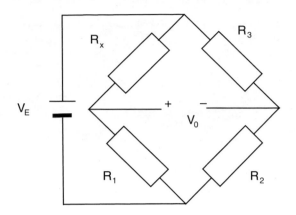

Therefore, $R_x = 100 + 1.80 = 101.8 \ \Omega$, substituting into the bridge circuit gives

$$V_0 = V_E \left[\frac{R_1}{R_x + R_1} - \frac{R_2}{R_2 + R_3} \right] = 5.00 \left[\frac{100}{101.8 + 100} - \frac{100}{100 + 100} \right] = -0.0223V = -22.3mV$$

Chapter 5

TEMPERATURE TRANSDUCERS

OBJECTIVES

- Explain the IPTS temperature scale.
- Perform temperature unit conversion.
- State common temperature measurement terminology
- Describe the principles of nonelectrical temperature gauges.
- Analyze the characteristics of RTDs, thermistors, thermocouples, and IC temperature sensors.
- Define errors due to lead resistance and self-heating effect in temperature measurement applications.
- Explain methods to linearize thermistor characteristics.

CHAPTER CONTENTS

INTRODUCTION

Temperature transducers have widespread applications in biomedical instrumentation. They can be used in direct body temperature measurement, in patient assessment, or to ensure patient safety by monitoring performance of machine parameters such as the heating fluid temperature of a blood warmer. Temperature transducers that are designed to provide temperature readings are called thermometers. This chapter covers concepts in temperature measurement and the principles of some commonly used temperature transducers.

REFERENCE TEMPERATURE AND TEMPERATURE SCALE

Unlike most other physical quantities, one cannot add temperatures together as one would add lengths to measure distances. We must rely on physical phenomenan to establish observable and consistent temperature references. For example, the freezing point and boiling point of water at one atmospheric pressure are assigned as $0°$ and $100°$, respectively, in the Celsius (or centigrade) scale and as $32°$ and $212°$ in the Fahrenheit scale. The entire temperature scale can be constructed by making interpolation of these fixed temperature references. Table 5–1 shows the reference temperatures on which the International Practical Temperature Scale (IPTS) is based. Interpolation of these references is performed by temperature transducers.

Common units of temperature measurement are degree Celsius ($°C$) in the Celsius scale, degree Fahrenheit ($°F$) in the Fahrenheit scale, and the

Table 5-1.
IPTS–68 Reference Temperatures

Reference Point	K	°C
Triple Point of Hydrogen	13.81	–259.34
Liquid/Vapor Phase of Hydrogen at 25/76 Std. Atm.	17.042	–256.108
Boiling Point of Hydrogen	20.28	–252.87
Boiling Point of Neon	27.102	–246.048
Triple Point of Oxygen	54.361	–218.789
Boiling Point of Oxygen	90.188	–142.962
Triple Point of Water	273.16	0.01
Boiling Point of Water	373.15	100
Freezing Point of Zinc	692.73	419.58
Freezing Point of Silver	1,235.08	961.93
Freezing Point of Gold	1,337.58	1,064.43

Kelvin (K) in the absolute scale. For a temperature of A°F, the equivalent temperature reading in the Celsius scale is B°C, where

$$B = \frac{5}{9}(A - 32) \tag{1}$$

or, in reverse, $A = \frac{9}{5}B + 32$.

The same temperature in Kelvin (C K) is given as

$$C = B + 273.15. \tag{2}$$

Example 1

The body temperature of a patient is measured to be 37.0°C, what are the temperature readings in the Fahrenheit and absolute scales.

Solution

From equation (1), $A = \frac{9}{5}B + 32 = \frac{9}{5} \times 37.0 + 32 = 98.6$°F.

From equation (2), $C = B + 273.15 = 37.0 + 273.15 = 310.2$ K.

NONELECTRICAL TEMPERATURE TRANSDUCERS

Fluid-in-glass thermometers have long been used to measure temperature. It has been the most popular type of thermometer in body temperature measurement until recently. Mercury-in-glass and petrolate-in-glass are the two most common types in this category. A fluid-in-glass thermometer is shown in Figure 5–1. It consists of a glass tube (or stem) with a uniform lumen connected to a reservoir. The top of the tube is sealed after air is removed. When the temperature increases, the fluid in the reservoir expands and pushes up the fluid level in the stem. The position of the fluid meniscus indicates the temperature under measurement. Two temperature references (e.g., water freezing and boiling points) are chosen to calibrate two points on the stem of the thermometer. Mercury-filled thermometers usually have a temperature measurement range from –40 to +900°C, while red-dyed petrolate can measure from –200 to +260°C. In medical applications, some glass thermometers are Teflon™ encapsulated to avoid shattering.

Bimetallic sensors are often used in temperature gauges as thermal

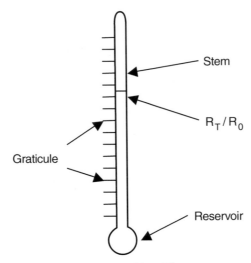

Figure 5–1. Fluid-in-Glass Thermometer.

switches. Two metals with different temperature expansion coefficients are bonded together to form a bimetallic strip. When the temperature changes, the differential expansion causes the strip to bend. The degree of bending can be calibrated and used in temperature measurement. Figure 5–2 shows a simple bimetallic strip, and Figure 5–3 shows a dial-type temperature gauge with the bimetallic strip formed into a helical coil to produce rotational motion with changes in temperature. Depending on the type of metals used, bimetallic gauges can measure temperature in the range of –40 to 1500°C.

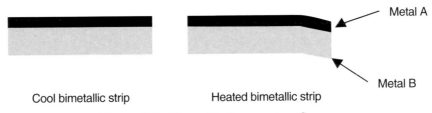

Figure 5–2. Bimetallic Temperature Sensor.

Another nonelectrical temperature sensor is constructed by sandwiching a liquid crystal material between an adhesive backing and a transparent Mylar™ film. The liquid crystal can be made to reflect different colors of light at different temperatures. Liquid crystal thermometers provide fast (1 to 2 seconds respond time) visual indication of temperature with a range from 0 to +60°C. Strip thermometers are available to measure body temperature.

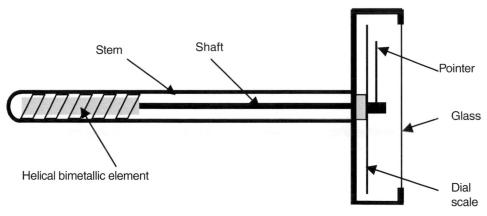

Figure 5–3. Dial-Type Temperature Gauge.

ELECTRICAL TEMPERATURE TRANSDUCERS

In general, electrical transducers can be divided into two types–passive and active. Resistance temperature devices and thermistors, both of which are passive transducers, are covered in this chapter. Thermocouples and integrated circuit sensors are covered as examples of active temperature transducers.

In addition to other instrumentation specification parameters covered in Chapter 2, some parameters that are commonly referred to in temperature measurement applications are:

- Operating range–the temperature between two limits within which the characteristics conform to the specifications.
- Stability–the quality of the sensor to maintain a consistent output when a constant input is applied. The shelf life of a disposable transducer is an indication of the stability of the sensor.
- Dissipation constant–the power in milliwatts required to raise the sensor by 1°C above the surrounding temperature. For example, a thermistor may be listed to have a dissipation constant of 1.0 mW/°C in still air.
- Respond time–the time required to reach a certain percentage of the steady state output followed by a step input. The time to reach 63.2% is referred to as one time constant. For most temperature transducers, approximately five time constants are necessary to reach 99% of the steady state output.

RESISTANCE TEMPERATURE DEVICES (RTD)

For a metal conductor, the resistance increases with temperature. Therefore, one can measure the resistance of a metal wire to determine its temperature. Figure 5–4 shows the normalized resistance-temperature characteristics of metal RTDs, including nickel, copper, platinum, and tungsten. R_T is the resistance of the metal wire in Ω at temperature T^oC, and R_0 is the resistance of the metal wire at T_0^oC. By selecting different metals, RTD can measure temperature from –200 to over +800°C. As shown in Figure 5–4, despite its low sensitivity, the platinum RTD shows an almost linear resistance-temperature relationship and therefore can be approximated by:

$$R_T = R_0 (1 + \alpha \Delta T) \qquad (3)$$

where $\Delta T = T - T_0$,
T_0 is usually specified at 0°C,
and α is the fractional change in resistance per unit temperature.

The temperature coefficient is defined as

$$\left(\frac{dR_T}{dT} \right)$$

which is equal to αR_0 from equation (3).

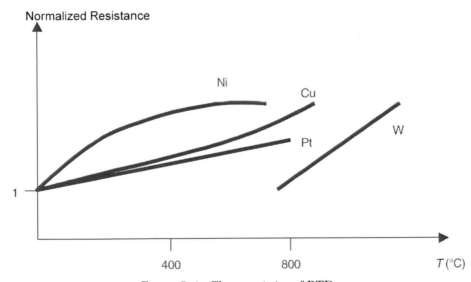

Figure 5–4. Characteristics of RTD.

Example 2

A platinum RTD is used in a bridge circuit as shown below. What is the bridge output V_0 at 10°C, given the excitation voltage $V_E = 2.0$ V, bridge resistance $R = R_0 = 100\Omega$ at 0°C, and $\alpha = 0.00385/°C$.

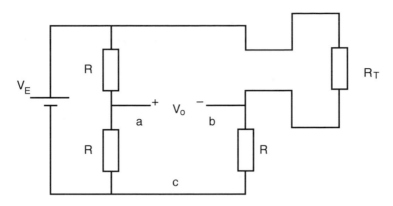

Solution

Let $\Delta R = R_T - R_0$,
at 10°C, $\Delta R = R_0 (1 + \alpha \Delta T) - R_0 = \alpha R_0 \Delta T = 0.00852*100*10 = 3.85\Omega$
for the Wheatstone bridge circuit.

$$V_0 = \left[\frac{R}{R + R_T} - \frac{R}{R + R} \right] = \left[\frac{R}{R + R + \Delta R} - \frac{1}{2} \right] = -\frac{\Delta R}{2R + \Delta R} \times \frac{V_E}{2}$$

Substituting $R = 100\Omega$, $\Delta R = 3.85\Omega$, and $V_E = 2.0$ V into the above gives
$V_0 = -18.9$ mV

Example 3

A piece of platinum RTD wire has a resistance of 100.0Ω at 0°C.

Find (a) its temperature coefficient and (b) its resistance at 180.0°C given that $\alpha = 0.00385/°C$ for platinum RTD.

Solution

(a) Temperature coefficient $= \alpha R_0 = 0.00385 \times 100 = 0.385\Omega/°C$
(b) Using equation (3), $R_{189} = 100 (1 + 0.00385*189) = 171.8 \ \Omega$

The value of α quoted in this example is according to the DIN Standard (European). In the United States, α is equal to 0.00392/°C for a standard platinum RTD. Usually, the RTD characteristics are specified in a lookup table of resistance against temperature supplied by the manufacturer.

LEAD ERRORS

It should be noted that RTDs in general have low sensitivities. That is, the output resistance changes only slightly for a relatively large change in temperature. For the platinum RTD in the above example, the temperature sensitivity (or temperature coefficient) is equal to $0.385V/^\circ C$. In temperature measurement using RTD, one must be aware of the errors introduced to the measurement from inadvertent additions and changes in the overall measured resistance.

Example 4

In a temperature measurement experiment using a platinum RTD, a pair of long lead wires are used to connect the RTD to an ohmmeter. If $\alpha = 0.00385/^\circ C$ and each lead wire has an overall resistance of 0.5Ω, find the lead error.

Solution

The lead wires add a total resistance of $0.5 + 0.5 = 1.0\Omega$ to the RTD. The temperature error T_E due to the lead resistance (or simply called lead error) is

$$T_E - \frac{1.0}{0.385} = 2.6^\circ C$$

which is a very significant error in medical applications.

Example 5

For the RTD application in Example 2, if each lead wire to the RTD has a resistance R_L of 0.50Ω, what is the bridge output?

Solution

With the lead resistance R_L, the effective resistance R_E across the bridge arm becomes $R_T + 2R_L$, substituting into

$$V_0 = \left[\frac{R}{R + R_E} - \frac{R}{R + R}\right] = \left[\frac{R}{R + R + \Delta R + 2R_L} - \frac{1}{2}\right] = -\frac{\Delta R + 2R_L}{2R + \Delta R + 2R_L} \times \frac{V_E}{2}$$

Substituting $R = 100\Omega$, $\Delta R = 3.85\Omega$, and $V_E = 2.0$ V into the equation

$$V_0 = -\frac{3.85 \times 2 \times 0.50}{2 \times 100 + 3.85 + 2 \times 0.50} \times \frac{2.0}{2} \text{ gives}$$

$V_0 = -23.7$ mV.

This result shows a -25% error compares to the bridge output $(-18.9$ mV$)$ without lead resistance in Example 3.

In any resistive transducer applications, lead resistance can introduce significant errors in the measurement. Lead errors can be accounted for if one knows the exact resistance of the lead wires. However, this may not be possible in some applications. Below are some methods used to minimize lead errors.

Three-Wire Bridge

One method to reduce the lead error is to use a 3-wire bridge circuit. Instead of using a conventional 2-wire RTD, a 3-wire RTD is used as shown

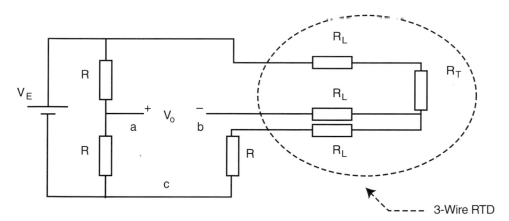

Figure 5–5. 3-Wire Wheatstone Bridge Circuit.

in Figure 5–5.

For the circuit in Figure 5–5, if we are using a high input impedance voltmeter to measure V_0, there will be no voltage drop across the middle lead (R_L) since the middle lead does not carry any current. Given $R_T = R + \Delta R$, the bridge output becomes

$$V_0 = \left[\frac{R + R_L}{R + R_T + R_L} - \frac{R}{R + R}\right] = \left[\frac{R + R_L}{2R + R_L + \Delta R} - \frac{1}{2}\right] = -\frac{\Delta R}{2R + 2R_L + \Delta R} \times \frac{V_E}{2}$$

Example 6

For the 3-wire RTD application in Figure 5–5, using the same circuit values as Example 5, that is, $R = 100\Omega$, $R_L = 0.05$, $\Delta R = 3.85\Omega$ (at 10°C), and $V_E = 2.0$ V, what is the bridge output?

Solution

Substituting $R = 100\ \Omega$, $\Delta R = 3.85\ \Omega$, $R_L = 3.85\ \Omega$, and $V_E = 2.0$ V into the equation.

$$V_0 = -\frac{\Delta R}{2R + 2R_L + \Delta R} \times \frac{V_E}{2}, \text{ which gives}$$

$$V_0 = -\frac{3.85}{2 \times 100 + 2 \times 0.50 + 3.85} \times \frac{2.0}{2} = -0.0188 \text{ V} = -18.8 \text{ mV.}$$

This result shows a mere 0.5% error compares to bridge output (−18.9 mV) without lead resistance (Example 2). This is a significant improvement to the 2-wire RTD bridge circuit in Example 5 (−25% error)!

To totally eliminate the error due to lead resistance, a 4-wire RTD with a high impedance voltmeter and constant current source connected as shown in Figure 5–6 is needed. The RTD resistance is simply calculated by divid-

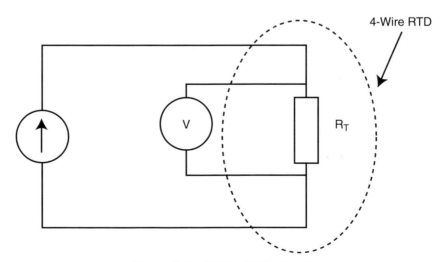

Figure 5–6. 4-Wire RTD Circuit.

SELF-HEATING ERRORS

An RTD is a resistor whose resistance changes with temperature. As we all know, when a current I passes through a resistor R, it will produce heat at a rate equals to I^2R. This heat will raise the temperature of the RTD and therefore will create an error in the measured temperature. Dissipation constants are specified for all resistive-type temperature transducers. The dissipation constant specifies the temperature error caused by the heat generated in the transducer due to externally applied current. The value of dissipation constant depends on the type of transducer element, its packaging, as well as the medium in which it is being used.

Example 7

A 100Ω platinum RTD in a bridge circuit is used to measure air temperature. The bridge excitation is 5.0 V and all the bridge resistors are 100Ω. Calculate the error due to self-heating if the dissipation constant of the RTD in still air is 5.0 mW/°C (or 0.20°C/mW).

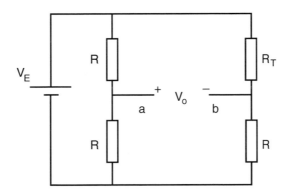

Solution

When the bridge is balanced, i.e. $R_T = R = 100Ω$.
The voltage V_T across R_T is 0.5 times the excitation voltage V_E. The power dissipated P_T in the RTD is therefore given by

$$P_T = \frac{V_T^2}{R_T} = \frac{V_E^2}{4R} = \frac{5.0^2}{4 \times 100} = 0.0625 \text{ W} = 62.5 \text{ mW.}$$

Therefore, self-heating error $= \dfrac{62.5 \text{ mW}}{5.0 \text{ mW/°C}} = 12.5°C,$

which means that the RTD will read 12.5°C higher than the correct temperature due to the self-heating effect.

From the above example, one can see that in order to reduce the self-heating error, one should reduce the excitation voltage or increase the bridge resistance.

THERMISTORS

Another common passive resistive temperature transducer is the thermistor. Thermistors are made from semiconductor materials such as oxide of nickel, manganese, iron, cobalt, or copper. As a thermistor is a semiconductor, it has nonlinear resistance temperature characteristics. Thermistors can have a positive or negative temperature coefficient and an operating range from −80 to +150°C. Thermistors have higher nominal resistance than RTD (ranges from 1 kΩ to 1 MΩ) as well as higher sensitivity (from 3 to 5%/°C). Although not as good as RTD, it has very good long-term stability (less than 0.2% drift in resistance per year). The most common type of thermistor used in medical instrument is the YSI 400 series thermistor (YSI stands for Yellow Spring Instrument, which is a manufacturer of temperature transducers), which has a negative temperature coefficient (Figure 5–7). The characteristics of a thermistor are available in manufacturer's lookup tables. Also, most negative temperature coefficient thermistors can be approximated by:

$$R_T = R_0 e^{\beta\left(\frac{1}{T} - \frac{1}{T_0}\right)} \qquad (4)$$

where R_T is the thermistor resistance in Ω at temperature T,
R_0 is the thermistor resistance in Ω at temperature T_0,
T and T_0 are absolute temperature in K (note that T is in °C in the RTD equation), and α is the thermistor material constant in the range of 2,500 to 5,000 K.

The temperature coefficient $\left(\dfrac{dR_T}{dT}\right)$ can be obtained by differentiating equation (4) with respect to temperature T, which gives:

$$\left(\frac{dR_T}{dT}\right) = R_0 \frac{d\left[e^{\beta\left(\frac{1}{T} - \frac{1}{T_0}\right)}\right]}{dT} = R_0 e^{\beta\left(\frac{1}{T} - \frac{1}{T_0}\right)} \frac{d}{dT}\left(\frac{\beta}{T}\right) = R_T\left(-\frac{\beta}{T^2}\right) = -\frac{R_T \beta}{T^2}$$

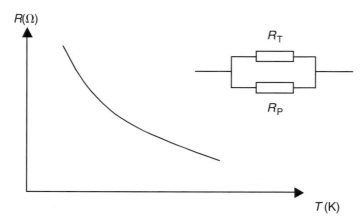

Figure 5-7. Thermistor Characteristics.

$$\left(\frac{}{dT}\right) = R_0 \ \frac{}{dT} = R_0e \qquad \frac{}{dT}\left(\frac{1}{T}\right) = R_T\left(-\frac{1}{T^2}\right) = -\ \frac{}{T^2}$$

Example 8

For a thermistor with $\beta = 4{,}000$ K, find (a) the thermistor resistance, and (b) the temperature coefficient at 37.0°C given the $R_0 = 7355\Omega$ at 0°C.

Solution

(a) Using equation (4)

$$R_T = 7{,}355 \ e^{\ 4000\left(\frac{1}{(37+273)}-\frac{1}{(0+273)}\right)} = 1280\Omega$$

(b) Temperature coefficient $= -\ \dfrac{R_T\beta}{T^2} = \dfrac{-1{,}280 \times 4{,}000}{(37+273)^2} = -53.3 \ {}^{\Omega}\!/_{K}$

    One of the major drawbacks for thermistor is its highly nonlinear characteristics. Much research was done to produce thermistors with linear resistance temperature characteristics. A rather efficient method to produce a piecewise linear characteristic within a narrow temperature region is achieved by connecting a parallel resistor R_P to the thermistor. This combination produces an approximate linear region centered around the temperature of interest T_m. The parallel resistor value R_P is derived from finding the point of inflexion $\left(\dfrac{d^2R}{dT^2}=0\right)$ of the resistor combination curve. Without going into the detailed derivation, R_P can be calculated from:

$$R_P = R_{Tm} \times \frac{\beta - 2T_m}{\beta + 2T_m} \qquad (5)$$

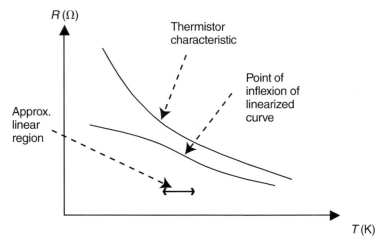

Figure 5–8. Thermistor Linearization.

The linearized characteristic using this method is shown in Figure 5–8. Note that this method reduces the overall sensitivity of the transducer.

Example 9

A YSI 400 thermistor is used for body temperature measurement. Choose a parallel resistor to the thermistor to linearize its resistance temperature characteristic around the temperature of interest.

Solution

The normal body temperature is about 37°C (= 310 K). From the manufacturer's lookup table of YSI 400 thermistor, R_{37} = 1,355 Ω and β = 4,000 K. Substituting into equation (5) gives

$$R_P = 1,355 \times \frac{4000 - 2 \times 310}{4000 + 2 \times 310} = 991 \ \Omega$$

Another method to obtain a linear relationship is by using two thermistors, Figure 5–9a shows a YSI 700 series thermistor combination, and Figure 5–9b shows one example of using this thermistor to produce a linear resistance temperature curve (Figure 5–10).

Note that there are three lead wires for a YSI 700 Series thermistor (one more than a 400 Series). There are other methods to linearize thermistor characteristics. However, newer microprocessor-based devices with large memory to store the entire thermistor lookup table have made linearlization

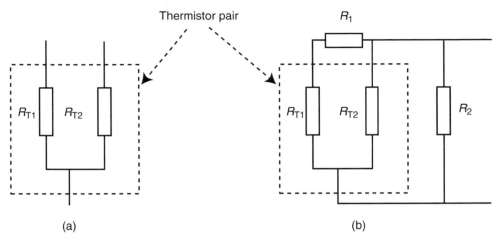

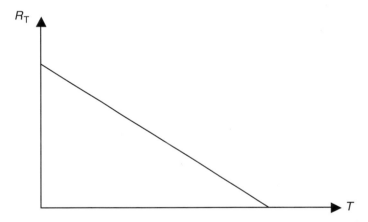

Figure 5–9. YSI 700 Series Thermistor and Application.

Figure 5-10. Linearized Characteristic of YSI 400 Series Thermistor Circuit.

less important. Different sizes and shapes of thermistor probes are designed for different applications.

THERMOCOUPLES

A thermocouple is an active temperature transducer that produces a small unique voltage according to the temperature. A thermocouple consists of two dissimilar metals joined together. Thomas Seebeck discovered this property in 1821.

Seebeck Effect

When two wires of dissimilar metals are joined at both ends and one end is at a higher temperature than the other, there is a continuous flow of cur-

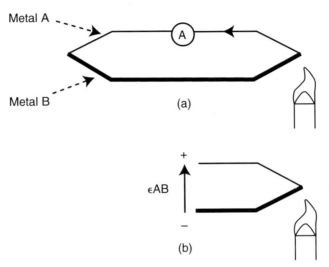

Figure 5–11. Seebeck Effect.

rent in the wire (Figure 5–11a). This current is called the thermoelectric current. When one junction is disconnected, a voltage called the Seebeck voltage can be measured across the two metal wires (Figure 5–11b).

For a small variation of the temperature difference between the hot and cold junctions, the Seebeck voltage ϵ_{AB} is proportional to the temperature variation ΔT with a proportional constant α called the Seebeck coefficient. This relationship is represented by

$$\epsilon_{AB} = \alpha\Delta T$$

The Seebeck coefficient is different for different thermocouples. It is small and varies with temperature. In addition, it has a nonlinear temperature characteristic. For example, the Seebeck coefficient for E-type (Chromel and Constanan) thermocouple varies from about 25 µV/°C at −200°C to 62 µV/°C at +800°C.

The thermoelectric sensitivity of a thermocouple material is usually given relative to a standard platinum reference. Since the Seebeck coefficient is temperature-dependent, the sensitivity is also temperature-dependent. Table 5–2 shows the sensitivities of some thermocouple metals referenced to platinum at 0°C. The sensitivity at 0°C of any combination of the materials can be obtained by taking the difference of the sensitivities of the materials forming the thermocouple. For example, the sensitivity of chromel and constanan (Type E thermocouple) is $-25 - (-35) = 60$ µV/°C. In temperature measurement, one of the junctions is kept at a known (or reference) temper-

Table 5–2.
Thermoelectric Sensitivity of Thermocouple Materials

	Copper	*Chromel*	*Constanan*	*Iron*	*Platinum*
Composition	Cu	90 Ni/10 Cr	60 Cu/40 Ni	Fe	Pt
Sensitivity, µV/°C	+6.5	+25	–35	+18.5	0

ature and the other junction is at the temperature to be measured. The reference temperature is often referred to as the cold temperature since thermocouples are usually used for high temperature measurements.

Thermocouples can be used to measure temperature from –200 to +2000

Table 5–3.
Characteristics of Thermocouples

Type	*Name*	*Temp Range*	*Output*, mV*
T	Copper/constanan	–200 to +300	4.25
J	Iron/constanan	–200 to +1,100	5.28
E	Chromel/constanan	0 to +1,100	6.30
K	Chromel/alumel	–200 to +1,200	4.10
S	Platinum/pt rhodium	0 to +1,450	0.64

* Output is measured at 100°C with reference at 0°C.

°C. In addition to its wide temperature range, it is rugged, accurate and can be made to be extremely small in size. The output characteristics of some common thermocouples are listed in Table 5–3 and shown in Figure 5–12.

Empirical Laws of Thermocouples

The following three empirical laws are important facts that enable thermocouples to be used as practical temperature measurement devices:

1. The law of homogeneous circuit
2. The law of intermediate metals

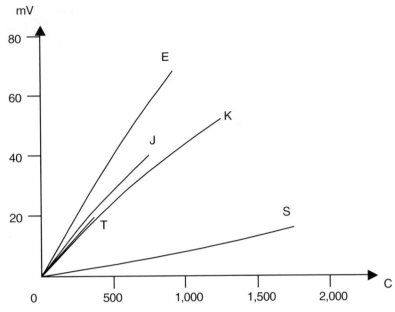

Figure 5–12. Thermocouple Output Characteristics.

3. The law of intermediate temperature

The law of homogeneous circuit states that for a thermocouple of metals

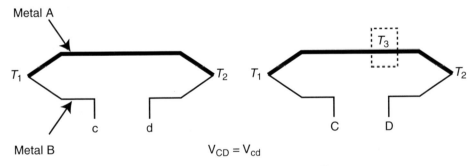

Figure 5–13. Law of Homogeneous Circuit.

A and B, the output voltage is not affected by the temperature along metal A or B. It is determined by the temperatures at the two junctions (Figure 5–13). This is required as the metals or lead wires between the thermocouple junctions will be at different temperatures than either of the junctions.

The law of intermediate metals states that the output voltage is not affect-

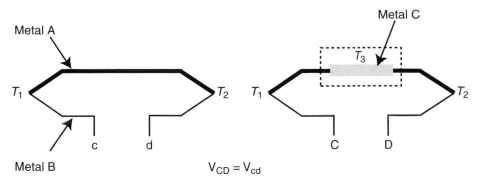

Figure 5–14. Law of Intermediate Metal.

ed by the use of a third metal in the circuit provided that the new junctions are at the same temperature (Figure 5–14). This allows lead wires (usually copper wires) of a voltmeter to be connected to the thermocouple circuit to measure its output voltage.

The law of intermediate temperature states that for the same thermocouple, the output voltage V_{31} where the temperature at the junctions are T_3 and

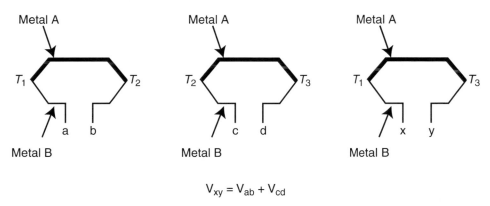

Figure 5–15. Law of Intermediate Temperature.

T_1, respectively, is equal to the sum of the output voltages of two separate measurements with junction temperatures T_3, T_2, and T_2, T_1 (i.e., $V_{31} = V_{32} + V_{21}$) (Figure 5–15). This allows using a standard thermocouple lookup table to calculate the junction temperature from the voltage measured.

In practice, the setup for temperature measurement using a thermocouple is as shown in Figure 5–16a. The empirical law of intermediate metal allows a third metal to connect the thermocouple to the voltmeter. It is important that the connections between the lead wires and the thermocouple metal wires be kept at the same temperature to avoid generating another voltage to upset the measurement. These connections are bonded to an isothermal block that has high thermal conductivity to ensure equal temperature at the connection points.

At the hot junction (temperature to be measured T_m), the junction voltage referenced to 0°C is equal to V_{m0}. At the isothermal block (at temperature T_r), the junction voltage referenced to 0°C is equal to V_{r0}. Using the empirical law of intermediate temperature, we can write:

$$V_{mr} + V_{r0} = V_{m0}, \text{ where } V_{mr} = V \text{ is the thermocouple output voltage, or}$$

$$V = V_{m0} - V_{r0} \tag{6}$$

If we know the reference temperature T_r and the output voltage, with the thermocouple lookup table, we can use equation (6) to find the hot junction temperature T_m.

Example 10

A J-type thermocouple is used to measure the temperature of an oven. If the temperature of the isothermal block is at 20.0°C and the output voltage measured is 9.210 mV, what is the temperature of the oven?

Solution

Step 1
Using a J-type thermocouple lookup table, find the junction voltage V_{r0} at T_r = 20°C. At 20.0°C, the junction voltage of a J-type thermocouple referenced to 0°C from the lookup table is 1.019 mV.
Step 2
Using equation (6), $V_{m0} = V + V_{r0} = 9.210 + 1.019 = 10.229$ mV.

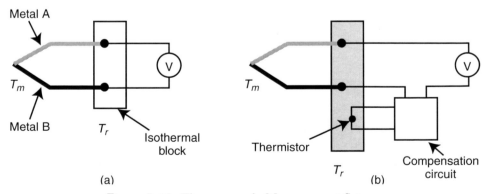

Figure 5–16. Thermocouple Measurement Setup.

The junction voltage at the hot junction referenced to 0°C is 10.229 mV.
Step 3
From the thermocouple lookup table, at $V_{m0} = 10.229$, $T_m = 190°C$.
Therefore, the temperature of the oven is 190°C.

The setup in Figure 5–16b includes a temperature sensor (thermistor) to measure the reference temperature. The compensation circuit produces a voltage according to the thermistor resistance. The output voltage becomes the algebraic sum of the compensation voltage and the junction voltage, which can be converted to the junction temperature.

Thermocouples are available in different package formats for different applications. The junction can be exposed, ungrounded, or grounded. An exposed junction is recommended for the measurement of static or flowing noncorrosive fluid where fast response time is required. An ungrounded junction is recommended for measurements in corrosive environments where it is desirable to have the thermocouple shielded from the corrosive environment by the protective sheath and electrically isolated and shielded. A grounded junction is recommended for the measurement of static or flowing corrosive fluid. The junction of a grounded thermocouple is welded to the protective sheath. As the magnitude of the thermocouple output voltage is usually very low, care must be taken to avoid errors due to electrical interference and voltaic effects.

INTEGRATED CIRCUIT TEMPERATURE SENSORS

The last temperature sensor to be discussed in this chapter is the IC temperature sensor. IC temperature sensors employ the temperature-dependent properties of the PN junction to measure temperature. IC temperature sensors are in general very accurate and linear. However, due to the fact that they are constructed from semiconductor materials, IC temperature sensors are not suitable for extreme temperature conditions. The operating range of IC temperature sensors is from -55 to $+150°C$. IC temperature sensors can be current type or voltage type. In a current type sensor, the sensor will produce a current proportional to the temperature. In a voltage type sensor, the output voltage is proportional to the temperature. An example of an IC temperature sensor is the National Semiconductor LM50, which has a temperature sensitivity of 10.0 mV/°C, $\pm0.8\%$ maximum nonlinearity and only requires a 4 to 10 V single power supply.

COMPARISON OF TEMPERATURE SENSORS'

CHARACTERISTICS

Table 5–4.
Comparison of Temperature Sensors Characteristics

	Thermistor	*Platinum RTD*	*Thermocouple*	*IC Sensor*
Sensitivity	3 to 5 KΩ/°C	0.00385/°C	7 to 60 µV/°C	1 µA/°C
Linearity	Poor	Good	Fair	Very good
Stability	Stable	Very stable	Stable	Less stable
Power Required	Yes	Yes	Self powered	Yes
Min. Practical Span	1°C	25°C	100°C	25°C
Temp. Range, °C	−100 to +250	−200 to +750	−100 to +2,000	−55 to +150
Reference Required	No	No	Cold junction	No
Ruggedness	Very rugged	Rugged	Very rugged	Rugged
Repeatability	Very good	Very good	Fair	Good
Hysteresis	Low	Low	High	Low

Chapter 6

MOTION TRANSDUCERS

OBJECTIVES

- State the relationships between displacement, velocity, and acceleration.
- Derive the principles of resistive, capacitive, and inductive displacement transducers.
- Describe application examples of resistive, capacitive, and inductive sensors in linear and angular displacement measurements.
- Explain the principles of Hall effect sensors.
- Describe application examples of Hall effect sensors in linear and angular displacement measurements.

CHAPTER CONTENTS

INTRODUCTION

The measurements of displacement, velocity, and acceleration are often performed in biomedical applications. Measuring the motion of the heart wall during open heart surgery, quantifying the frequency and magnitude of hand tremor for a patient suffering from Parkinson disease, and monitoring the position of a surgical retractor are a few examples of the applications. The displacement x (in m), velocity v (in m/s), and acceleration a (m/s^2) of an object are related by the following equations, where t is the time in seconds:

$$v = \frac{dx}{dt}$$

$$a = \frac{dv}{dt} = \frac{d^2x}{dt^2}$$

Therefore, if the displacement versus time of an object is recorded, its velocity and acceleration can be calculated. In a similar manner, if the angle versus time is recorded, the angular velocity and angular acceleration can be computed. This chapter focuses on the measurement of displacement including linear (or translational) and angular displacement.

RESISTIVE DISPLACEMENT TRANSDUCERS

A passive displacement transducer is a device such that a displacement causes a related change in a circuit parameter such as resistance, inductance, and capacitance.

For a resistive wire, the resistance R is given by

$$R = \frac{\rho L}{A} \tag{1}$$

where ρ = the resistivity of the wire material,
L = the length of the wire, and
A = the cross-sectional area of the wire.

An example of a linear displacement transducer using the above property is shown in Figure 6–1a, where the displacement to be measured is linked to the wiper of the potentiometer. In this example, the measured resistance is directly proportional to the displacement. A practical displacement transducer is shown in Figure 6–1b. Figure 6–2 shows an example of a resistive angular motion transducer.

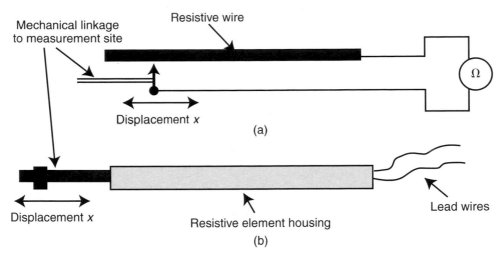

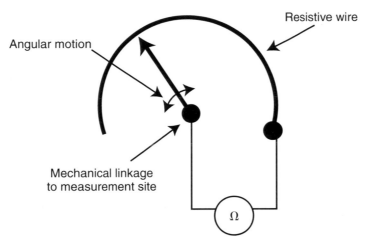

Figure 6–1. Linear Displacement Transducer.

Figure 6–2. Resistive Angular Motion Transducer.

INDUCTIVE DISPLACEMENT TRANSDUCERS

The inductance L of a solenoid is given by

$$L = N^2 \mu \frac{A}{l} \qquad (2)$$

where N = the number of turns of the solenoid,
μ = the effective permeability of the material inside the solenoid core,
A = the cross-sectional area, and
l = the length of the solenoid.

A displacement transducer can be made by linking the change in displacement with one of the parameters in equation (2). A simple example is shown in Figure 6–3a, where the ferromagnetic core of the solenoid is connected to the object of which the motion is to be measured. The effective permeability of the solenoid is changed by the displacement of the core in the solenoid. The direction and magnitude of the displacement can thus be found by measuring the inductance of the solenoid. Another example is shown in Figure 6–3b, where the displacement is measured by measuring the changes in magnetic flux caused by the motion of the magnetic material.

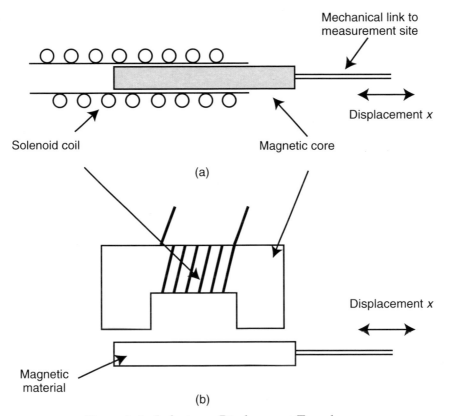

Figure 6–3. Inductance Displacement Transducer.

Figure 6–4a shows a displacement transducer called the linear variable differential transformer (LVDT). It consists of a primary winding L1 and two secondary equal but oppositely wound windings L2 and L3. When L1 is connected to an AC excitation and the core is right at the middle position, the induced voltages of the two secondary windings are of equal magnitude and hence cancel each other. The output of the LVDT is therefore zero. When the core is off-centered, the induced voltage of winding L1 is different from that of L2. A nonzero output voltage *Vo* appears at the output. *Vo* is proportional to the distance of the core away from the center position. The input-output characteristic is as shown in Figure 6–4b. In addition to its linear characteristic, an LVDT theoretically has infinitely small resolution. Since *Vo* is a sinusoidal voltage, the output is always positive. A phase detector is therefore required to determine on which side of the center the magnetic core is located.

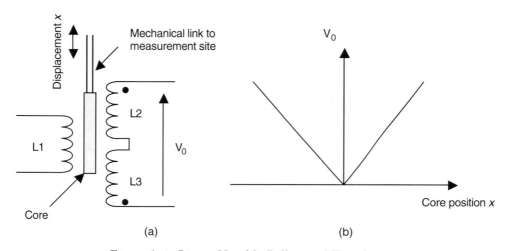

(a) (b)

Figure 6–4. Linear Variable Differential Transformer.

CAPACITIVE DISPLACEMENT TRANSDUCERS

For a parallel plate capacitor, the capacitance C is given by:

$$C = \frac{\epsilon A}{d} \tag{3}$$

where ϵ = the permittivity of the dielectric,
A = the overlapping area of the plates, and
d = the distance between the two plates.

A capacitive displacement transducer element converts a change in either the permittivity ϵ, the area A, or the plate separation d into a change in the value of the capacitance C. The change in capacitance will in turn cause a change in an electrical signal. For example, one of the plates can be moved together with the object to be measured to provide a signal according to the displacement of the object (Figure 6–5a). In Figure 6–5b, the permittivity ϵ is changed by the movement of the dielectric linked to the displacement to be measured. Figure 6–5c shows how the change in the overlapping area A can be tied to the displacement. A modification of that can be used for angular displacement measurement (Figure 6–5d).

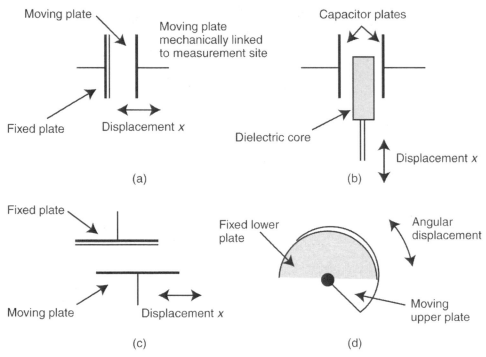

Figure 6–5. Capacitive Displacement Transducers.

HALL EFFECT SENSORS

Hall effect sensors are found in many medical devices. For example, they are used as a proximity sensor in the door switch of an infusion pump. Figure 6–6 illustrates the setup of a Hall effect sensor. The Hall element is a rectangular plate of metal or semiconductor material such as bismuth or tellurium. When the current carrying plate is placed in a magnetic field perpendicular to the plate, a voltage (called the Hall voltage) will be induced at the side faces of the plate in a direction perpendicular to the current in the plate. The Hall voltage E_h is given by the equation:

$$E_h = \frac{KIB}{t} \tag{4}$$

t

where I = the current flowing through the Hall plate,
B = the magnetic field perpendicular to the plate,

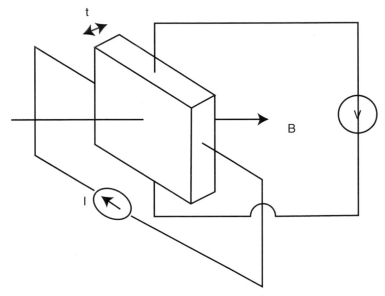

Figure 6–6. Hall Effect Transducer.

t = the thickness of the plate, and
K = the Hall coefficient, which is dependent on the material.

In practice, the current I is often held constant. From equation (4), E_h is proportional to the magnetic field strength B perpendicular to the plate. Hall effect sensors are commonly used in magnetic field measurements with sensitivity of a few mV per kGauss. A Hall effect sensor can easily be adapted to become a position or displacement sensor. Figure 6–7 shows several setups using Hall sensors as displacement transducers.

In Figure 6–7a, the Hall sensor is positioned between the two north poles of the magnets and supplied by a constant current. If the magnets are identical, the magnetic field strength is zero right at the middle and therefore the output of the sensor (Hall voltage) is zero. The magnetic field strength at both sides of the center varies with the distance from the center. By mechanically connecting the object to be measured to the sensor, the motion of the object can be monitored by measuring the Hall voltage. In the setup as shown in Figure 6–7b, the Hall effect sensor is placed stationary between the poles of

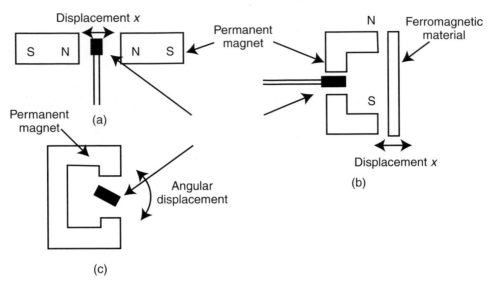

Figure 6–7. Applications of Hall Effect Devices.

a magnet. The magnetic flux in the magnet and therefore the magnetic field at the Hall sensor varies with the air gap between the magnet and the ferromagnetic plate. Motion of the object can thus be measured by the Hall sensor by connecting the ferromagnetic plate to the object. In Figure 6–7c, the magnetic field between the poles is constant. However, when the Hall effect sensor rotates, the magnetic field perpendicular to the surface of the sensor varies by a factor equal to sin θ, where θ is the angle between the magnetic axis and the surface of the sensor. In essence, a displacement sensor can be constructed by linking the object to a setup such that the Hall effect sensor element is exposed to changing magnetic field strength caused by the motion of the object.

Chapter 7

FLOW TRANSDUCERS

OBJECTIVES

- Explain the differences between laminar and turbulent flow.
- State Bernoulli's equation and Poiseuille's law.
- Define viscosity and Reynolds number.
- Derive the Venturi tube equation and explain the principle of operation of Venturi tube, orifice, pitot tube, and rotameter flow meters.
- Explain the operation of turbine and paddle wheel flowmeters, hot wire anemometers, electromagnetic and ultrasound flow sensors.

CHAPTER CONTENTS

INTRODUCTION

The cardiovascular system consists of the heart, which generates pressure to circulate blood through a network of blood vessels around the body. The blood pressure and flow velocity are different at different locations of the circulatory system. Chapter 4 covers pressure transducers that can be used to measure blood pressure, while this chapter covers flow transducers to measure blood flow velocity. Physiological parameters in the flow measurement category include, blood flow, respiratory gas flow, and urine flow.

Flow measurement includes measuring the velocity v (m/s), volume flow rate Q (L/s), or mass flow rate F (kg/s). The mass flow rate is defined as the mass m of the fluid that flows through a cross section of the vessel per unit time t. Since mass is equal to volume V times density ρ, the mass flow rate is given by

$$F = \frac{m}{t} = \frac{\rho \times V}{t} = \frac{\rho \times A \times l}{t} = \rho \times A \times v = \rho \times Q \quad (1)$$

where A = the cross section of the vessel, and
l = the distance of the fluid path.

LAMINAR AND TURBULENT FLOW

There are two types of fluid flow: laminar flow and turbulent flow. Laminar (or streamline) flow is smooth flow such that neighboring layers of the fluid slide by each other smoothly. It is characterized by the fact that each particle of the fluid follows a smooth path and the paths do not cross over one another; such a path is called a streamline. Laminar flow is usually slower flow. When the velocity of the flow increases, the flow eventually becomes turbulent. Turbulent flow is characterized by flow with eddies. Eddies absorb more energy and create large internal friction, which increases the fluid viscosity. Laminar and turbulent flows are shown in Figures 7–1a and 7–1b, respectively.

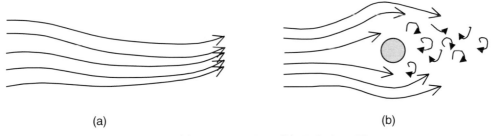

(a)   (b)

Figure 7–1. (a) Laminar Flow, (b) Turbulent Flow.

For an incompressible fluid continuously flowing through a vessel (Figure 7–2), the mass of the fluid flowing through section 1 per unit time is the same as that in section 2. Therefore,

$$\frac{m}{t} = \rho_1 \times A_1 \times v_1 = \rho_2 \times A_2 \times v_2$$

since $\rho_1 = \rho_2$, the equation becomes

$$A_1 \times v_1 = A_2 \times v_2 \tag{2}$$

which shows that the fluid velocity is higher when the cross section is smaller.

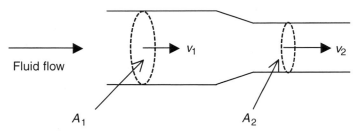

Figure 7–2. Fluid Flow Through Pipe with Varying Diameter.

BERNOULLI'S EQUATION

In the early eighteenth century, Daniel Bernoulli developed the Bernoulli's equation, which expresses the relationships between the velocity, pressure, and elevation of liquid flowing in a pipe with nonuniform cross section and varying height. Consider the setup shown in Figure 7–3. Assuming the flow is laminar, the fluid is incompressible, and the viscosity is negligible (i.e., there is no energy loss in the flow), equating the fluid energy at points 1 and 2 produces the following equation, which is called the Bernoulli's equation.

$$P_1 + \frac{1}{2}\rho v_1^2 + \rho g h_1 = P_2 + \frac{1}{2}\rho v_2^2 + \rho g h_2 \tag{3}$$

where ρ = the density of the fluid, and
g = the acceleration due to gravity.

The equation shows that the quantity $P + \frac{1}{2}\rho v^2 + \rho g h$ is constant at any point in a lossless fluid flow. Although any fluid flow in real life has certain energy loss, the Bernoulli's equation provides an estimate of the trade-off between the pressure, flow, and elevation of the fluid in a vessel.

Bernoulli's equation ignores the friction (called viscosity in fluid analysis) within a flowing fluid. This friction creates thermal energy, which is loss in the form of heat. This is why a pump is required (to input energy into the sys-

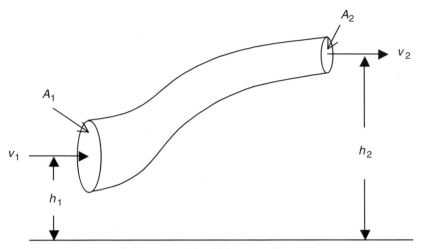

Figure 7–3. Fluid Flow in a Pipe.

tem) to move the fluid through a pipe. Viscosity exists in both liquids and gases. In laminar flow, the fluid layer in immediate contact with the wall of the pipe is stationary due to the adhesive force between the molecules. The stationary layer slows down the flow of the layer in contact due to viscosity; this layer in turns slows down the next layer and so on. Therefore, the velocity of the fluid varies continuously from zero at the pipe wall to a maximum velocity at the center of the pipe as shown in Figure 7–4. The viscosity of different fluids can be expressed quantitatively by the coefficient of viscosity η. The values of η for different fluids stated in Table 7–1 are at 20°C except for blood and blood plasma, which are measured at 37°C (body temperature).

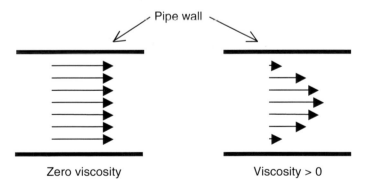

(length of arrow indicates the magnitude of flow velocity)

Figure 7–4. Velocity Flow Profile of Fluid in a Pipe.

Table 7–1.
Coefficient of Viscosity for Different Fluids

Fluid	Coefficient of viscosity η ($\times 10^{-3}$ Pa.s)
Water	1.0
Ethyl alcohol	1.2
Glycerine	1500
Air	0.018
Whole blood	~ 4
Blood plasma	~ 1.5

For an incompressible fluid, the volume flow rate Q of the fluid under-going laminar flow in a uniform cylindrical pipe can be expressed by the Poiseuille's law

$$Q = \frac{\pi r^4 (P_1 - P_2)}{8\eta L} \tag{4}$$

where r = the radius of the pipe,
L = the length of the pipe section,
P_1 and P_2 =, respectively, the pressure of the fluid at the beginning and the end of the section, and
η = the coefficient of viscosity.

Poiseuille's law shows that the flow rate is directly proportional to the pressure gradient and to the fourth power of the radius, but inversely proportional to the viscosity of the fluid. From equation (4), one can easily note that if there is a stenosis in the blood vessel (decreased radius of the vessel), the blood pressure must increase substantially to maintain the same blood flow.

When the flow velocity is high, the flow will become turbulent and Poiseuille's law will become invalid. The average flow rate at a given pressure under turbulent flow is less than that of laminar flow given by equation (4) since the turbulence creates extra friction in the fluid. The onset of turbulence is often abrupt and is characterized by the Reynolds number *Re*, where

$$Re = \frac{2\rho \bar{v} r}{\eta} \tag{5}$$

where ρ = the density of the fluid,
$\bar{v}$ = the average velocity,
r = the radius of the pipe, and
η = the coefficient of viscosity.

Experiments have shown that when *Re* exceeds about 2,000, the flow becomes turbulent.

Example

The average blood velocity in a vessel of radius 3.0 mm is about 0.4 m/s. Determine whether the blood flow is laminar or turbulent given that the density of blood is 1.05×10^3 kg/m^3 and the coefficient of viscosity of blood is 4.0×10^{-3} N.s/m^2.

Solution

Using equation (5), the Reynolds number is:

$$\text{Re} = \frac{2 \times 1.05 \times 10^3 \times 0.4 \times 3.0 \times 10^{-3}}{4.0 \times 10^{-3}} = 1,056$$

which is less than 2,000

The flow is therefore laminar.

FLOW TRANSDUCERS

There are many flow transducers available. This section describes a number of common flow transducers that may be found in medical instrumentation.

Venturi Tube

Figure 7–5 shows the construction of a circular, horizontal Venturi tube flowmeter. For an incompressible fluid flowing inside a pipe, assuming it is a frictionless flow, we can apply the Bernoulli's equation at points 1 and 2 of the fluid in the tube.

$$P_1 + \rho gh_1 + \frac{\rho v_1^2}{2} = P_2 + \rho gh_2 + \frac{\rho v_2^2}{2}$$

as the tube is horizontal, substituting $h_1 = h_2$ and rearranging the equation gives

$$P_1 - P_2 = \frac{\rho}{2}\left(v_2^2 - v_1^2\right) \tag{6}$$

As the fluid is incompressible, the volume flow of fluid Q passing through section 1 and section 2 of the pipe are equal, i.e., $Q_1 = Q_2$.

But $Q = \dfrac{\pi D^2}{4}\, v$, where D is the diameter of the pipe and v is the flow

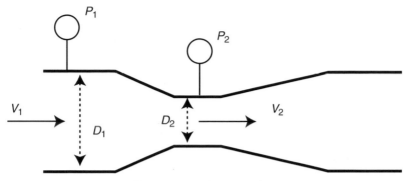

Figure 7–5. Venturi Tube.

velocity. Therefore

$$Q = \frac{\pi D_1^2}{4} v_1 = \frac{\pi D_2^2}{4} v_2$$

$$\Longrightarrow v_1 = \frac{D_2^2}{D_1^2} v_2 \tag{7}$$

Substituting equation (7) into equation (6) yields

$$P_1 - P_2 = \frac{\rho}{2}\left[1 - \left(\frac{D_2}{D_1}\right)^4\right]v_2^2 \tag{8}$$

$$\Rightarrow v_2 = \sqrt{\frac{P_1 - P_2}{\left[1 - \left(\frac{D_2}{D_1}\right)^4\right]} \times \frac{2}{\rho}}$$

Therefore, the volume flow rate Q becomes:

$$Q = \frac{\pi D_2^2}{4} v_2 = \frac{\pi D_2^2}{4}\sqrt{\frac{P_1 - P_2}{\left[1 - \left(\frac{D_2}{D_1}\right)^4\right]} \times \frac{2}{\rho}} = \frac{\pi D_2^2 D_1^2}{4}\sqrt{\frac{(P_1 - P_2)}{(D_1^4 - D_2^4)} \times \frac{2}{\rho}} \tag{9}$$

Equation (9) shows that the volume flow rate can be found by measuring the fluid pressures and pipe diameters at points 1 and 2 of the Venturi tube.

Orifice Plate

A variation of the Venturi tube is the orifice plate (Figure 7–6). The circular opening of the plate inside the pipe creates a reduction in the diameter of the fluid flow path downstream of the orifice opening. The differential pressure $\Delta P = P_1 - P_2$ is measured to determine the flow velocity v and the volume flow rate Q. Lookup tables of Q against ΔP are usually provided by

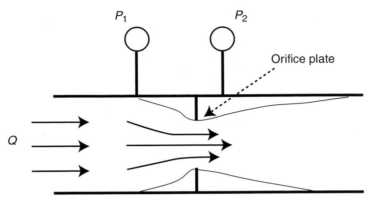

Figure 7–6. Orifice Plate Flowmeter.

the manufacturers.

Pitot Tube

A Pitot tube determines the velocity of the fluid by measuring the differences between the static pressure Ps in the flow and the impact pressure Pt. A Pitot tube has two concentric pipes as shown in Figure 7–7. The inner pipe has an opening at the outer wall on the side parallel to the direction of fluid flow and therefore measures the static pressure in the flow. The opening of the outer pipe is facing the flow and therefore detects the total pressure

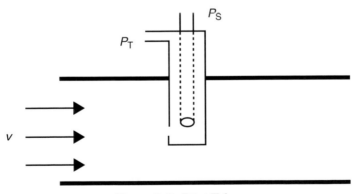

Figure 7–7. Pitot Tube.

developed by the moving fluid.

By the Bernoulli's equation, the total pressure is given by $P_T = P + \rho g h + \dfrac{\rho v^2}{2}$, and the static pressure is $P_S = P + \rho g h$. The differential pressure is therefore given by:

$$\Delta P = P_T - P_S = \frac{\rho v^2}{2}$$

Compared with the orifice plate or the Venturi tube, a Pitot tube can easily be installed in the field by drilling a hole on the pipe and inserting the element through the hole.

Rotameter

A rotameter (or variable area flowmeter) consists of a float in a uniformly tapered tube as shown in Figure 7–8. An upward flow creates an upward force on the float. The float will go up or down until the upward force is equal to the weight of the float. The volume flow rate Q can be shown to be proportional to the area of the round gap between the float and the tube. The volume flow rate is usually calibrated and marked on the side of the tube. Rotameters are commonly used as reliable and maintenance-free indicators

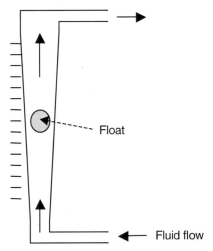

Figure 7–8. Rotameter.

of gas flow such as oxygen or medical gases.

Turbine Flowmeters

A turbine (or vane or paddle wheel) installed in a pipe will rotate at a speed proportional to the fluid flow velocity. A typical example of this class of flowmeter is a spirometer. Spirometers are used in respiratory gas flow measurements (Figure 7–9). The vane of a spirometer is made of very light material supported by bearings to reduce its resistance to the gas flow. Gas flow causes the vane to rotate at a speed proportional to the flow velocity. Through a train of gears, the volume of the gas flow through the vane is indi-

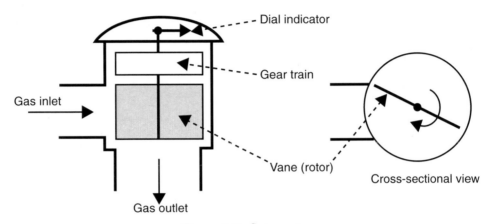

Figure 7–9. Spirometer.

cated on the readout dial.

Electromagnetic Flowmeters

When a conductive fluid flows across a magnetic field, an electromotive force (emf) is induced between the two electrodes placed orthogonal to the magnetic field and the direction of flow (Figure 7–10). The induced emf is proportional to the average flow velocity of the conductive fluid in the tube. For a steady flow, factors such as fluid density, viscosity, turbulence, or Reynolds number, which normally affect other flow measurement methods, do not affect the output signal. In addition, since none of the components of the flowmeter is inside the fluid flow path, flow measurement without creating obstruction to the flow is possible.

Ultrasound Flowmeters

An ultrasound flowmeter using the Doppler principle consists of an ultra-

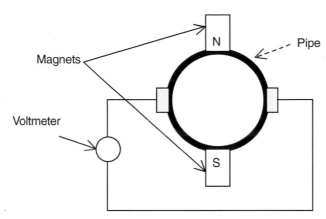

Figure 7–10. Electromagnetic Flowmeter.

sound transmitter and a receiver as shown in Figure 7–11a. Particles such as blood cells in the fluid reflect the ultrasound signal from the transmitter to the receiver. The frequency shift of the ultrasound signal received by the receiver is dependent on the velocity of the reflecting particles traveling in the fluid.

An ultrasound flowmeter using the transit time principle consists of two ultrasound transmitter and receiver pairs placed in the fluid path is shown in Figure 7–11b. As the sound traveling upstream is slower than that traveling downstream, the time difference measured between the upstream and downstream transit times is used to derive the flow velocity of the fluid in the pipe. The principles and construction of ultrasound blood flow devices will be covered in Chapter 27.

Figure 7–12 shows the construction of an ultrasound vortex flowmeter.

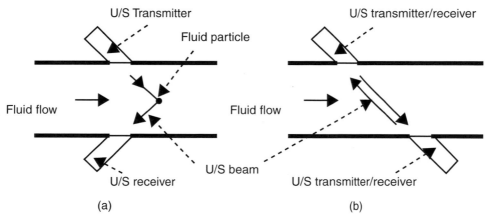

Figure 7–11. Ultrasound Flowmeters (a) Doppler, (b) Transit Time.

When the flowing fluid hits the wedge located at the center of the vessel, vortices are formed; these vortices create turbulence in the fluid, which can be detected by an ultrasound transmitter and receiver setup. The number of

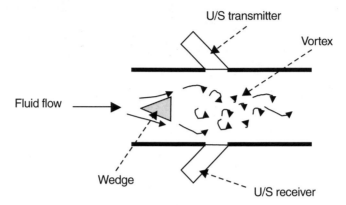

Figure 7–12. Ultrasound Vortex Flowmeter.

vortices formed is proportional to the velocity of the fluid.

Thermal Flowmeters

A thermal flowmeter with a heating element and two temperature sensors (e.g., thermistors) placed at equal distance to the element is shown in Figure 7–13a. The heater heats the fluid in contact with the heating element. When there is no flow, the sensors are at the same temperature. The flow of the fluid causes a temperature imbalance. The flow rate as well as the direction of flow are determined by the temperature difference between the two

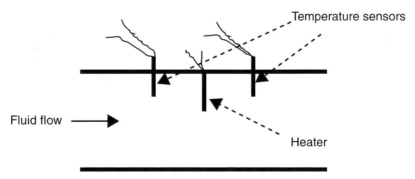

Figure 7–13. Thermal Flowmeter.

temperature sensors.

Hot Wire Anemometer

Another type of thermal flowmeter is the anemometer. In a hot wire anemometer, a wire heated by an electrical current is placed in the fluid flow path. The fluid flows pass the wire cools it to a lower temperature. The rate of heat removal from the hot wire is a function of the fluid flow rate. Figure 7–14 shows a hot wire anemometer for respiratory gas flow measurement. When the gas flow rate becomes higher, it removes heat from the hot filament at a faster rate. To maintain a constant temperature on the filament, the flowmeter responses by increasing the filament heating current. The gas flow velocity is therefore a function of the filament current. To obtain the flow direction, another hot wire is placed behind a flow diverting pin at the same level as the first wire. The upstream wire will be cooled more rapidly than

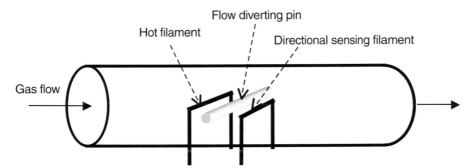

Figure 7–14. Hot Wire Anemometer.

the downstream wire.

A variation of the hot wire anemometer is the hot film anemometer, which replaces the heated wire with a heated metal film. The hot film provides a larger contact area between the gas and the heated element to

Chapter 8

OPTICAL TRANSDUCERS

OBJECTIVES

- Identify the frequency band of medical optics in the electromagnetic spectrum.
- Differentiate between photon and thermal optical detectors.
- Differentiate between radiometry and photometry; define and list the parameters and units of measurements.
- Define blackbody, graybody, selective radiators, and color temperature.
- Analyze the characteristics of common photosensors.
- Study the construction and principles of operation of a charged-couple device image sensor.

CHAPTER CONTENTS

1. Introduction
2. Thermal and Quantum Events
3. Definitions
4. Types of Photosensing Elements
5. Application Examples

INTRODUCTION

With the rapid advancement of optical instrumentation and communication systems, optical transducers (also known as photodetectors) have been undergoing rapid development in the past decade. Many photodetectors have found applications in medical instrumentation. Photodetectors may be used to measure energy, flux, intensity, et cetera, of an electromagnetic radiation. Electromagnetic radiation from low (e.g., 2.4 GHz or $\lambda = 12.5$ cm in telemetry) to high frequencies (e.g., 3×10^{22} Hz or $\lambda = 10^{-14}$ m in Gamma radiation) are used in various medical applications. Radiometry is the measurement of quantities associated with radiant energy, whereas photometry is the measurement of quantities associated with visible light. Visible light falls within a narrow band ($\lambda = 380$ to 780 nm) in the electromagnetic spectrum (Figure 8–1). This chapter covers the principles and construction of some common optical transducers used in medicine.

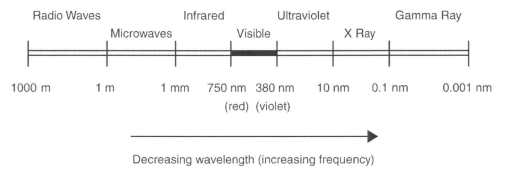

Figure 8–1. Electromagnetic Spectrum.

QUANTUM AND THERMAL EVENTS

There are two different mechanisms in radiant energy transduction: quantum (photon) event and thermal event. In a quantum event, photons are absorbed by the sensing element, which generates an electrical output according to the amount and rate of absorption of the light quanta. Quantum event is governed by the equation:

$$E = hf = \frac{hc}{\lambda} \tag{1}$$

where h = the Planck's constant = 6.625×10^{-34} Js,
f = frequency of electromagnetic radiation, Hz,
λ = wavelength of electromagnetic radiation, m,
c = speed of light = 3.00×10^{10} ms^{-1} for all frequencies in a vacuum but lower in other media, e.g., 2.25×10^{10} ms^{-1} in water for a 589 nm light source.

As the electrons must gain sufficient energy in order to jump over the energy gap, a minimum photon energy E_{min} is required to initiate the event. Therefore, radiation with wavelengths longer than λ_{max} ($= \dfrac{hc}{E_{min}}$) will not produce a quantum event (define λ_{max} as the maximum wavelength to produce a quantum event).

In a thermal event, radiant energy is first absorbed by the sensing element to produce heat energy; the heat generated in turn causes a change in an electrical value. Unlike quantum events, thermal events happen at all wavelengths. The sensitivity of a thermal photosensor also depends on the wavelength of the incident radiation.

The spectral response of a photosensor is often provided in the device specifications by the manufacturer. In addition, filters can be used to modify the spectral response of a sensor.

DEFINITIONS

Thermal and Photon Detectors

Photodetectors can be divided into two classes: thermal detectors and photon detectors. The sensing element of a thermal detector first converts the electromagnetic radiation to heat and then to an electrical value. This change in electrical value is often proportional to the received energy. That is, they are using the thermal event of transduction. Photon detection is achieved by quantum events that stimulate the sensing element to produce an electrical signal proportional to the rate of absorption of light photons.

Radiometry and Photometry

Radiometry is the measurement of quantities associated with radiant energy. The units of measurements and definitions of some radiometric parameters are listed below:

- Radiant Energy–Energy traveling in the form of electromagnetic waves.
- Radiant Density–Radiant energy per unit volume.
- Radiant Flux–The time rate of flow of any parts of the radiant energy spectrum.
- Radiant Flux Density at a surface–The quotient of radiant flux to the area at that surface. Radiant emittance (M) refers to radiant flux density leaving a surface while irradiance (E) refers to radiant flux density incident on a surface.

- Radiant Intensity–The radiant flux from the source per unit solid angle.
- Radiance–The radiance in a direction at a point on a surface is the quotient of the radiant intensity leaving, passing through, or arriving at the surface to the area of the orthogonal projection of the surface on a plane perpendicular to the given direction.

In photometry or lighting engineering applications when only the visible part (for human eyes, $\lambda = 380$ to 780 nm) of the electromagnetic spectrum is of interest, the term "radiant" is changed to "luminous" for the measurement quantities. For example:

- Luminous Energy–radiant energy of the electromagnetic radiation in the visible spectrum (from 380 to 780 nm).
- Luminous Flux–The time rate of flow of the luminous part (380 to 780 nm) of the radiant energy spectrum.

The quantities, symbols, and SI units of these parameters are tabulated in Table 8–1.

Table 8-1.
Standard Units of Radiometry and Photometry

Radiometric Parameter	SI unit	Photometric Parameter	SI Unit	Equation
Radiant Energy (Q)	J	Luminous Energy (Q)	lm.s	
Radiant Density (Ω)	J/m^3	Luminous Density (Ω)	lm.h/cm^3	$\Omega = \dfrac{dQ}{dV}$
Radiant Flux (Φ)	W	Luminous Flux (Φ)	lm	$\Phi = \dfrac{dQ}{dt}$
Radiant Flux Density at a Surface	W/m^2	Luminous Flux Density at a Surface	lm/m^2	
• Radiant Emittance (M)		• Luminous Emittance (M)		$M = \dfrac{d\phi}{dA}$
• Irradiance (E)		• Illuminance (E)		$E = \dfrac{d\phi}{dA}$
Radiant Intensity (I)	W/sr	Luminous Intensity (I)	cd	$I = \dfrac{d\phi}{d\omega}$
Radiance (L)	W/(sr.m^2)	Luminance (L)	nit	$L = \dfrac{d^2\phi}{d\omega(dA\cos\theta)}$

Blackbody, Graybody, and Selective Radiators

The radiant energy from a practical source is often described by comparing it with a blackbody radiator. A blackbody is defined as an entity that absorbs all incident radiation, with no transmission or reflection. A blackbody also radiates the most power at any given wavelength than any other source operating at the same temperature. The ratio of the output power of a radiator at wavelength λ to that of a blackbody at the same temperature and the same wavelength is known as the spectral emissivity $\epsilon\,(\lambda)$ of the radiator. When the spectral emissivity of a radiator is constant for all wavelengths, it is called a graybody. No known radiator has a constant spectral emissivity over the entire electromagnetic spectrum. However, some materials exhibit near graybody characteristics within a certain range of wavelengths (e.g., a carbon filament in the visible region). Non-graybody radiators are called selective radiators. The emissivity of a selective radiator is different at different wavelengths.

The color temperature of a selective radiator is equal to that temperature at which a blackbody must be operated in order that its output characteristic be the closest possible to a perfect color match with the output of the selective radiator (Figure 8–2). Note that color matching does not imply equal radiant output.

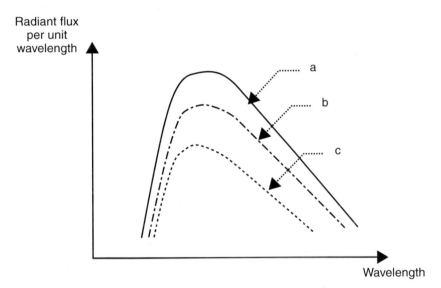

Figure 8–2. Radiant Curves for (a) Blackbody, (b) Graybody, and (c) Selective Radiator at the Same Color Temperature.

Although the match is never perfect, color temperature values are used to represent spectral distribution of light sources. For example, sunlight and the output of a tungsten filament incandescent lamp have color temperatures of 6500 K and 3000 K, respectively. Table 8–2 shows the visible color corresponds to the absolute temperature (K) of a blackbody radiator.

Table 8–2.
Color Temperature of a Blackbody Radiator

Temperature (K)	Color
800–900	Red
3000	Yellow
5000	White
8000–10000	Blue
60000–100000	Brilliant sky blue

TYPES OF PHOTOSENSING ELEMENTS

Some examples of photosensors are discussed in this section. Photoresistive sensors, thermopiles, and pyroelectric sensors are primarily thermal event detectors, while photoconductors, photoemissive sensors, photodiodes, phototransistors, and charge-coupled devices are quantum event detectors.

Photoresistive Sensors

For a semiconductor material, the electron and hole mobility, and hence its resistivity, varies with temperature. This property of temperature-dependent resistivity of semiconductor material can be used to detect thermal energy from a radiant source. The resistivity increases with temperature for lightly doped silicon but decreases at high doping level.

Thermopiles

A thermopile is made up of a number of thermocouples connected in series (Figure 8–3). Radiant energy is first converted to heat, creating a differential temperature between the hot and cold junctions of the thermocouples. Each thermocouple will generate a small voltage (on the order of μVs) according to this temperature difference. The output of the thermopile is the summation of all the voltages from the thermocouples in the cell. The sensitivity of the thermopile is proportional to the number of thermocouple elements in series. Miniature thermopiles, such as Si/Al thermopile, are fabricated from microelectronic technology.

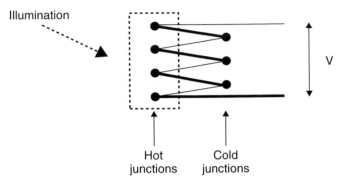

Figure 8–3. Thermopile Composed of Four Thermocouples.

Pyroelectric Sensors

In a pyroelectric sensor, a conductive material is deposited on the opposite surfaces of a slice of ferroelectric material, such as triglycine sulfate (TGS). The conductor on the sensing side is transparent to the light source to be measured. The ferroelectric material absorbs radiation and converts it to heat. The resulting rise in temperature changes the polarization of the material. The current I flowing through the external resistor connected across the two conductive surfaces is proportional to the rate of change of temperature of the sensor. Pyroelectric sensors with cooling can detect radiant power down to 10^{-8} W with λ_{max} of up to 100 μm.

Photoconductive Sensors

In a semiconductor, electrons can be raised from the valence band to the conduction band by absorbing energy from light photons. The presence of these photon-induced electrons increases the conductivity of the semiconductor material. In order to raise the electron from the valence band to the conduction band, it must absorb enough energy from the photon to overcome the band gap energy E_G. Therefore, to create the photoconductive effect, the energy of the light photon should be greater than E_G and hence the wavelength of the radiation must be smaller than λ_{max} given by equation (2):

$$\lambda_{max} \leq \frac{hc}{E_G} \tag{2}$$

For high-precision applications, the sensing element often must be cooled to reduce noise from thermionic electrons, which decrease the signal to noise ratio of the sensor.

Photoemissive Sensors

The phenomenon that electrons are liberated to the free space from the surface of a material when excited by light photons is called photoelectric effect. For high-efficiency conversion, the potential barrier or work function E_0 of the material must be much smaller than the photon energy. The efficiency or quantum yield of the sensor is defined as the ratio of the number of emitted electrons to the number of absorbed photons. Materials with low E_0, such as NaKCsSb or cesium oxide on GaAs substrate, have high quantum yields and therefore are good materials for photocathodes (photoemissive elements). In a simple photoelectric tube (Figure 8–4), under light illumination, electrons are liberated from the photocathode and conducted through the external circuit. If the wavelength is shorter than the work function, the photoelectric current produced in a vacuum photoelectric tube changes linearly with the level of illumination. In a gas-filled tube (e.g., filled with low-pressure argon), collisions of the electrons with gas atoms may produce secondary electrons emissions, resulting in higher sensitivity photodetection.

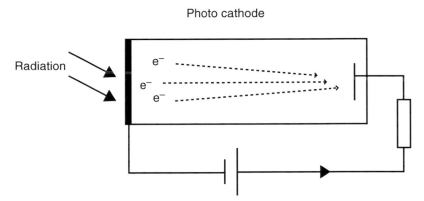

Figure 8–4. Photoelectric Tube.

Photodiodes

A diode is constructed of an n-type semiconductor (e.g., phosphorus doped silicon) in contact with a p-type semiconductor (e.g., boron doped silicon). Under normal conditions, electrons readily break away from the impurity in the n-type material to become free electrons. In the p-type semiconductor, mobile holes are created instead. Despite the presence of mobile electrons in the n-type and mobile holes in the p-type semiconductor, the individual semiconductors are both neutral in charge (i.e., the number of electrons is the same as the number of protons). However, when the two types of semiconductors are put together, the electrons from the n-type semiconductor will migrate across to fill the holes in the p-type semiconductor, forming a P-N junction (Figure 8–5). This migration of electrons also creates a net positive charge in the n-type and a negative charge in the p-type semiconductor. These charge layers create a net electric field and will eventually prevent further electrons from traveling across the junction. The electric field at the junction acts as a diode, creating a barrier for electrons to move from the n-type to p-type but not the other way around.

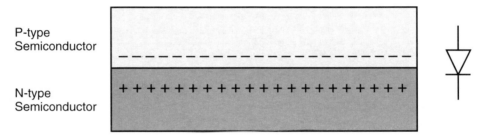

Figure 8–5. Semiconductor P-N Junction.

When light is incident upon the P-N junction of a semiconductor, a photon with sufficient energy will free a number of electrons from the atom. The number of free electrons (or accumulation of charges) can be found by measuring the voltage across the photodiode (photovoltaic mode) or by measuring the reverse bias current of the photodiode (photoconductive mode). The voltage-current characteristic of a typical photodiode and its equivalent circuit are shown in Figure 8–6 where v is the voltage across the diode and i is the diode current. The current source represents the current produced when the junction is exposed to radiation. Notice that when the output is short-circuited (i.e., v = 0), the short-circuit current is negative and its magnitude depends on the wavelength and the intensity of the incident illumination.

In the photoconductive mode of operation, a reverse bias voltage is applied to the photodiode as shown in Figure 8–7 (i.e., v is negative). The magnitude of this reverse bias current i will increase with the intensity I of the illumination. Although the reverse bias current is almost the same for a constant illumination, a higher reverse bias voltage will produce a faster response time. However, dark current (noise) increases with the magnitude of the applied bias voltage. Diodes in photoconductive modes operate in quadrant A of the photodiode characteristic curve (Figure 8–6).

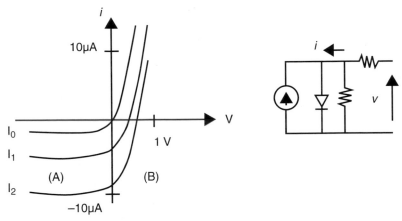

Figure 8–6. Current-Voltage Characteristic of Photodiode
with Illumination Intensity $I_0 < I_1 < I_2$.

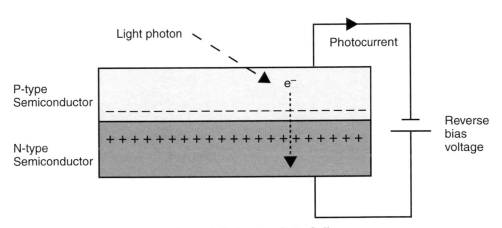

Figure 8–7. Photovoltaic Cell.

In photovoltaic mode of operation, no bias voltage is required. The free electrons created in the p-type semiconductor, being moved by the positive electric field, will cross the junction into the n-type semiconductor. These electrons will accumulate at the junction and create a potential difference (photovoltaic) between the p-type and n-type semiconductors. A photocurrent will flow if an external path is established between the semiconductors (Figure 8–8). This is often referred to as a solar cell. The magnitude of the photocurrent increases with the light intensity. Since dark current is a function of the bias magnitude, photovoltaic mode is ideal for low signal level detection. However, it is less suitable for high-frequency application because of its slow respond time. Diodes in photovoltaic modes operate in quadrant

B of the photodiode characteristic curve (Figure 8–6). Other than silicon, semiconductor materials such as gallium arsenide, and copper indium diselenide are common materials for photodiodes.

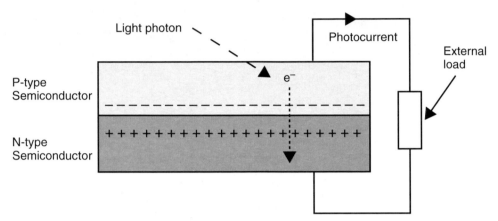

Figure 8–8. Photovoltaic Cell (Solar Cell).

Phototransistors

A phototransistor can provide amplification of the photocurrent within the sensing element. The basic construction of the phototransistor is similar to that of a bipolar transistor except that the base normally has no connection and is exposed to the illumination being measured. For the phototransistor connection shown in Figure 8–9, the emitter current is given by:

$$i_E = (i_\lambda + i_R)(h_{fe} + 1)$$

where i_λ = light-induced base current,
i_R = reverse leakage current, and
h_{fe} = forward current transfer ratio.

If $i_\lambda >> i_R$ and $h_{fe} >> 1$, the above equation can be simplified to

$$i_E \approx i_\lambda h_{fe} \tag{3}$$

Equation 3 shows a linear high gain characteristic, which converts luminous intensity to a relatively large emitter current.

Charge-Coupled Device (CCD)

Charge-coupled devices (CCDs) are often used in digital image acquisitions. The sensing elements of a CCD are MOS capacitors. Figure 8–10 illus-

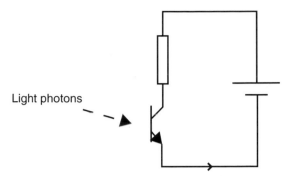

Figure 8–9. Phototransistor Circuit.

trates the cross section of a buried channel MOS capacitor. A typical buried channel MOS capacitor has a n-type semiconductor layer (about 1 μm) above a p-type semiconductor substrate with an insulation formed by growing a thin oxide layer (about 0.1 μm) on top of the n-type layer. A conductive layer (metal or heavily doped semiconductor) is then deposited on top of the oxide to serve as the metal gate.

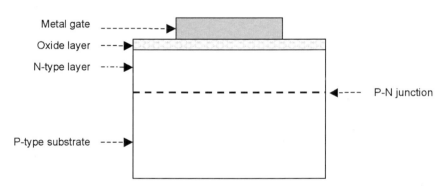

Figure 8–10. Buried Channel MOS Capacitor.

When light photons are allowed to incident on the P-N junction, electron-hole pairs are formed. Similar to a photodiode, the electrons will migrate to the n-type side of the junction and will be trapped in the "buried channel" (Figure 8–11). To create separation between adjacent pixels, a p-type stop region on each side of the metal gate is formed to confine the charges under the gate. The amount of trapped charge is proportional to the number of incident light photons.

A CCD consists of an array of these individual elements (pixels) built on a single substrate. A 256 × 256 array CCD contains 2^{16} number of MOS capacitor elements. To understand the operation of CCDs, we can represent

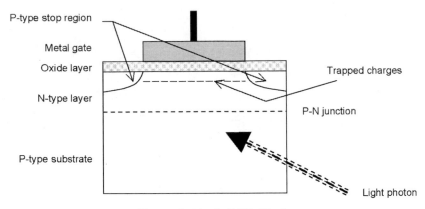

Figure 8–11. A CCD Pixel.

a MOS capacitor element by a bucket and the amount of trapped charges by the level of water in the bucket. When light of nonuniform intensity incidents on the CCD array for a predetermined duration of time (usually controlled by a timer-controlled shutter), the amount of charges created and trapped in each MOS capacitor is proportional to the number of light photons received by the capacitor. Figure 8–12 shows a 1 × 3 CCD linear array at the top and its water bucket analogy at the bottom. A larger amount of light photons creates a brighter CCD pixel, which is represented by a higher water level in the bucket.

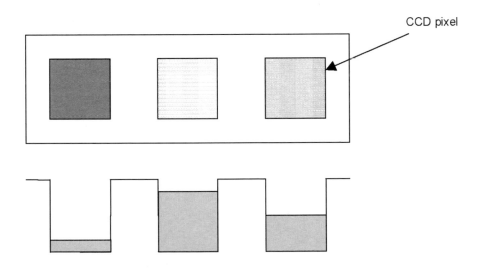

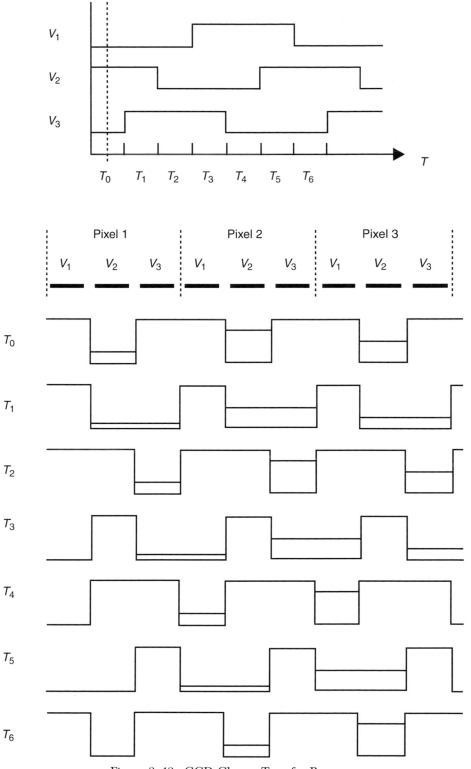

Figure 8–13. CCD Charge Transfer Process.

The process of reading the amount of charge in each pixel involves moving the charges from the site of collection to a charge-detecting circuit located at one end of the linear array. Reading out the charges in a CCD array is a sequential process. This process is illustrated in Figure 8–13.

In general, each pixel has three gates; each gate is connected to a time-controlled bias voltage V_1, V_2, and V_3 as shown (upper diagram of Fig. 8–13). Consider the charges stored in pixel number 2. At time T_1, V_3 becomes positive. As a result, some charges below the V_2 electrode migrate to the region under V_3. At time T_2, the V_2 electrode is turned off; the rest of the charges under the V_2 electrode have now all migrated to the region under V_3. Similar charge shifts happen at time T_3, T_4, T_5, and T_6. After time T_6 (one shift cycle), the charges under pixel 2 has been shifted to pixel 3. Note that all charge packets in the array move (or shift) simultaneously one pixel to the right. For an N-pixel linear array, N shift cycles are required to read out the entire array.

Figure 8–14 shows the physical layout of a 3×2 (6 pixels) CCD array. The pixels are represented by the rectangular boxes. In this particular con-

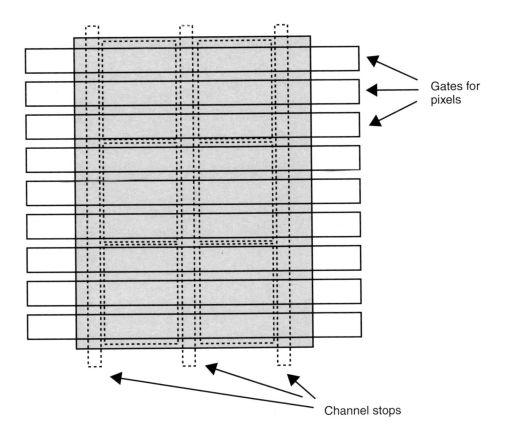

Gates for pixels

Channel stops

figuration, reading out the charges is achieved by shifting the charges in the vertical direction.

CCDs used in imaging are usually in square or rectangular arrays. An N × M array (Figure 8–15) can be considered to be made up of M linear arrays, each with N pixel elements. Reading out the array requires simultaneously shifting all rows of charge packets one pixel downward toward the serial register. The charge packets are then transferred from the serial register to the output amplifier one row at a time.

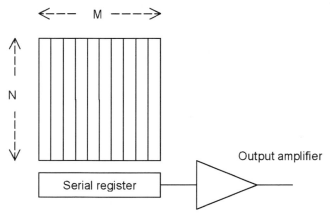

Figure 8–15. Two-Dimension CCD Array.

The unwanted charge accumulated in CCD pixels due to thermally generated electrons instead of light photons is called the dark current. Dark current contributes to noisy picture, especially when the input light level is low (i.e., low signal to noise ratio). As this noise is due to thermal effects, dark current can be reduced by cooling the CCD to a lower temperature. Quantum efficiency (*QE*) measures the efficiency of incident photon detection. It is defined as the ratio of the number of detected electrons *N* divided by the number of incident photons *M* times the expected number of electrons *R* generated from each photon.

$$QE = \frac{N}{M \times R} \times 100\%$$

APPLICATION EXAMPLES

There are many applications of optical sensors in medicine. A few examples are:

- LED-photodiode pair in infusion pump fluid drop sensors
- LED and photosensors in pulse oximeters
- Thermopiles in tympanic thermometers
- Photodetectors in capnometers
- CCD cameras in endoscopic video systems
- Ambient light sensors in monitor screen dimmers
- Flat panel detectors in digital x-ray systems

Chapter 9

ELECTROCHEMICAL TRANSDUCERS

OBJECTIVES

- Differentiate galvanic and electrolytic electrochemical cells.
- Describe the construction of a galvanic cell and analyze the function of each component with respect to the electrochemical reactions.
- Define standard half-cell potential and compute cell potential under nonstandard conditions.
- Explain how galvanic cells can be used as electrolyte analyzers.
- Analyze the constructions and the electrochemical reactions of reference electrodes including hydrogen, calomel, and Ag/AgCl standard electrodes.
- Analyze the constructions and electrochemical reactions of ion selective electrodes including pH, pK, and pCO_2.
- Define amperometry and potentiometry.
- State the principles of enzyme biosensors.
- Describe the principles of batteries and fuel cells.

CHAPTER CONTENTS

125

INTRODUCTION

Electrochemistry plays an important role in understanding as well as measuring biopotential signals. This chapter covers the principles of galvanic cells and electrode potentials. Reference electrodes including hydrogen, Ag/AgCl, and calomel electrodes are studied. Application examples such as K^+, pH, pO_2, and pCO_2 electrodes are discussed to illustrate the principles of ion selective electrodes. Enzyme sensors for glucose and cholesterol measurement are introduced to illustrate this growing field of biosensors. The principles of energy storage cells and fuel cells are also discussed.

ELECTROCHEMISTRY

Electrochemistry is the study of the interconversion processes concerning the relationship between electrical energy and chemical changes. An electrochemical cell is a device that permits the interconversion of chemical and electrical energy. There are two types of electrochemical cells: galvanic and electrolytic cells. In a galvanic cell, also known as a voltaic cell, chemical energy is converted to electrical energy. The reverse happens in an electrolytic cell, where electrical energy is converted to chemical energy. In the context of medical instrumentation, we consider only galvanic cells in this chapter.

Galvanic (Voltaic) Cells

In a galvanic cell, the electrical energy produced is the result of a spontaneous redox reaction between the substances in the cell. Redox reaction is a chemical reaction involving oxidation (losing electrons) and reduction (gaining electrons). Consider the simple redox reaction by placing a zinc rod into a solution of copper sulfate. One would immediately notice a black dull deposit forming on the shiny zinc surface. The chemical equation of this spontaneous reaction is:

$$Zn(s) + Cu^{2+} \rightarrow Zn^{2+} + Cu(s)$$

In this chemical reaction, copper ions from the solution are reduced to fine particles of copper metal, which grow to form a spongy layer on top of the zinc metal. The blue color of the copper sulfate solution gradually becomes paler (from its blue color), indicating that hydrated copper ions are used up in the reaction. The redox equation can be separated into an oxidation equation and a reduction equation as shown below. Each of these is called a half-reaction.

$$Zn(s) \rightarrow Zn^{2+} + 2e^- \qquad \text{(oxidation)}$$

$$Cu^{2+} + 2e^- \rightarrow Cu(s) \qquad \text{(reduction)}$$

The free-energy change of the overall redox reaction is –212 kJ when the reactants and products are in their standard states (i.e., pure metal and 1 M ionic concentration). This large negative free-energy indicates a strong tendency for electrons to be transferred from the zinc metal to the copper ions. The free-energy change in a reaction depends only on the nature and state of the reactants and products and not on how the process takes place.

Consider the setup in Figure 9–1, where the zinc rod is separated from the copper sulfate solution. In the setup, the zinc rod is immersed in a solution of zinc sulfate and a copper rod is immersed in a solution of copper sulfate. The two compartments of the cell are separated by a porous partition such as a piece of porcelain or clay. The zinc and copper rods become electrodes to provide surfaces at which oxidation and reduction half-cell reactions can take place.

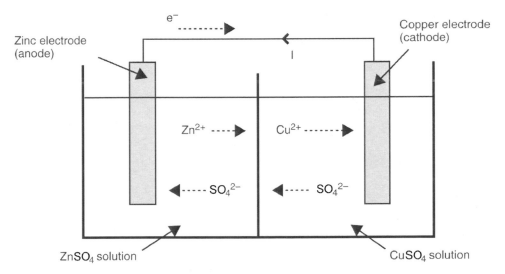

Figure 9–1. Galvanic Cell with Porous Partition.

If the zinc and copper electrodes are connected by an external conductor, electrons will leave the zinc metal and travel through this external conductor to the copper electrode. These electrons reduce the copper ions in the solution adjacent to the copper electrode to form atomic copper, which deposits on the surface of the copper electrode. In this galvanic cell, the anode (the electrode at which oxidation takes place) is the zinc electrode and the cathode (the electrode at which reduction takes place) is the copper electrode. The positive ions (in this case Zn^{2+}) which migrate toward the cathode, are called cations, whereas the negative ions (SO_4^{2-}), which migrate toward the anode, are called anions.

When the external circuit is broken and a voltmeter of high-input impedance is connected across the cathode and anode, the voltmeter reading represents the electrical potential difference of the galvanic cell. The cell voltage depends on the type of metal and its electrolyte concentration in each of the two half-reaction compartments. The potential difference measured between the cathode and the anode for this zinc-copper cell at 1 M ionic concentration and 25°C is 1.10 V (note that the cathode is positive and the anode is negative).

The purpose of the porous partition is to prevent direct transfer of electrons in the solution from the zinc metal to the copper ions. Without the porous partition, there will be no electron flow in the external circuit as the copper ions are able to migrate in the solution to the zinc electrode and capture the electrons directly from the anode. The porous partition in Figure 9–1 can be replaced by a "salt bridge" as shown in Figure 9–2. A salt bridge is a tube filled with a conductive solution such as potassium chloride (KCl). In the salt bridge, K^+ migrates toward the cathode and Cl^- toward the anode. A salt bridge provides physical separation between the galvanic cell compartments and establishes electrical continuity within the cell. In addition, it reduces the liquid-junction potential. Liquid-junction potential is a voltage

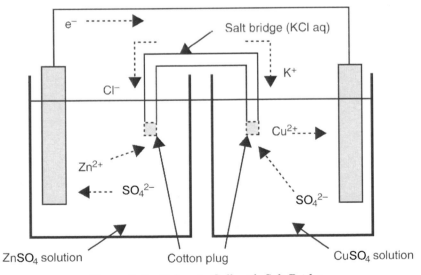

Figure 9–2. Galvanic Cell with Salt Bridge.

produced where two dissimilar solutions are in contact and when the rates of migration of the cations and anions are not the same across the contact region (or the junction). The ions in the salt bridge are chosen such that cations and anions migrate across the junction at almost equal rates, thus minimizing the liquid-junction potential. Calculation of the cell voltage is simplified if no liquid-junction potential is present.

The Zn-Cu galvanic cell we have discussed so far in which electrons must travel through an external circuit before reaching the cathode compartment is called a Daniell cell. The galvanic cells described in Figures 9–1 and 9–2 are both Daniell cells. Galvanic cells can be depicted by a line notation called a cell diagram. The cell diagram of the Daniell cell is:

$$Zn(s) \mid ZnSO_4(aq) \mid CuSO_4(aq) \mid Cu(s)$$

In this cell diagram, the anode is at the left and the vertical lines represent the junctions. When the salt bridge is present, the junction is represented by a double vertical line:

$$Zn(s) \mid ZnSO_4(aq) \parallel CuSO_4(aq) \mid Cu(s)$$

This can be further simplified by showing only the reacting ions in the solution phases:

$$Zn(s) \mid Zn^{2+} \parallel Cu^{2+} \mid Cu(s)$$

Standard Electrode Potentials

Consider the two half-reactions of the Daniel cell:

$$Zn(s) \rightarrow Zn^{2+} + 2e^- \qquad \text{(oxidation)}$$

$$Cu^{2+} + 2e^- \rightarrow Cu(s) \qquad \text{(reduction)}$$

If we reverse the first half-reaction, it becomes a reduction reaction:

$$Zn^{2+} + 2e^- \rightarrow Zn(s) \qquad \text{(reduction)}$$

It is not possible to measure the absolute potential of a single electrode (or half-cell) as all measuring devices can measure only the difference in potential. However, we can use a standard reference electrode to establish the half-cell potentials of different electrodes. The standard electrode potentials are measured against a hydrogen electrode under standard conditions, that is, all concentrations are 1 M, partial pressure of gases of 1 atmosphere, and temperature at 25°C. The potential of this standard reference hydrogen electrode is given a value of zero volt. Figure 9–3 shows the setup of a standard reference hydrogen electrode used to measure the standard electrode potential of a metal Me.

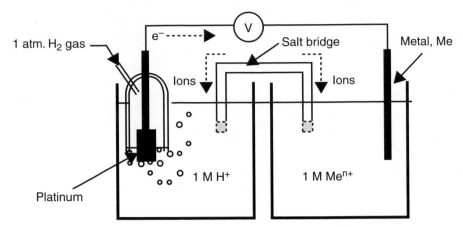

Figure 9–3. Measurement of Standard Electrode Potential.

By convention, the half-cell reaction is written as a reduction reaction and the potential measured is denoted as the standard reduction potential E^0:

$$Me^{n+} + ne^- \rightarrow Me(s) \quad \text{(reduction)}$$

Table 9–1 lists the standard electrode potentials of some half-cell reactions.

Table 9–1.
Standard Electrode Potentials

Half-Reaction (Reduction)	E^0 (V)
$Li^+ + e^- \rightarrow Li(s)$	–3.05
$Na^+ + e^- \rightarrow Na(s)$	–2.71
$Al^{3+} + 3e^- \rightarrow Al(s)$	–1.66
$Zn^{2+} + 2e^- \rightarrow Zn(s)$	–0.76
$Fe^{2+} + 2e^- \rightarrow Fe(s)$	–0.44
$2H^+ + 2e^- \rightarrow H_2(g)$	0.00
$AgCl(s) + e^- \rightarrow Ag(s) + Cl^-$	+0.22
$Hg_2Cl_2(s) + 2e^- \rightarrow 2Hg(l) + 2Cl^-$	+0.27
$Cu^{2+} + 2e^- \rightarrow Cu(s)$	+0.34
$Fe^{3+} + e^- \rightarrow Fe^{2+}$	+0.77
$Ag^+ + e^- \rightarrow Ag(s)$	+0.80
$O_2(g) + 4H^+ \rightarrow H_2O(l)$	+1.23
$Cl_2(g) + 2e^- \rightarrow 2Cl^-$	+1.36

Note that the sign of the standard potential may be positive or negative. A more negative standard potential implies higher reducing strength of the reaction. The standard oxidation potential has the same magnitude but opposite polarity to the standard reduction potential. For example, the oxidation potential of the copper half-reaction is −0.34 V:

$$Cu(s) \rightarrow Cu^{2+} + 2e^-$$

The potential of a galvanic cell E^0_{cell} is the sum of the standard reduction potential for the reaction at the cathode $E^0_{cathode}$ and the standard oxidation potential for the reaction at the anode $(-E^0_{anode})$. Therefore, in the case of the Daniell cell,

$$E^0_{cell} = E^0_{cathode} + (-E^0_{anode}) = 0.34 \text{ V} + (+0.76 \text{ V}) = 1.10 \text{ V}$$

Example 1

Find the standard voltage produced by the cell

$$Ag(s) \mid AgCl \mid Cl^- \parallel Cu^{2+} \mid Cu(s)$$

Solution

The separate half-reactions of the cell are:

$$Ag(s) + Cl^- \rightarrow AgCl(s) + e^- \qquad E^0_{ox} = -E_0 = -0.22 \text{ V}$$
$$Cu^{2+} + 2e^- \rightarrow Cu(s) \qquad E^0 = +0.34 \text{ V}$$

For the galvanic cell:

$$2Ag(s) + 2Cl^- + Cu^{2+} \rightarrow 2AgCl(s) + Cu(s)$$
$$E^0_{cell} = +0.34 - 0.22 = +0.12 \text{ V}$$

Example 2

Find the standard voltage produced by the cell

$$Pt(s) \mid Fe^{2+}, Fe^{3+} \parallel Cl^- \mid Cl2(g) \mid Pt(s)$$

Solution

The separate half-reactions of the cell are:

$$Fe^{2+} \rightarrow Fe^{3+} + e^- \qquad E^0_{ox} = -E_0 = -0.77 \text{ V}$$
$$Cl2(g) + 2e^- \rightarrow 2Cl- \qquad E^0 = +1.36 \text{ V}$$

For the galvanic cell:

$$2Fe^{2+} + Cl2(g) \rightarrow 2Fe^{3+} + 2Cl^-$$

$$E^0_{cell} = +1.36 - 0.77 = +0.59 \text{ V}$$

Nernst Equation

Consider a hypothetical half-cell reaction:

$$aOx + ne^- \rightarrow bRed$$

When it is under nonstandard condition (i.e., concentration other than 1 M and T is not equal to 25°C), the cell voltage can be quantitatively estimated by the Nernst equation:

$$E = E^0 - \frac{2.303RT}{nF} \log Q$$

where R = the gas constant = 8.314 J K^{-1} mol^{-1},
T = the temperature in Kelvin,
F = the Faraday constant = 96,485 C mol^{-1}, and
Q = the reaction quotient = $\frac{[Red]^b}{[Ox]^a}$ where concentrations are in mol^{-1}.

At 25°C, the Nernst equation can be simplified to:

$$E = E^0 - \frac{0.0592}{n} \log \frac{[Red]^b}{[Ox]^a}$$

Note that the concentration for solid and liquid is given a value of 1 in the equation.

Example 3

a) Find the half-cell potential of a copper electrode immersed in a 0.010 M Cu^{2+} solution at 25°C.
b) If the above half-cell is connected to a standard zinc half-cell, what would be the cell potential?

Solution

a) The half cell reaction is

$$Cu^{2+} + 2e^- \rightarrow Cu(s)$$

At standard condition, $E^0 = +0.34$ V.

$$E = 0.34 - \frac{0.0592}{2} \log \frac{1^1}{0.010^1} = 0.34 - \frac{0.0592}{2} \log 100 = 0.34 - 0.0592 = +0.28 \text{ V}$$

b) Since $E_{anode} = E^0_{zinc} = -0.76$ V, the cell potential is

$$E_{cell} = E_{cathode} + (-E_{anode}) = +0.28 + 0.76 = +1.04 \text{ V}$$

The cell potential is $+1.04$ V (instead of $+1.10$ V under standard condition).

Example 4

When the copper half-cell in Example 3 is connected to a nonstandard zinc half-cell at 25°C, the cell potential is measured to be $+0.98$ V. What is the Zn^{2+} concentration in the solution?

Solution

The zinc half-cell reaction ($E^0 = -0.76$ V) is

$$Zn^{2+} + 2e^- \rightarrow Zn(s)$$

Since $E_{cell} = E_{cathode} + (-E_{anode})$

$$E_{zinc} = E_{cathode} - E_{cell} = 0.28 - 0.98 = -0.70 \text{ V}$$

and

$$E^0_{zinc} = -0.76 \text{ V}$$

Using the Nernst equation

$$E = E^0 - \frac{0.0592}{n} \log \frac{[Red]^b}{[Ox]^a}$$

$\Rightarrow$
$$-0.76 = -0.70 - \frac{0.0592}{1} \log \frac{1^1}{x^1}$$

$\Rightarrow$
$$2.027 = \log \frac{1}{x}$$

$\Rightarrow$
$$x = 0.0094 \text{ M}$$

The concentration of Zn^{2+} in the solution is 0.0094 M.

We have shown in Example 4 that the concentration of a cation in a solution can be measured by using a reference electrode and a metal indicator electrode of the same cation. Consider the example of a silver indicator electrode to find the concentration of Ag^+ in a solution. The half-reaction and the standard potential are:

$$Ag^+ + e^- \rightarrow Ag(s) \qquad\qquad E^0 = +0.80 \text{ V}$$

Using the Nernst equation, the half-cell potential is:

$$E = +0.80 - \frac{0.0592}{1} \log \frac{1}{[Ag^+]} = +0.80 - 0.0592 \log \frac{1}{[Ag^+]}$$

From the above equation, if the half-cell potential E is known, then the concentration of *Ag⁺* can be calculated.

Note that if more than one ion are reduced (or oxidized) at the same time, such a metal indicator electrode will fail to provide the correct measurement. For example, a copper electrode will measure both Cu^{2+} and Ag^+ ions in the solution. Furthermore, many metals react with dissolved oxygen from the air and therefore deaerated solution must be used.

A metal electrode can also be used to measure the concentration of an anion if the cations of the metal form a precipitate with the anions. Consider a silver electrode in a saturated solution of AgCl.

$$AgCl(s) \leftrightarrow Ag^+(aq) + Cl^-(aq)$$

The solubility product K_{sp} is given by

$$K_{sp} = [Ag^+]\,[Cl^-] \Rightarrow [Ag^+] = \frac{K_{sp}}{[Cl^-]}$$

Substituting $[Ag^+]$ into the Nernst equation gives

$$E = +0.80 - \frac{0.0592}{1} \log \frac{1}{[Ag^+]} = +0.80 - 0.0592 \log \frac{[Cl^-]}{K_{sp}}$$

The concentration of Cl^- can therefore be calculated if the half-cell potential E is known.

REFERENCE ELECTRODES

Example 4 shows that one can use the Nernst equation to determine the concentration of an analyte (in this case Zn^{2+} ion concentration) in the solution of a half-cell by measuring the potential difference of the cell when the potential of the other half-cell is known. A typical cell used in potentiometric analysis is denoted by:

Reference Electrode || Analyte | Indicator Electrode

The cell voltage is the potential difference between the indicator electrode and the reference electrode. An indicator electrode is a half-cell whose potential varies in a known way with the concentration of the analyte, whereas a reference electrode is a half-cell with a known constant potential that is independent of the analyte. In addition to the standard hydrogen electrode mentioned above, two other commonly used reference electrodes are discussed in this section. They are the silver/silver chloride (Ag/AgCl) electrode and the calomel electrode.

Hydrogen Reference Electrode

The hydrogen electrode is a gas-ion electrode. A gas-ion electrode uses a gas in contact with its anion or cation in a solution. The gas is bubbled into the solution and electrical contact is made by means of a piece of inert metal, usually platinum. Figure 9–4 shows the construction of a hydrogen electrode. The cell diagram and electrode half-reaction of this hydrogen half-cell are:

$$Pt(s) \mid H_2(g) \mid H^+ \mid\mid \qquad\qquad 2H^+ + 2e^- \rightarrow H_2(g)$$

Under standard condition (1 atm. and 25°C), the hydrogen half-cell

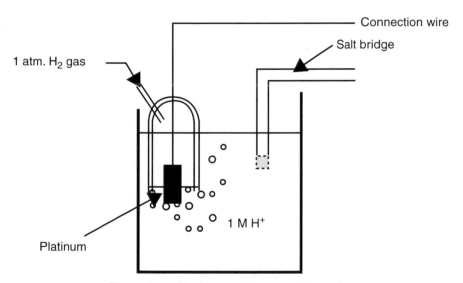

Figure 9–4. Hydrogen Reference Electrode.

potential is assigned a value of 0 V.

Silver/Silver Chloride Reference Electrode

A silver/silver chloride (Ag/AgCl) electrode consists of a piece of silver coated with AgCl immersed in a solution of potassium chloride (KCl) saturated with AgCl. Figure 9–5 shows a reference Ag/AgCl electrode (dotted line) replacing the hydrogen electrode in Figure 9–3 to measure the standard electrode potential of a metal Me or the ionic concentration of the metal in the solution. The cell diagram of this half-cell is:

$$\text{Ag(s)} \mid \text{AgCl(sat'd)} \mid \text{Cl}^- \parallel$$

The half-cell reaction and the standard reduction potential E^0, respectively, are:

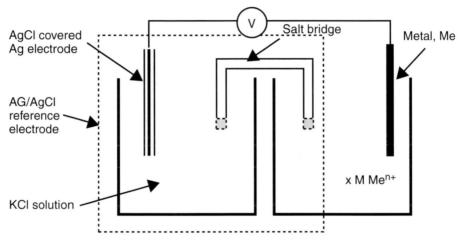

Figure 9–5. Measurement Using a Ag/AgCl Reference Electrode.

$$\text{AgCl(s)} + \text{e}^- \rightarrow \text{Ag(s)} + \text{Cl}^- \qquad E^0 = 0.22 \text{ V}$$

Applying the Nernst equation to this half-cell reaction at 25°C, the half-cell potential of the Ag/AgCl electrode is

$$E = E^0 - \frac{0.0592}{n} \log \frac{[\text{Ag(s)}] \, [\text{Cl}^-]}{[\text{AgCl(s)}]} = E^0 - 0.059 \log [\text{Cl}^-]$$

This potential depends on the concentration of the chloride ion in the KCl solution. Instead of using a standard 1 M solution, in order to maintain a constant concentration (to keep E constant), a saturated solution of KCl (approx. 4.6 M) is used. With a saturated KCl solution and at 25°C, the half-cell voltage becomes 0.20 V.

Figure 9–6 shows a typical commercial Ag/AgCl reference electrode. The salt bridge is replaced by a porous plug at the base of the electrode to allow passage of ions and completion of the electrical circuit. The air vent allows the electrolyte to drain slowly through the porous plug. The presence of some solid KCl and AgCl at the bottom maintains a solution saturated

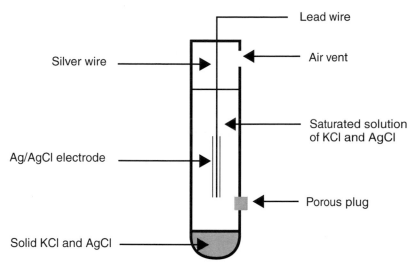

Figure 9–6. Ag/AgCl Reference Electrode.

with KCl and AgCl.

Calomel Reference Electrode

A calomel electrode consists of a platinum electrode in contact with mercury, mercury chloride (also known as calomel), and a KCl solution of known concentration. The half-cell is denoted by the cell diagram:

$$Hg(l) \mid Hg_2Cl_2(s) \mid Cl^-(x\ M) \parallel$$

where $x =$ the molar concentration of KCl in the solution.

The half-reaction and standard reduction potential (1 M Cl$^-$ ions) is given by:

$$Hg_2Cl_2(s) + 2e^- \rightarrow 2Hg(l) + 2Cl^- \qquad E^0 = 0.27\ V$$

In practice, saturated KCl (4.6 M) is often used. The advantage is that the concentration, and therefore the potential, will not change even when some of the solution evaporates. At 25°C, a saturated calomel electrode (SCE) has a potential of 0.24 V. Figure 9–7 shows the construction of a laboratory calomel electrode. Similar to the Ag/AgCl reference electrode, the salt bridge is replaced by a porous plug in a commercial calomel reference electrode (Figure 9–8).

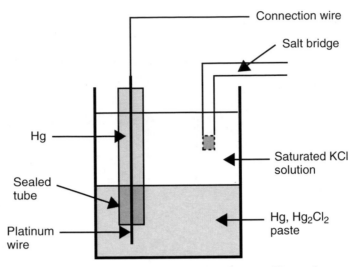

Figure 9–7. Laboratory Calomel Reference Electrode.

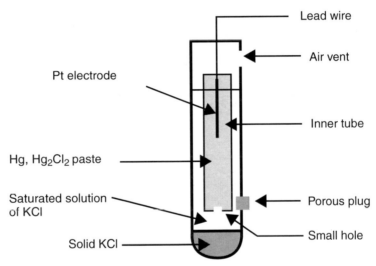

Figure 9–8. Commercial Calomel Reference Electrode.

ION SELECTIVE ELECTRODES

An ion selective electrode (ISE) is an indicator electrode that produces a voltage when it is in contact with a solution of a particular ion. In general, this is achieved by using a membrane that is selective for the ion being analyzed. An ion selective electrode is also known as a membrane indicator electrode.

pK Electrode

An example of an ISE is a K^+ electrode or pK electrode. The ion selective membrane of a pK electrode is a hydrophobic synthetic material containing ionophores such as valinomycin. The membrane is impermeable to H^+, OH^-, K^+, Cl^-, et cetera. Ionophores are antibiotics produced by bacteria, which are used to facilitate the movement of cations across the synthetic membrane. Valinomycin (an ionophore) can bind K^+ tightly but has a 1,000 times lower affinity for Na^+. The valinomycin-K^+ complex can readily pass through the membrane, from a solution of high K^+ concentration to a solution of low K^+ concentration. In the case of a solution of 0.1 M KCl and a solution of 0.01 M KCl separated by the membrane, potassium ions (K^+) are transported via the valinomycin-K^+ complex from the high concentration solution into the low concentration solution. However, as Cl^- ions cannot pass through, a slight positive potential will develop on the low concentration side of the membrane with respect to the high concentration side. This potential eventually stops the net transfer of the K^+ ions across the membrane. The potential across the membrane is the difference in potential E_1 and E_2 at the surfaces of membrane due to different concentration of K^+ at both sides of the membrane. At 25°C this membrane potential is given by:

$$E_{membrane} = E_1 - E_2 = \frac{0.0592}{n} \log \frac{[K^+_1]}{[K^+_2]} = 0.059 \log \frac{0.01}{0.1} = -0.059 \text{ V}$$

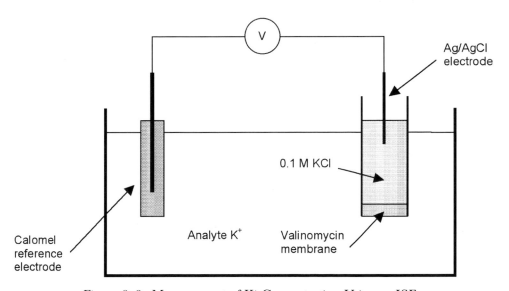

Figure 9–9. Measurement of K^+ Concentration Using an ISE.

where n is the charge on the ion; for K^+, $n = 1$.

Figure 9–9 shows the galvanic cell setup to measure the concentration of the analyte K^+ in the solution. The indicator electrode consists of a reference Ag/AgCl electrode in a solution with a known KCl concentration (e.g., 0.1 M KCl). A calomel electrode is used as the other reference electrode.

The cell diagram of this cell can be denoted as:

$$\text{Hg(l)} \mid \text{Hg}_2\text{Cl}_2\text{(s)} \mid \text{Cl}^-\text{(sat'd)} \parallel K^+_{analyte} \mid \text{membrane} \mid K^+(0.1 \text{ M}), \text{Cl}^- \mid \text{AgCl(s)} \mid \text{Ag(s)}$$

The cell galvanic potential of this setup is:

$$E_{cell} = E_{reference} + E_{indicator} = E_{calomel} + E_{Ag/Ag/Cl} + E_{membrane}$$

Since both $E_{calomel}$ and $E_{Ag/Ag/Cl}$ are known,

$$E_{cell} = C + \frac{0.0592}{1} \log \frac{[K^+_{analyte}]}{[0.1]} = C' + 0.059 \log [K^+_{analyte}] = C' - 0.059pK$$

where $pK = -\log[K^+]$.

A plot of the cell potential E_{cell} versus pK at 25°C is a straight line with a negative slope of 0.059.

pH Electrode

Another example of an ISE is the glass membrane pH electrode. The membrane of this electrode is usually a thin (0.1 mm) sodium glass with a composition of 72% SiO_2, 22% Na_2O, and 6% CaO. The silicon and the oxygen in the glass membrane form a negatively charged structure with mobile positive ions to balance the charge. When the glass is soaked in an aqueous solution, the aqueous solution exchanges H^+ for Na^+ at the glass surface. The amount of Na^+–H^+ exchanged is proportional to the H^+ concentration in the solution.

When the two sides of the glass membrane are soaked in two solutions of different H^+ concentrations, a potential E_{glass} develops across the glass membrane. At 25°C,

$$E_{glass} = \frac{0.0592}{1} \log \frac{[H^+_1]}{[H^+_2]}$$

If one of the solutions has a known constant H^+ concentration, the concentration of H^+ in the other solution can be determined.

Figure 9–10 shows a setup to measure the pH of a solution. The cell diagram of this cell can be denoted as:

$$\text{Hg(l)} \mid \text{Hg}_2\text{Cl}_2\text{(s)} \mid \text{Cl}^-\text{(sat'd)} \parallel H^+_{analyte} \mid \text{glass} \mid H^+(0.1 \text{ M}), \text{Cl}^- \mid \text{AgCl(s)} \mid \text{Ag(s)}$$

Similar to pK electrode, the cell potential is:

$$E_{cell} = C' + 0.059 \log [H^+_{analyte}] = C' - 0.059 pH$$

where $pH = -\log[H^+]$.

A plot of the cell potential E_{cell} versus pH at 25°C is a straight line with a negative slope of 0.059.

In a base solution, sodium glass starts to react with alkali metals such as Na^+ in addition to H^+. A sodium glass membrane electrode will start to produce noticeable error (referred to as alkaline error) at pH above 9. Therefore, to measure solution with pH greater than 9, a lithium glass membrane (72%

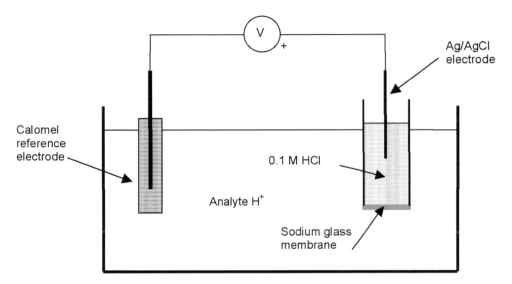

Figure 9–10. Measurement of pH Using a Glass Membrane Electrode.

SiO_2, 22% Li_2O, and 6% CaO) is used instead.

The reference electrode and the H^+ sensing glass membrane electrode in most industry models are combined into a single probe. Ag/AgCl electrodes may also be used (to replace the calomel electrode) as the reference electrode. A voltmeter connected to the electrode is usually calibrated to provide a direct readout of the measured pH. As pH is affected by temperature, pH meter is often calibrated by using two known buffers with known temperature characteristics.

pCO₂ Electrodes

In pCO₂ measurement, a membrane permeable to CO_2 (e.g., silicon rubber) is used to separate the sample solution (e.g., blood) from a buffer (e.g., sodium bicarbonate). As the CO_2 diffuses from the sample into the buffer, the pH of the buffer is lowered. The change in pH in the buffer, measured by a pH electrode, correlates to the pCO_2 in the sample. A voltmeter is often connected across the pH electrode and a reference electrode (Figure 9–11) to

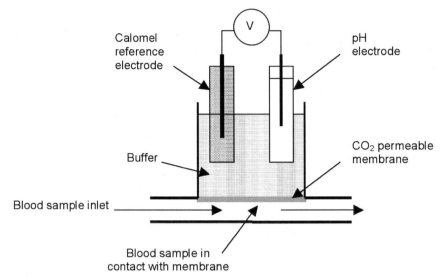

Figure 9–11. Measurement of pCO_2 in Blood.

produce a reading calibrated to read pCO_2.

pO_2 Electrodes

In a pO_2 electrode, a constant voltage source is applied across and the current flowing through the electrode is measured. The magnitude of the current is a function of the pO_2 level in the sample solution. This electro-chemical method is known as amperometry (measurement of current flowing through the electrodes with an applied voltage) in contrast to potentiometry (measurement of voltage between the electrodes with almost no current flow). An amperometric cell is also known as a polarographic cell.

Figure 9–12 shows a Clark polarographic oxygen electrode designed to measure pO_2 in a solution. The indicator electrode is a platinum cathode in a buffer solution of KCl. The anode is a Ag/AgCl electrode. An oxygen-permeable membrane (such as Teflon™ or polypropylene) separates the buffer and the sample solution. When a voltage is applied across the anode and the cathode, oxygen molecules diffused through the membrane are reduced at the platinum cathode to form OH^- ions. The half-reactions at the electrodes are:

$$Ag(s) + Cl^-(aq) \rightarrow AgCl(s) + e^- \qquad \text{Anode}$$

$$O_2 + 2H_2O + 4e^- \rightarrow 4OH^- \qquad \text{Cathode}$$

The magnitude of the current flowing out from the cathode is proportional to the dissolved O_2 level in the sample solution.

The cathode of a pO_2 electrode is usually made from an inert metal such as gold or platinum. To increase the respond time, oxygen must diffuse rapidly through the membrane and reach the cathode quickly. To achieve this, the membrane is made to be very thin (about 20 μm) and the cathode is in the form of a disk placed very close to the membrane (with separation about 10

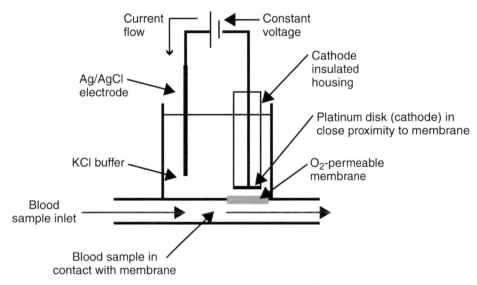

Figure 9–12. Measurement of pO_2 in Blood Serum.

μm).

A galvanic oxygen cell operates on the same principle, except that it does not have an external voltage source. Instead of measuring its current, the cell voltage is monitored. The cell potential is directly proportional to the concentration of oxygen of the gas outside the membrane.

pH, pCO_2, and pO_2 are the three analytes in blood gas analysis. In practice, the membranes of these electrodes must be kept clean and replaced regularly. Two point calibrations of the electrodes should be performed at 37°C and corrected to 37°C saturated vapor pressure.

BIOSENSORS (ENZYME SENSORS)

An oxygen sensor (e.g., Clark oxygen electrode) can be used indirectly to measure glucose or cholesterol concentration in blood. In serum glucose measurements, glucose in blood serum is first broken down by the enzyme glucose oxidase. This process consumes oxygen (see reactions below). The concentration of glucose is proportional to the amount of O_2 consumed, which can be measured using an oxygen electrode. The reaction is:

$$Glucose + O_2 + H_2O \rightarrow gluconic\ acid + H_2O_2$$

In cholesterol measurement, the cholesterol ester in the blood serum is first broken down into cholesterol by the enzyme cholesterol esterase and then into cholest-4-ene-3-one and H_2O_2 by the enzyme cholesterol oxidase. The latter reaction consumes oxygen. The amount of O_2 consumed is proportional to the concentration of the blood serum cholesterol.

$$Cholesterol\ esters + H_2O \rightarrow cholesterol + fatty\ acid$$

$$Cholesterol + O_2 \rightarrow cholest\text{-}4\text{-}ene\text{-}3\text{-}one + H_2O_2$$

In addition to measuring the oxygen consumed, an alternative method is to measure the amount of hydrogen peroxide produced from the reaction, which is proportional to the concentration of glucose or cholesterol in the blood serum. The hydrogen peroxide is separated by an ion selective membrane (such as cellulose acetate membrane) and oxidized to give oxygen according to the reaction:

$$H_2O_2 \rightarrow O_2 + 2H^+ + 2e^-$$

The amount of O_2, which is proportional to the concentration of glucose, is measured by an oxygen sensor.

In general, an enzyme sensor consists of three layers:

1. The first (outer) layer allows the analyte (e.g., glucose) to pass from the sample solution (e.g., blood serum) into the electrode.
2. The second layer contains an enzyme (e.g., glucose oxidase) to produce H_2O_2.
3. The inner layer collects and oxidizes H_2O_2 to form O_2. An O_2 sensor in this layer generates a current proportional to the concentration of the analyte.

Other analytes may be measured using this type of biosensor as long as an enzyme can be found that specifically oxidizes the analyte to produce hydrogen peroxide.

BATTERIES AND FUEL CELLS

Some galvanic cells are used in the industry and home as power sources. These energy storage cells are often referred to as batteries. A common battery is the Leclanché cell, also known as dry cell, or zinc-carbon cell. This galvanic cell consists of a zinc can, which serves as the anode; a central carbon rod is the cathode. The anode and the cathode are separated by a paste of manganese oxide, carbon, ammonium chloride, and zinc chloride moistened with water. At the anode, zinc is oxidized and at the cathode, MnO_2 is reduced. The half-reactions are:

$$Zn(s) \rightarrow Zn^{2+} + 2e^- \qquad \text{Anode}$$

$$e^- + NH_4^+ + MnO_2(s) \rightarrow MnO(OH)(s) + NH_3 \qquad \text{Cathode}$$

An external conductor connecting the anode and the cathode allows the flow of electrons from the anode to the cathode through an external load.

A lead acid cell is another example of an energy storage galvanic cell. The anode of the cell consists of a frame of lead filled with some spongelike lead. When the lead is oxidized, Pb^{2+} ions immediately precipitate as $PbSO_4$ and deposit on the lead frame. The cathode is also a lead frame filled with PbO_2. The half-reactions are:

$$Pb(s) + HSO_4^- \rightarrow PbSO_4(s) + H^+ + 2e^- \qquad \text{Anode}$$

$$2e^- + PbO_2(s) + 2H^+ + HSO_4^- \rightarrow PbSO_4(s) + 2H_2O \qquad \text{Cathode}$$

When an external conductor is connected between the anode and the cathode, a current is drawn. The solid $PbSO_4$ is produced at both electrodes as the cell discharges; H^+ and HSO_4^- are removed from the solution at the same time.

A lead acid cell can be recharged by imposing a slightly larger reverse voltage on the cell. This reverse voltage forces the electrons to flow into the anode and out of the cathode to reverse the reactions, converting $PbSO_4$ back into Pb at the anode and into PbO_2 at the cathode. Cells that are specifically designed for reuse are called secondary cells, whereas those for single use are called primary cells. Some common primary and secondary cells and their nominal open circuit voltages are listed in Table 9–2.

A fuel cell is a galvanic cell in which the reactants are continuously fed into the cell to produce electricity. Figure 9–13 shows one type of hydrogen-oxygen fuel cell. The electrodes are made of porous carbon impregnated with platinum (as a catalyst). Hydrogen is oxidized at the anode and oxygen is reduced at the cathode. The half-reactions are:

$$H_2(g) + 2OH^- \rightarrow 2H_2O + 2e^- \qquad \text{Anode}$$

Table 9–2.
Common Primary and Secondary Cells

	Type	Nominal cell voltage
Primary Cells	Zinc-carbon	1.5 V
	Zinc-air	1.4 V
	Alkaline	1.5 V
	Lithium-manganese dioxide	3.0 V
Secondary Cells	Lead-acid	2.1 V
	Nickel-cadmium	1.2 V
	Nickel metal-hydride	1.2 V
	Lithium-ion	3.6 V

$$4e^- + O_2(g) + 2H_2O \rightarrow 4OH^- \qquad \text{Cathode}$$

Hydrogen and oxygen are combined to produce water (steam). The process produces an electron flow when an external load is connected between the anode and the cathode. The overall reaction is:

$$2H_2(g) + O_2(g) \rightarrow 2H_2O$$

For the hydrogen-oxygen fuel cell, if the water is present as a liquid, then $E^0 = 1.23$ V; if it is a gas, then $E^0 = 1.18$ V. This is the voltage of a single cell. Practical fuel cells are built from a number of single cells in series or parallel

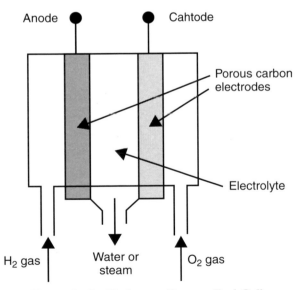

Figure 9–13. Hydrogen-Oxygen Fuel Cell.

to provide the desired voltage and power output.

There are many types of fuel cells using different electrolytes (e.g., alkaline, solid polymer, phosphoric acid) and different fuels (e.g., methane, carbon monoxide) "burned" at the anode. However, oxygen from air is the oxidant at the cathode in most of these cells. Fuel cells are considered as the energy conversion of choice in the future as it has no objectionable by-products and relatively high efficiencies (above 80% theoretical efficiency).

Chapter 10

BIOPOTENTIAL ELECTRODES

OBJECTIVES

- State the mechanism of ion flow in the body.
- Define biopotential and its origin.
- Explain the formation of cell membrane potential and action potential.
- List the characteristics of ideal biopotential electrodes.
- Explain half-cell potentials, offset potential, and their significance in biopotential measurements.
- Analyze the characteristics of perfectly polarized and perfectly nonpolarized electrodes.
- Sketch and analyze the electrical equivalent circuit of Ag/AgCl skin electrodes.

CHAPTER CONTENTS

1. Introduction
2. Origin of Biopotentials
3. Biopotential Electrodes

INTRODUCTION

An Italian physiologist and physicist, Luigi Galvani, was the first to explore electrical potentials of the body, now commonly called biopotentials. The element that produces electrical events in biological tissue is the ion in the electrolyte solution, as opposed to the electron in the electrical circuit. A biopotential, then, is an electrical voltage caused by a current flow of ions through biological tissues. The devices that pick up these biopotentials are referred to as biopotential electrodes. Biopotential electrodes are a form of transducer.

ORIGIN OF BIOPOTENTIALS

There are two fundamental mechanisms of ion flow in the body: diffusion and drift. Fick's law states that if there is a high concentration of particles in one region and they are free to move, they will flow in a direction that equalizes the concentration. The resulting movement of these charges is called diffusion.

The movement of charged particles (such as ions) that is due to the force of an electric field (the forces of attraction and repulsion) constitutes particle drift. Each cell in the body has a potential voltage across its membrane and the cell content, known as the single-cell membrane potential V_m. The membrane potential forms the basis for the biopotentials of the body. Some of the biopotentials of interest include the electrocardiogram (ECG), electroencephalogram (EEG), electrooculogram (EOG), electroretinogram (ERG), and electromyogram (EMG).

The potential is the result of the diffusion and drift of ions across the high-resistance semipermeable cell membrane. The ions are predominantly sodium [Na^+] ions moving into the cell, and potassium [K^+] ions moving out of it (Figure 10–1). Because of the semipermeable nature of the membrane, Na^+ ions are partially restricted from passing into the cell. As a result, the concentration of Na^+ outside the cell is higher than that inside.

In addition, a process called sodium-potassium pump keeps sodium largely outside the cell and potassium ions inside. In the process, potassium is pumped into the cell while sodium is pumped out. The rate of sodium pumping out of the cell is about two to five times that of potassium pumping into cells. In the presence of the offsetting effects of diffusion and drift and the sodium-potassium pump, the equilibrium concentration point is established when the net flow of ions is zero. As there are more positive ions moved outside the cells (Na^+) than positive ions moved into the cells (K^+), the inside of the cell is less positive than the outside and more negative ions are present within the cell. Therefore, the cell is negative with respect to the outside; the cell becomes polarized. This potential difference between the inside and outside of the cell at equilibrium is called the resting potential. The magnitude of the resting potential is –70 mV to –90 mV.

If, for any reason, the potential across the cell membrane is raised, say, by voluntary or involuntary muscle contractions, to a level above a stimulus

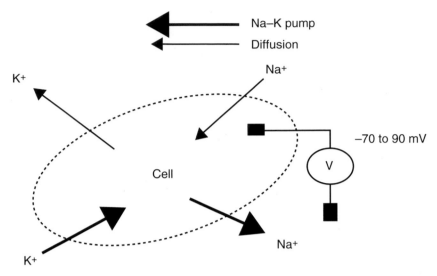

Figure 10–1. Mechanism of Cell Resting.

threshold, the cell membrane resistance changes. Under this condition, the nature of the cell membrane changes and becomes permeable to sodium ions. The sodium ions will start to rush into the cell. The inrush of positively charged sodium ions caused by this change in cell membrane resistance gives rise to a change in ion concentrations within and without the cell. The result is a change in the membrane potential called the action potential (Figure 10–2).

During this time, the potential inside the cell is 20 to 40 mV more positive than the potential outside. The action potential lasts for about 1 to 2 milliseconds. As long as the action potential exists, the cell is said to be depolarized. Under certain conditions, this action potential disturbance is propagated from one cell to the next, causing the entire tissue to become depolarized. Eventually the cell equilibrium returns to its normal state (i.e., to its polarized state) and the –90 mV cell membrane potential is resumed. The time period when the cell is changing its polarization is called the refractory period. During this time, the cell is not responsive to any stimulation.

When cells are stimulated, they generate a small action potential. If a large group of cells is stimulated simultaneously, the resultant action potentials can be readily detected. For example, when the heart contracts and relaxes, the polarization and repolarization of the heart cells create a resultant action potential. This action potential can be monitored by external machines using electrodes placed on the surface of the body. This sequence of polarization and repolarization gives rise to a complete waveform known as the electrocardiogram.

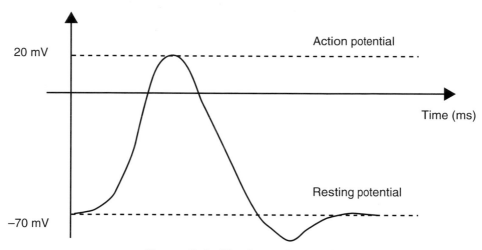

Figure 10–2. The Action Potential.

BIOPOTENTIAL ELECTRODES

Biopotential electrodes are transducers that pick up the body electrical signals via the body electrolytes. An electrode provides the interface that is needed between the ionic current flowing in the body and the electron current flowing in the machine. In other words, the electrode allows the machine to measure the electrical effects in tissue by making a transformation between ionic conduction to electron conduction at the tissue-electrode interface. Ideally, the amount of current flowing through the electrode is zero; hence the purpose of the electrode is to measure the potential at the tissue due to the flow of ions across the biological tissue. But practically speaking, some small amount of current will flow through the electrode.

An ideal electrode is characterized by a number of features, including:

- absence of distortion or electrical noise
- immunity to external interference
- inertness of the electrode in the presence of tissue and bodily fluid
- absence of interference with or influence on the tissue
- absence of interference with or influence on the movement of the subject
- ease of making contact with the biological source
- invariance of the contact even during long periods of time
- absence of discomfort to the subject
- repeatability of results
- low cost, durability, small size, and low weight

The Tissue-Electrode Interface

Given the listed preferred characteristics, biopotential measurement using a pair of electrodes should not be considered as simply connecting two pieces of wire to two conductors and placing them onto a patient. Biopotential measurement at the tissue-electrode interface in the clinical setting is a rather complicated process. The electrode is the metal that makes contact with the electrolyte, and the electrolyte is interfaced to the biological tissue through which ions are free to flow. The tissue-electrode interface has a significant effect on the quality of the biopotential signal measured by the medical device.

Electrode Half-Cell Potential

In Chapter 9, it was discussed that if two dissimilar metals are submerged into a solution of electrolyte, a potential difference can be measured between the two metals. Each of these metals with the electrolyte creates a half-cell potential. In biopotential measurements, each electrode-tissue interface therefore will create a half-cell potential.

In electrophysiology studies (study of the electrical activities within the human body) the difference in half-cell potentials that can be detected between two electrodes is referred to as the "offset potential" of the electrode pair. Under ideal conditions, when measuring biopotential using a pair of identical electrodes, the offset potential is zero as the half-cell electrode potential at each electrode-tissue interface will cancel out each other. However, in practice, the offset potential is never zero as the half-cell potentials at different locations are never identical. Offset potential on the order of ± 0.1 V is very common in body surface biopotential measurements.

Polarized and Nonpolarized Electrodes

As with any redox reaction, at any electrode/electrolyte interface, the electrode tends to discharge ions into the solution, and the ions in the electrolyte tend to combine with the electrode. That is,

Metal $\rightarrow$ electrons + metal ions (oxidation reaction)

Electrons + metal ions $\rightarrow$ metal (reduction reaction)

The net result of these reactions at the tissue-electrode interface is the creation of a charge gradient, the spatial arrangement of which is called the electrode double layer. Electrodes in which no net transfer occurs across the metal-electrolyte interface are said to be perfectly polarized or perfectly nonreversible electrodes; that is, only one of the two chemical reactions described above can occur. An example of this is shown in Figure 10–3A. Electrodes in which unhindered transfer of charge is possible are said to be perfectly nonpolarized or perfectly reversible; that is, both of the equations referred to above can occur with equal ease. An example of this is shown in Figure 10–3B. Perfectly nonpolarized electrodes are the ideal electrode of use since they allow for the best ion-electron interface. However, practical electrodes used in clinical situations have properties that lie between these ideal limits.

(A) METALLIC ELECTRODE

Perfectly Polarized Electrodes: Only one reaction occurs with ease.

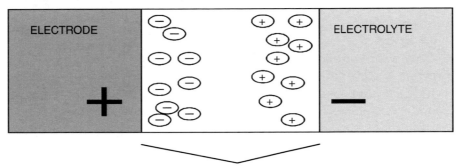

ELECTRODE DOUBLE LAYER FORMS

Potential exists between the electrode and electrolyte due to the formation of the electrode double layer.

(B) SILVER/SILVER CHLORIDE ELECTRODE

Perfectly Nonpolarized Electrodes: Both reactions occur with ease.

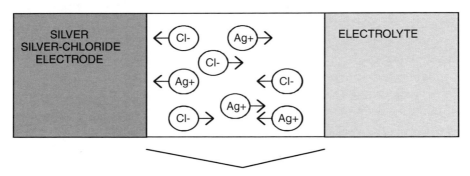

Silver chloride forms free silver ions (Ag+) and chloride ions (Cl-) which prevent the formation of the electron double layer

Figure 10–3. Perfectly Polarized and Perfectly Nonpolarized Electrode.

Silver/Silver-Chloride Electrodes

The silver/silver-chloride (Ag/AgCl) electrode is an important electrode in biopotential measurement since its interface characteristic is close to a perfectly nonpolarized electrode. Silver/silver-chloride electrodes may be manufactured in one of two ways: the electrode may consist of a solid silver surface coated with a thin layer of solid silver-chloride, or it may consist of silver powder and silver-chloride powder compressed into a solid pellet. In either case, the presence of the silver-chloride allows the electrode to behave as a near-perfect nonpolarizable or reversible electrode.

When the electrode is submerged in an electrolyte such as potassium chloride (KCl) containing chloride ions (Cl^-), dissociation of silver ions (Ag^+) from the electrode into the solution and association of the chloride ions (Cl^-) from the solution to the electrode will form free ionic and charge movement between the electrolyte and the electrode. This free ionic flow effect prohibits the formation of the electrode double layer. The net result is a low-impedance, low-offset potential interface between the silver and the electrolyte. Another advantage of the Ag/AgCl electrode is, since silver-chloride is almost insoluble in a chloride-containing solution (i.e., the body that contains chloride ions), very few free silver ions exist. Therefore, tissue damage as a result of the silver ions is negligible.

Electrical Equivalent Circuit

One of the most common electrodes used in biopotential measurement is the surface (or skin) electrode. A typical example of surface electrode is the electrode used in electrocardiogram acquisition. In such application, the electrodes are placed on the surface of the skin over the chest; each pair of electrodes is placed at some specified location and connected via lead wires to the input of a differential amplifier (Figure 10–5). The difference in potential at the two electrode sites is amplified and displayed.

An approximate, electrical equivalent circuit of a tissue-electrode interface is shown in Figure 10–4. In this model, the impedance to ion flow between the tissue and the electrode through the skin is modeled as a 1,000 Ω resistor, often referred to as the skin resistance (R_{se}). The double-layer impedance may be regarded as a 10 µF capacitor (C_d) in parallel with a reasonably high value resistor (R_d), typically 10 kΩ. V_{hc} represents the half cell electrode potential; about 0.3 V for a typical Ag/AgCl electrode and KCl electrolyte.

Figure 10–5 shows the configuration and its electrical equivalent circuit of a pair of electrodes attached to the patient's body and connected to a differential amplifier. The upper and lower branches represent the two elec-

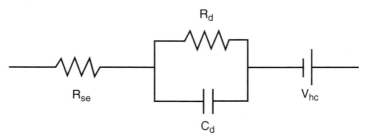

Figure 10–4. Electrical Equivalent Circuit of Single Electrode Tissue Interface.

trode-tissue interfaces; a 2 MΩ resistance represents the input impedance of the differential amplifier; the impedance to ion flow in the tissue between the electrodes is modeled by a 100 Ω resistance.

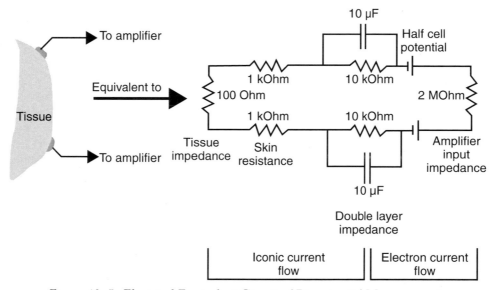

Figure 10–5. Electrical Equivalent Circuit of Biopotential Measurement.

Note that in practice, the half-cell potential of the two electrodes will not be identical; therefore, a nonzero DC offset voltage will appear at the input of the differential amplifier and hence will appear as an amplified DC offset voltage at the output of the amplifier. In some applications, this DC offset can be eliminated by using a high pass filter. The value of the double layer capacitance (C_d) is larger for a polarized electrode and smaller for a nonpolarized electrode (as there is little static charge accumulated at the electrode-electrolyte interface).

Floating Surface Electrode

At the electrode-tissue interface, any mechanical disturbances will create electrode noise. This is especially true of surface electrodes because the electrode double layer acts as a region of charge gradient. Figure 10–6A shows a Ag/AgCl electrode resting directly on the skin surface with a thin layer of electrode gel. Electrode gel is a jelly pastelike solution containing chloride ions; its primary function is to provide a good electrical conduction interface between the electrode and the tissue. Any relative movement between the electrode and skin surface will create a disturbance to the charge gradient distribution in the gel. Any disturbance on this charge gradient causes a change in capacitance and thus a change in the measured electric potential. The result of this disturbance is referred to as motion artifacts in electrophysiological measurements.

The electrical stability of the electrode may be considerably enhanced by mechanically stabilizing the electrode-electrolyte interface. This is achieved by using indirect-contact floating electrodes that interpose an electrolyte jelly paste or gel between the electrode and the tissue. This gel substantially reduces any electrical noise arising from mechanical disturbances in the double-layer charge gradient. Figure 10–6B illustrates the stabilization of the double layer by using a gel-filled electrode housing. In this configuration, any movement between the electrode housing and the skin surface will cause little or no disturbance to the electrode double layer as it is at a distance away from the location of movement. A gel-filled foam between the electrode and tissue will have a similar effect. In the case of internal electrodes, which are usually constructed of stainless steel, the electrode-tissue interface is already enhanced and stabilized by the presence of extracellular fluid.

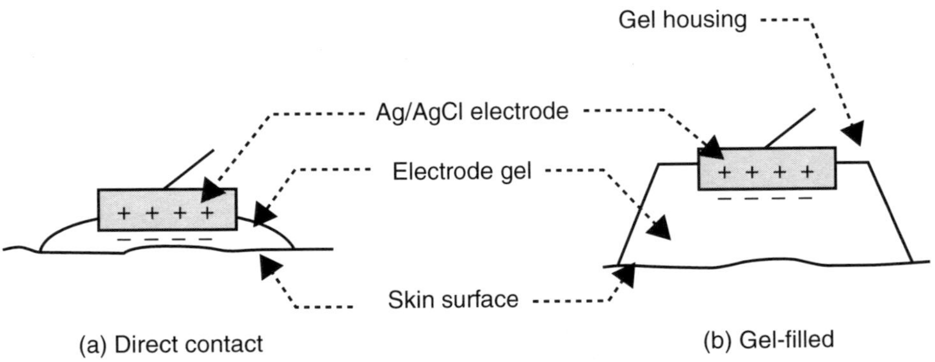

Figure 10–6. Gel-filled Electrode Housing to Minimize Motion Artifact.

Other Biopotential Electrodes

The Ag/AgCl surface electrode described above is only one of the many different types of electrodes used in biopotential signal measurements. For example, metal (e.g., copper) electrodes can be used in measuring surface ECG. Other than surface electrodes, invasive electrodes are commonly used to measure signals deep inside the body or in a small localized region in the tissue. Figure 10–7A shows a needle electrode for measuring electromyogram. It measures the localized electrical activity when inserted into a muscle fiber. Figure 10–7B is a fine-wire electrode for similar applications but can allow more movement by the subject as it is more flexible than a needle electrode.

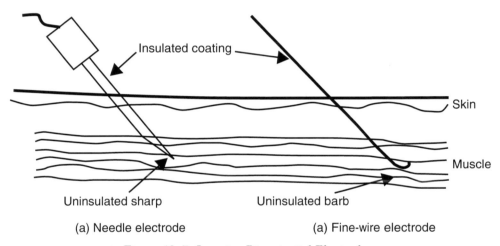

(a) Needle electrode　　　　(a) Fine-wire electrode

Figure 10–7. Invasive Biopotential Electrodes.

Chapter 11

BIOPOTENTIAL AMPLIFIERS

OBJECTIVES

- State the characteristics of an instrumentation amplifier.
- Define common mode and differential mode input.
- Derive the differential gain, common mode gain, and common mode rejection ratio of an instrumentation amplifier.
- Explain the use of a differential amplifier in minimizing common mode signals.
- List common sources of noise and interference affecting biopotential measurements in health care environment.
- Analyze methods to reduce noise and interference including lead shielding, input guarding, right leg driven circuits, and filters.
- Explain interference due to magnetic induction and describe means to reduce such interference.
- List sources of conductive interference and explain the principles of surge suppressors.

CHAPTER CONTENTS

INTRODUCTION

A biopotential signal is often small in amplitude, mixed with other signals, and subjected to external interference. In addition to amplifying the signal, a biopotential amplifier is designed to extract the desired signal from interfering sources as well as to prevent external noise to corrupt the signal. This chapter studies the principles and design of biopotential amplifiers to achieve these objectives.

INSTRUMENTATION AMPLIFIER

Figure 11–1 shows a simple operational amplifier equivalent circuit with gain $= A$, input voltage $V_i = V_2 - V_1$, output $V_o = AV_i$, input impedance Z_i, and output impedance Z_o.

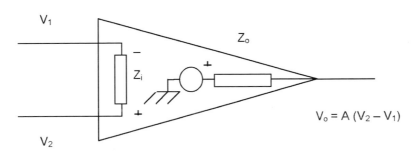

Figure 11–1. Operational Amplifier.

An ideal operational amplifier should have the following characteristics:
- Infinite open loop gain, or $A = \infty$
- Infinite input impedance, or $Z_i = \infty$
- Zero output impedance $Z_o = 0$
- Infinite bandwidth and no phase distortion

In reality, there is no ideal operational amplifier. However, in circuit analysis, when compared to other circuit parameters, a good operational amplifier may be considered to be ideal, which, to a great extend, simplifies the analysis process.

In biopotential measurements, a special amplifier called the instrumentation amplifier is often used. An instrumentation amplifier (Figure 11–2) is a closed-loop, differential input amplifier designed with the purpose of accurately amplifying the voltage applied to its inputs. Ideally, an instrumentation

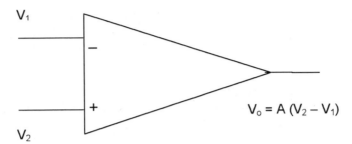

Figure 11–2. Instrumentation Amplifier.

amplifier responds only to the difference between the two input signals and has very high input impedance between its two input terminals and between each input to ground. The characteristics of a good instrumentation amplifier are:

- Very large input impedance
- Very low output impedance
- Constant differential gain with zero nonlinearity
- High common mode rejection
- Very wide bandwidth with no phase distortion
- Low DC offset voltage or drift
- Low input bias current and offset current
- Low noise

Figure 11–3 shows a single Op-Amp differential amplifier.

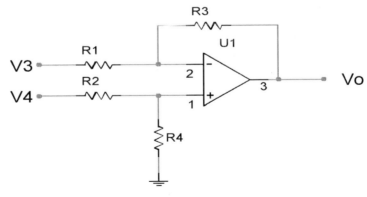

Figure 11–3. Differential Amp Stage of Instrumentation Amplifier.

The voltage V_+ at the noninverting input terminal of the amplifier is given by:

$$V_+ = \frac{R_4}{R_2 + R_4} V_4 \qquad (1)$$

For an Op-Amp in its active nonsaturated state, the voltages at the input terminals of the amplifier must be the same, i.e., $V_+ = V_-$. The current flowing through R_1 and R_3 are given by:

$$i_{R1} = \frac{V_3 - V_-}{R_1}$$

$$i_{R3} = \frac{V_- - V_o}{R_3}$$

Since the input impedance of the Op-Amp is very large, there is no current flowing into the input of the amplifier; the currents flowing through R_1 and R_3 are the same, therefore:

$$\frac{V_- - V_o}{R_3} = \frac{V_3 - V_-}{R_1} \qquad (2)$$

Solving equations (1) and (2) using $V_- = V_+$ yields:

$$V_0 = \left[\frac{R_4}{R_1} \frac{(R_1 + R_3)}{(R_2 + R_4)} \right] V4 - \left[\frac{R_3}{R_1} \right] V3 \qquad (3)$$

If $\dfrac{R_1}{R_3} = \dfrac{R_2}{R_4}$, equation (3) can be simplified to:

$$V_o = \frac{R_3}{R_1} (V_4 - V_3) = - \frac{R_3}{R_1} (V_3 - V_4) \qquad (4)$$

Equation (4) is the characteristic of a true differential amplifier with differential gain DG equal to $-R_3/R_1$ and common mode gain CMG (when $V_3 = V_4$) equal to zero. The common mode rejection ratio (CMRR) of this amplifier is therefore equal to infinity:

$$\text{CMRR} = \left| \frac{\text{DG}}{\text{CMG}} \right| = \frac{R_3/R_1}{0} = \infty$$

The input impedance of this amplifier between the inverting and noninverting input to ground is $R_1 + R_3$ and $R_2 + R_4$, respectively. Since these resistances must be much smaller than the input impedance of the Op-Amp, typical input impedance of this differential amplifier stage is usually chosen to be below 100 kΩ. To overcome this shortcoming, another amplifier stage shown in Figure 11–4 is required to increase the input impedance of the instrumentation amplifier. Below is the analysis of this impedance matching stage of the amplifier:

162   *Biomedical Device Technology: Principles and Design*

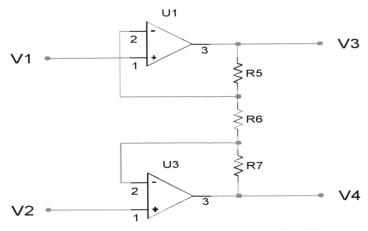

Figure 11–4. Input Stage of Instrumentation Amplifier.

For an ideal Op-Amp, due to its large input impedance, no current flows into the input terminals; therefore, the currents flowing through R_5, R_6, and R_7 are identical and can be written as:

$$i = \frac{V_3 - V_4}{R_5 + R_6 + R_7} \qquad (5)$$

Since the voltages at the two input terminals of an active nonsaturated Op-Amp are identical, the current flowing through the resistor R_6 is equal to:

$$i = \frac{V_1 - V_2}{R_6} \qquad (6)$$

Therefore,

$$V_3 - V_4 = \frac{R_5 + R_6 + R_7}{R_6}(V_1 - V_2)$$

The differential gain of this stage is therefore $= \dfrac{R_5 + R_6 + R_7}{R_6}$. From equation (6), when $V_1 = V_2$, $i = 0$. Since there is no current flowing through the R_5, $V_3 = V_1$; similarly, we can show that $V_4 = V_2$. If the common mode voltage at the input is V_{cm}, the same common voltage will appear at the outputs V_2 and V_3 of the Op-Amps. Therefore, the common mode gain for this circuit is equal to unity. The common mode rejection ratio for this stage is given by:

$$CMRR = \frac{|DG|}{|CMG|} = \frac{R_5 + R_6 + R_7}{R_6}$$

As the signals inputs are directly connected to the input terminals of the Op-Amp, the input impedance of the circuit is equal to the input impedance of the Op-Amp. Figure 11–5 shows the combination of these two amplifier stages forming a classical instrumentation amplifier (IA). The theoretical differential gain, common mode gain, common mode rejection ratio, and input impedance of this classical IA are:

$$DG = -\left(\frac{R_5 + R_6 + R_7}{R_6}\right)\frac{R_3}{R_1}$$

CMG = zero,
CMRR = infinity, and
Z_{in} = infinity.

However, these values are not achievable due to nonideal Op-Amp characteristics (such as nonzero input bias and offset current). In practice, a good IA can have CMRR > 100,000 and Z_{in} > 100 MΩ.

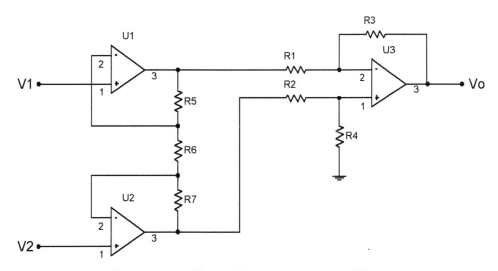

Figure 11–5. Classical Instrumentation Amplifier.

DIFFERENTIAL AND COMMON MODE SIGNALS

Consider the instrumentation amplifier shown in Figure 11–6a with voltage signals V_1 and V_2 connected to the input terminals of the amplifier. These input signals can be represented by their common mode and differential mode signals, V_c and V_d, respectively (Figure 11–6b). The mathematical relationships between these voltages are shown by the following equations:

$$Vc = \frac{V_1 + V_2}{2}$$

$$V_d = V_1 - V_2$$

or,

$$V_1 = V_c + \frac{1}{2} V_d$$

$$V_2 = V_c - \frac{1}{2} V_d$$

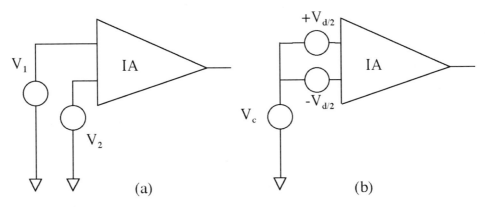

Figure 11–6. Common Mode and Differential Mode Inputs.

If the amplifier is an ideal instrumentation amplifier with a differential gain of A, the output is equal to AV_d. The common mode signal V_c will not appear at the output (since the common mode gain is zero).

Example 1

Referring to the amplifier in Figure 11–2, suppose the voltage measured at V_1 with respect to ground is 4.0 mVdc, the voltage a V_2 with respect to ground is 2.5 mVdc, and if the differential gain A_d of the differential amplifier is 500, the output voltage V_{out} of the differential amplifier is:

Solution

$$V_{out} = A_d (V_2 - V_1) + 500 (4.0 - 2.5) \text{ mVdc} = 500 \times 1.5 \text{ mVdc} = 750 \text{ mVdc}$$

Example 2

For an instrumentation amplifier with differential gain $A_d = 1,000$, common mode gain $A_c = 0.001$, what is output voltage V_{out} if the differential input is a 1.5 mV 1 Hz sinusoidal signal and the common mode input is 2.0 mV 60 Hz noise?

Solution

$V_d = 1.5 \sin (2\pi t)$ mV, $V_c = 2.0 \sin (120\pi t)$ mV
$V_{out} = A_d V_d + A_c V_c = [1,000 \times 1.5 \sin (2\pi t) + 0.001 \times 2.0 \sin (120\pi t)]$mV
$\quad\quad = [1,500 \sin (2\pi t) + 0.002 \sin (120\pi t)]$ mV
$\quad\quad = 1.5 \sin (2\pi t)$ V $+ 2.0 \sin (120\pi t)$ μV
This example illustrates the function of the differential amplifier to amplify the differential (desired) while suppressing the common mode signal (noise).

Example 3

In an experiment with the Op-Amp in Figure 11–6b, if $V_{out} = 10$ V when $V_d = 1.0$ mV and $V_c = 0.0$, and $V_{out} = 50$ mV when $V_d = 0.0$ and $V_c = 5.0$ V, find the differential gain A_d, the common mode gain A_c, the common code rejection ratio CMRR, and CMRdB.

Solution

$A_d = V_{out}/V_d = 10/0.001 = 10,000$, $A_c = V_{out}/V_c = 0.05/5 = 0.01$
CMRR $= A_d/A_c = 10,000/0.01 = 1,000,000$
The CMRR expressed in dB (that is, CMRdB) is given as:
CMRdB $= 20 \log$ (CMRR) $= 20 \log (1,000,000) = 120$dB.

NOISE IN BIOPOTENTIAL SIGNAL MEASUREMENTS

Biopotential signals are produced as a result of action potentials at the cellular level. In physiological monitoring, a biopotential signal is often the resultant electrical potentials from the activities of a group of tissues. We have learned in earlier chapters that a biopotential signal is usually small in magnitude and surrounded by noise. One of the many problems with the amplification of small signals is the concurrent amplification of noise and the presence of interference. Interference and noise are simply defined as any signal other than the desired signal. In physiological signal measurements, there are two different sources of noise and interference:

1. Artificial sources from the surrounding environment such as electromagnetic interference or mechanical motion. For example, artifacts on an ECG strip caused by fluorescent lighting or unshielded power supply voltages are considered artificial interference.
2. Natural biological signal sources from the patient. For example, in ECG measurement, any signals other than ECG that arise from other biopotentials of the body are considered as natural noise. These include muscle artifact from the patient or electrical activity of the brain. While brain activity is noise when measuring ECG, ECG signal is considered as noise when brain wave (EEG) is measured.

One of the functions of a biopotential amplifier and its associated electronic circuitry is to amplify those biopotential signals of interest while rejecting or minimizing all other interfering signals.

An example of a common form of interference in biopotential measurements is shown in Figure 11–7. The ECG signal is corrupted by 60 Hz power noise induced on the body of the patient. Noise from power line interference may have an amplitude of several millivolts, which can be larger than the signal of interest. Fortunately, the power line induced 60 Hz noise is on the entire body of the patient and therefore appears equally at both the inverting and noninverting input terminals of the biopotential amplifier. Such common mode signal can be substantially reduced by using a good instrumentation amplifier with a large common mode rejection ratio. Filters can also be used to remove the undesirable signal if the bandwidth of the interfering signal is not overlapping that of the desired signal.

In order to obtain a good signal in a noisy environment, it is important to have a signal level much larger than the noise level. The ratio of signal to noise level is an important parameter in signal analysis and processing.

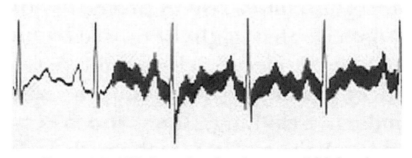

Figure 11–7. 60Hz Power Line Interference on ECG Signal.

Signal to noise ratio (SNR) in decibel is defined as:

$$SNR(dB) = 20 \times \log \frac{V_s}{V_n}$$

where V_s and V_n are the signal and noise voltage, respectively.

When dealing with medical instrumentations, the most common external noise source is from the power lines or equipment in the patient care area. Interference from 60 Hz power can be induced by electric or magnetic fields. A 60 Hz electric field can induce current on lead wires as well as on the patient's body. A changing magnetic field (e.g., from 60 Hz power lines) can induce a voltage or current on a conductor loop. Other than 60 Hz power line interference, much equipment (e.g., switching regulators, electrosurgical units) emits electromagnetic noise into the surrounding area. These EMI can be of low or high frequencies (e.g., 500 kHz from an electrosurgical unit), which may create problems if it is not dealt with properly. EMI can be radiated as well as conducted through cables or conductor connections. For example, high-frequency harmonics from switching power supplies can be transmitted through the power grid to other equipment in the vicinity. Switching transient, which may cause damage to electronic components, can be transferred in the same way.

In general, the design of the first stage of medical devices, which usually includes the patient interface and the instrumentation amplifier, is critical to maintain a healthy SNR. The remainder of this chapter discusses the mechanism of interference and some practical noise suppression measures.

INTERFERENCE FROM EXTERNAL ELECTRICAL FIELD

A typical electromedical device measuring biopotential from the patient has conductor wires connecting the device to a patient. The patient and the device are usually working in an environment filled with electric field produced by 120 V power lines and line-powered devices. Figure 11-8 shows such an arrangement. Using an ECG as an example, terminals A and B are the input of the instrumentation amplifier and G is the ground connecting point of the device.

Under typical operating conditions, through capacitive coupling, the electric field produced by the 120 V power sources will induce current flowing into the lead wires as well as into the patient's body to ground. The following sections examine the effects of such induced currents on the output and methods to reduce these interferences.

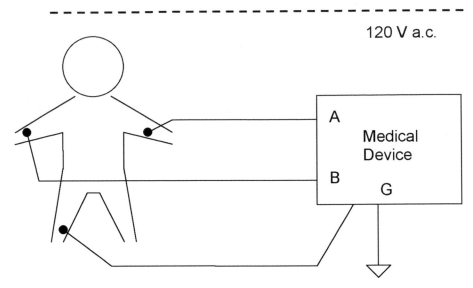

Figure 11–8. Connection of Medical Device to Patient.

Currents Induced on Lead Wires

Consider that the medical device is an electrocardiograph (ECG) with skin electrodes attached to the patient as shown in Figure 11–9. Z_1, Z_2, and Z_G represent the impedances of the skin electrode interfaces and electrodes. C_1 and C_2 are the coupling capacitors between the 120 V power line and the lead wires. These capacitance values depend on the length of the conductors and their distance from the 120 V power sources. Due to these capacitive couplings, displacement currents (I_{d1} and I_{d2}) will flow in the wires to ground. Similarly, C_3 is the coupling capacitor between the power line and the chassis of the device. As the chassis is grounded, the displacement current I_{d3} will flow through the chassis to ground.

C_b is the coupling capacitor between the power line and the body of the patient. A displacement current I_{db} will flow into the body of the patient.

Assuming the input impedances of the instrumentation amplifier (IA) are very large, the displacement currents I_{d1} and I_{d2}, which are 60 Hz induced currents, will flow through the skin-electrode interfaces, into the patient's body and out through the skin-electrode interface (Z_G) to ground. This current path will create a voltage across the input terminals A and B of the IA given by:

$$V_A - V_B = (I_{d1}Z_1 + I_{dB}Z_G) - (I_{d2}Z_2 + I_{dB}Z_G) = I_{d1}Z_1 - I_{d2}Z_2$$

(note the cancellation of the common mode voltage $I_{dB}Z_G$ by the differential amplifier).

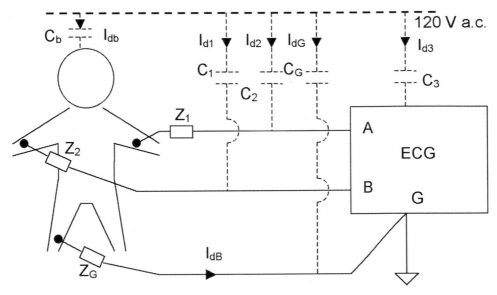

Figure 11–9. Interference from Power Line.

If similar electrodes and lead wires are used and they are placed close together, one can simplify this expression by making $I_{d1} = I_{d2} = I_d$. In this case:

$$V_A - V_B = I_d (Z_1 - Z_2) \tag{7}$$

Example 4

In an ECG measurement using the setup in Figure 11–9, if the displacement current I_d due to power line interference is 9 nA and difference in the skin-electrode impedances of the two limb electrodes are 20 kΩ, find the 60 Hz interference voltage across the input terminals of the ECG machine.

Solution

Using the above derived equation:

$$V_A - V_B = I_d (Z_1 - Z_2) = 9 \text{ nA} \times 20 \text{ kΩ} = 180 \text{ μV}$$

With a typical ECG signal amplitude of 1 mV, this represents 8% of the desired signal. This electromagnetic interference creates a 60 Hz signal riding on the 1 mV amplitude ECG waveform (Figure 11–7).

Example 5

For Example 4, if the displacement current I_{db} through the patient's body is $0.2\mu A$, what is the common mode voltage at the input terminals of the ECG machine given that the skin-electrode impedance Z_G at the leg electrode is $50\ k\Omega$ and the body impedance Z_b is 500Ω?

Solution

The common mode voltage V_{cm} at the input terminals of the ECG machine is due to the current flowing through the body impedance and the skin-electrode impedance.

$$V_{cm} = (I_{db} + I_{d1} + I_{d2})\,(Z_G + Z_b)$$

Since I_{db} is much larger than I_{d1} and I_{d2} and Z_G is much larger than Z_b, we can write

$$V_{cm} = I_{db}Z_G = 0.2\ \mu A \times 50\ k\Omega = 10\ mV.$$

This common mode voltage is 10 times the typical amplitude of an ECG signal! Fortunately, this 60 Hz common mode signal will not appear at the output due to the high common mode rejection signal of the instrumentation amplifier.

From equation (7), in order to reduce the interference signal (power line 60 Hz interference in this case), it is desirable to reduce I_{d1} and I_{d2} or ensure that the skin-electrode impedances are the same (so that $Z_1 - Z_2 = 0$). The latter can be achieved by using identical electrodes and ensuring that proper skin preparation is done before the electrodes are applied. One attempt to reduce or even eliminate I_{d1} and I_{d2} is to use shielded lead wires as shown in Figure 11–10a. When the entire length of the lead wires is surrounded by a grounded sheath, the coupling capacitors between the power line and each lead wire are eliminated (i.e., $I_d = I_{d1} = I_{d2} = 0$). Therefore, from equation (7), $V_A - V_B = 0$. However, the shield, which is in close proximity to the lead wires, creates coupling capacitances C_{s1} and C_{s2} with each of the wires. From the equivalent circuit shown in Figure 11–10b, one can show that the voltage across the input terminals of the ECG machine due to the nonzero common mode voltage on the patient body (see Example 5 for estimation of body common mode voltage) is equal to:

$$V_A - V_B = \left(\frac{Z_{s1}}{Z_1 + Z_{s1}} - \frac{Z_{s2}}{Z_2 + Z_{s2}}\right) V_{cm} \qquad (8)$$

where Z_{s1} and Z_{s2} are the impedances due to capacitances C_{s1} and C_{s2}, respectively.

Equation (8) becomes zero only if $\dfrac{Z_1}{Z_2} = \dfrac{Z_{s1}}{Z_{s2}}$. If this condition is not met, V_{cm} will appear at the output no matter how good the common mode rejection ratio of the ECG is.

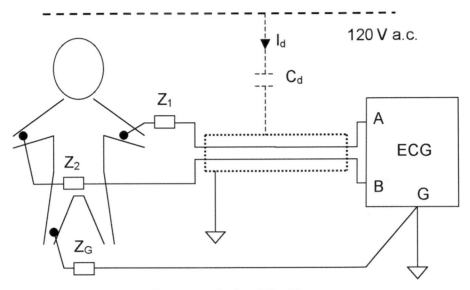

Figure 11–10a. Lead Shielding.

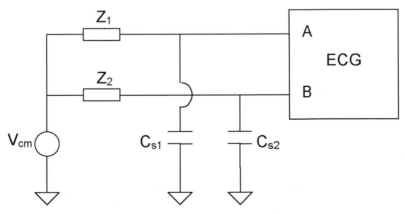

Figure 11–10b. Lead Shielding–Equivalent Circuit.

To prevent this, a second shield (called the guarding shield) is placed between the first shield and the lead wires, and the guarding shield is connected to the patient's body (e.g., the right leg) via an electrode. This setup is shown in Figure 11–11a and its equivalent circuit is shown in Figure 11–11b. Note the potential of the guarding shield is at the same level as that of the patient body (i.e., at V_{cm}). Therefore, V_{cm} will not show up across the input terminals of the ECG as there is no current flow around the loops of Z_1–$Z_{s'1}$–Z_G and Z_1–$Z_{s'2}$–Z_G in the circuit. ($Z_{s'1}$ and $Z_{s'2}$ are the impedances of the coupling capacitors $C_{s'1}$ and $C_{s'2}$, respectively, between the guarding shield and the lead wires.)

By using the input guarding method, the induced lead current I_d and the common mode voltage V_{cm} will not appear across the input terminals of the instrumentation amplifier of the ECG.

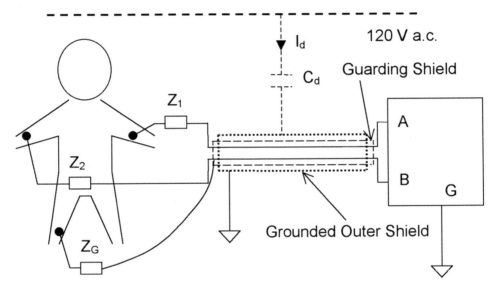

Figure 11–11a. Input Guarding.

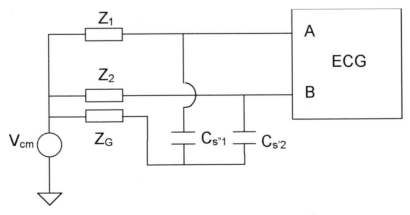

Figure 11–11b. Input Guarding–Equivalent Circuit.

Right-Leg-Driven Circuit

So far, we have been assuming that the ECG input stage is an ideal instrumentation amplifier (i.e., with infinite input impedance and zero common mode gain). Under these ideal conditions, all common mode signals at the input terminals of the IA are rejected. Let's consider a more realistic situation when the input impedance of the instrumentation amplifier has a finite value.

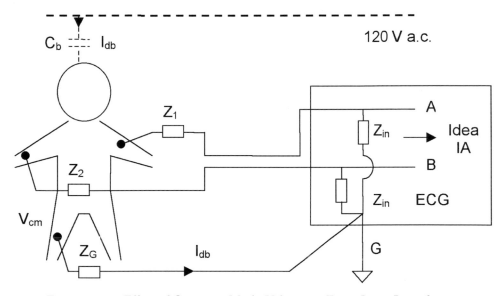

Figure 11–12. Effect of Common Mode Voltage on Finite Input Impedance.

An ECG machine with a nonideal instrumentation amplifier can be represented by an ideal IA coupled to finite input impedances Z_{in} to ground at each of its input terminals (Figure 11–12). The differential input voltage of this configuration is given by:

$$V_A - V_B = \left(\frac{Z_{in}}{Z_1 + Z_{in}} - \frac{Z_{in}}{Z_2 + Z_{in}} \right) V_{cm}$$

If Z_{in} is much greater than Z_1 and Z_2, we can simply the equation to:

$$V_A - V_B = \frac{Z_2 - Z_1}{Z_{in}} V_{cm} \tag{9}$$

This differential input voltage ($V_A - V_B$) to the IA due to nonzero common mode voltage V_{cm} will be amplified no matter how large the CMRR is (or how small the CMG). To reduce this voltage, we can either choose an IA with very large Z_{in}, use perfectly matching electrodes with good skin preparation (i.e., make $Z_1 = Z_2$) or reduce V_{cm}. A practical method using active cancellation to reduce V_{cm} is the right leg driven circuit shown in Figure 11–13.

Example 6

An instrumentation amplifier with input impedances of 5 MΩ between each input terminal to ground is used as the first stage of an ECG machine. If the difference in the skin-electrode impedance is 20 kΩ and the common mode voltage induced from power lines on the patient's body is 10 mV, calculate the magnitude of the 60 Hz interference appearing across the input terminals of the IA.

Solution

Substituting the value into equation (9), the voltage across the input of the ideal IA is:

$$V_A - V_B = \frac{20 \text{ k}\Omega}{5 \text{ M}\Omega} 10\text{mV} = 40\mu\text{V}$$

Since this is a differential input signal to the IA, it will be amplified and

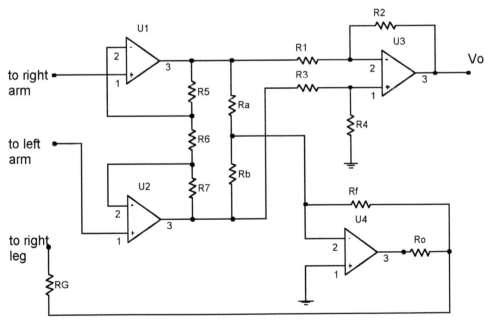

Figure 11–13. Instrumentation Amplifier with Right-Leg-Driven Circuit.

appear at the output of the ECG machine. Compared to the typical ampli-tude of an ECG signal (1 mV), this is a noticeable noise level.

The Op-Amps U1, U2, and U3 form a classical instrumentation amplifi-er (see also Figure 11–5). The inputs are connected to the left and right arm electrodes of the patient. The output voltage V_o of U3 is the amplified biopo-tential signal between these two limb electrodes. V_o is coupled to the next stage of the ECG machine. U4 with R_f and R_o forms an inverting amplifier with input taken from the output of U1 and U2. This circuit extracts the com-mon mode voltage from the patient's body, inverts it, and feeds it back to the patient via the right leg electrode. It creates an active cancellation effect on the common mode voltage induced on the patient's body and thereby reduces the magnitude of V_{cm} to a much smaller value. Figure 11–14 redraws the right leg driven circuit to facilitate quantitative analysis of this circuit

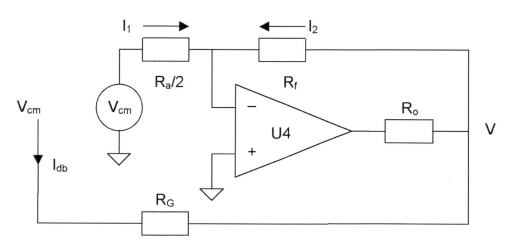

Figure 11–14. Equivalent Circuit of Right-Leg-Driven Circuit.

For the right-leg-driven (RLD) circuit in Figure 11–13, R_a is chosen to be equal to R_b. We have also proven earlier that the same common mode volt-age V_{cm} at the patient's body appears at the output of U1 and U2. Therefore, we can represent this part of the circuit by a voltage source V_{cm} and a resis-tor with resistance equal to the parallel resistance of R_a and R_b (equal to $R_a/2$ as $R_a = R_b$). At the right leg electrode, the voltage at the electrode is also V_{cm} (electrode connecting to the patient's body), and there is an induced 60 Hz current I_{db} flowing from the patient into the ECG machine. This equivalent circuit is shown in Figure 11–14.

At the noninverting input terminal of U4, due to the large input imped-ance of the amplifier, there is no current flowing into or out of the Op-Amp.

Therefore $I_1 + I_2 = 0$.

But $I_2 = (V - 0)/R_f$ and $I_1 = (V_{cm} - 0)/R_a/2$, therefore

$$\frac{V}{R_f} + \frac{2V_{cm}}{R_a} = 0 \Rightarrow V = -\frac{2R_f}{R_a} V_{cm} \qquad (10)$$

From the lower branch of the circuit:

$$V_{cm} = R_G I_{db} + V \qquad (11)$$

Combining equations (10) and (11) gives:

$$V_{cm} = \frac{R_G}{1 + \frac{2R_f}{R_a}} I_{db} \qquad (12)$$

From equation (12), we can see that if we want to have a small V_{cm}, we must make the denominator as large as possible. That is, the ratio of R_f/R_a should be very large.

Example 7

For the RLD circuit in Figure 11–13, using the values in Example 5 (i.e., I_{db} = 0.2 μA, R_G = 50 kΩ: 1) find the common mode voltage V_{cm} on the patient's body if R_f = 5 MΩ and R_a = 25 kΩ. 2) Using this new V_{cm} value, calculate the magnitude of the 60 Hz interference appearing across the input terminals of the IA in Example 6.

Solution

1) Substituting values into equation (12) gives:

$$V_{cm} = \frac{50 \text{ k}\Omega}{1 + \frac{2 \times 5 \text{ M}\Omega}{25 \text{ k}\Omega}} 0.2 \text{ μA} = 125 \text{ }\Omega \times 0.2 \text{ μA} = 25 \text{ μV}$$

Using the right-leg-driven circuit, we have reduced the V_{cm} from 10 mV to 25 μV, a 400 times reduction!

2) Substituting values into equation (9), the voltage across the input of the ideal IA is:

$$V_A - V_B = \frac{20 \text{ k}\Omega}{5 \text{ M}\Omega} 25 \text{μV} = 0.1 \text{μV}$$

This magnitude of noise is negligible when compared to a 1 mV level of the ECG signal.

The function of R_o is used to limit the current flowing into the Op-Amp when there is a large V_{cm}. R_o, usually of resistance equal to several MΩ, is primarily for the protection of the electronic circuits during cardiac defibrillation.

An alternative configuration of the RLD circuit is shown in Figure 11–15. Interested readers may go through a similar derivation to determine the common modes signal level using this feedback configuration.

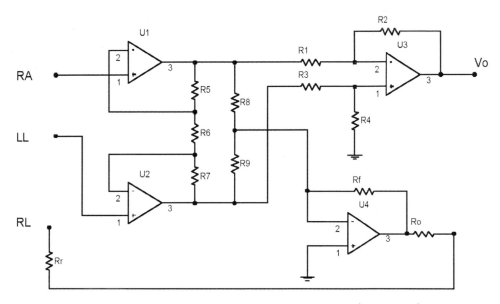

Figure 11–15. Instrumentation Amplifier with RLD (alternative).

INTERFERENCE FROM EXTERNAL MAGNETIC FIELD

Another source of interference is magnetic induction from changing magnetic fields. This can be from power lines and devices that create magnetic fields such as large motors or transformers. If such magnetic field passes through a conductor loop, it will induce a voltage V_i proportional to the rate of change of the magnetic flux Φ, that is

$$V_i \propto \frac{d\phi}{dt} \text{ or } V_i \propto \frac{d(B \times A)}{dt} \tag{13}$$

where Φ is the product of the magnetic field B and the area A of the conductor loop perpendicular to B.

Figure 11–16a shows the magnetic field interference during an ECG measurement procedure. The conductor loop is formed by the lead wires and the patient's body. If the magnetic field is generated from the ballast of a fluorescent light fitting, a 60 Hz differential signal will appear across the input terminals of the ECG machine. From equation (13), one can minimize the magnitude of interference by reducing loop area *A*. A simple approach is to place the lead wires closer together to reduce the magnetic induction area. Another method is to twist the wires together (as shown in Figure 11–16b) so that the fluxes cancel each other (flux generated in a loop is in opposite polarity to the flux generated in the adjacent loops). Unwanted magnetic field can also be shielded but often it is relatively expensive to produce a practical magnetic shield to protect the device from magnetic field interference.

We so far have been using 60 Hz power line signals as examples of elec-

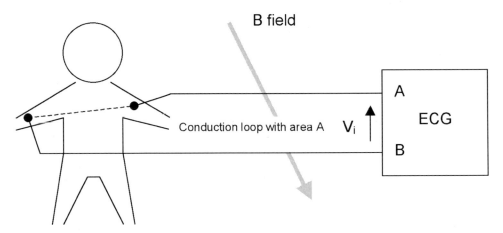

Figure 11–16a. Interference Due to Magnetic Field.

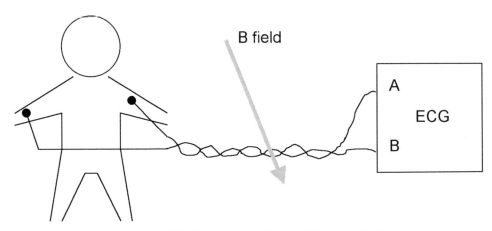

Figure 11–16b. Interference Due to Magnetic Field.

tromagnetic interference (EMI). Other than power frequency interference, there are many other sources of interference that radiate EMI to the surrounding area. In medical settings, electrosurgical units that produce 500 kHz EMI, and radio broadcasting and cellular phones that produce EMI in the GHz range are just a few of the many examples.

CONDUCTIVE INTERFERENCE

Other than EMI, which is often considered as radiated noise, interference can also be caused by unwanted signals conducted to the device via lead wires, power cables, et cetera. Some of these conductive interference sources are discussed in the following sections.

High Frequency and Harmonics

This interference appears as high frequency riding on the 60 Hz power voltage. It is usually caused by poorly designed switch-mode regulators that return the high-frequency signal into the power lines. These harmonics and high frequency affect devices connected to the same power grid. They can be eliminated by placing power line filters at the input of the power supply of a device.

Switching Transients

Switching transients are produced when high voltage or high current is turned on and off by a switch or a circuit breaker. During the interruption of a switch or power breaker, arcing occurs across the contact of the switch. This arcing may generate an overvoltage and a short duration of high-frequency oscillation. Switching transients can damage sensitive electronic equipment if the device is not properly protected. Switching transient damage can be prevented by using power line filters and surge protectors.

Lightning Surges

When lightning strikes a conductive cable (such as a power line, a telephone cable, or network cable) connected to a device, the high voltage and high power surge will be transmitted through the power grid into the medical device and cause component damage. Surge protection devices with adequate power capacities are required to protect electromedical devices from lightning damage.

Defibrillator Pulses

Medical devices are designed to be safe to patients and operators. Under normal operation, patients and users are not subjected to any electrical risk from the medical device. However, there are times a patient can present electrical risk to a device. An example of such an occurrence is when a patient may need to be defibrillated while an ECG monitor is still connected to the patient. In this case, a high voltage pulse of several thousand volts may be transmitted through the lead wires into the ECG monitors. Special high voltage protection circuits (referred to as defibrillation protection circuits) are built into devices that are subject to such risks. Figure 11–17 shows the defibrillator protection components of an ECG machine. In the case of a high voltage applied to the ECG lead wires, the voltage limiting device will clamp the voltage, to say 0.7 V, to protect the instrumentation amplifiers and other electronic components in the machine. The resistance R limits the current flowing into the voltage limiting device.

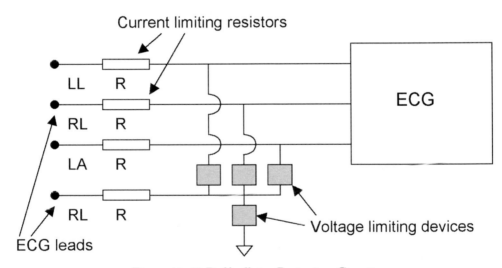

Figure 11–17. Defibrillator Protection Circuit.

The voltage limiting device can be two parallel diodes arranged as in Figure 11–18a, two zener diodes in series, or a gas discharge lamp. All these devices can limit the voltage level at the input of the ECG machine. The transfer function of the voltage limiting circuit (consisting of the voltage limiting device together with the current limiting resistor) is shown in Figure 11–18b.

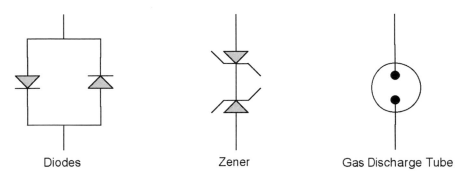

Diodes   Zener   Gas Discharge Tube

Figure 11–18a. Examples of Voltage Limiting Devices.

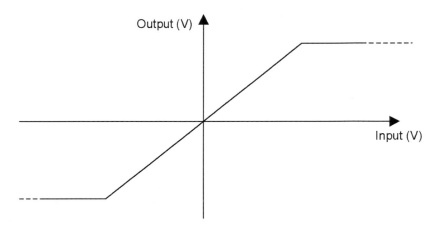

Figure 11–18b. Characteristics of Voltage Limiting Circuits.

For the defibrillator protection circuit shown in Figure 11–17, since the ECG signal is at the most a few millivolts, one can use a silicon diode (with turn-on voltage = 0.7 V) as the voltage limiter. Under normal measurement conditions, the voltage at the input of the ECG machine will be equal to the ECG signal (about 1 mV amplitude). During defibrillation, although the voltage on the patient's body can be several thousand volts, the voltage at the input terminals of the ECG machine will be limited to 0.7 V, thereby protecting the electronic components in the ECG from being damaged by the high voltage of the defibrillator.

Chapter 12

ELECTRICAL SAFETY
AND SIGNAL ISOLATION

OBJECTIVES

- State the nature and causes of electrical shock hazards from medical devices.
- Explain the physiological and tissue effects of risk current.
- Differentiate micro and macro shocks.
- Define leakage current and identify its sources.
- List user precautions to minimize risk from electrical shock.
- Compare grounded and isolated power supply systems.
- Analyze the principles and shortfalls of grounded and isolated power systems in term of electrical safety.
- Explain the function of the line isolation transformer in an isolated power system.
- Explain the purpose of signal isolation and identify common isolation barriers.
- Describe other measures to enhance electrical safety.
- Evaluate the IEC601-1 leakage measurement device and its applications.

CHAPTER CONTENTS

1. Introduction
2. Electrical Shock Hazards
3. Macroshock and Microshock
4. Prevention of Electrical Safety Hazards

INTRODUCTION

Concerned with the increasing use of medical procedures that penetrate the skin barrier (e.g., catheterization), a number of studies published in the early 1970s suggested the occurrences of electrocution of patients from low-level electrical current passing directly through the heart (microshock). It was also demonstrated from animal studies that a 60 Hz current with level as low as 20 µA directly flowing through the heart can cause ventricular fibrillation.

Although the actual occurrence of death due to microshock in hospitals has never been documented, the potential of such occurrence is believed to be present. In the interest of electrical safety and risk reduction, hospitals have implemented both infrastructure and procedural measures to prevent such electrical shock hazards. Special considerations were given in designing medical devices to make them electrically safe. This chapter discusses these safety measures and device designs to prevent electrical shock to patients.

ELECTRICAL SHOCK HAZARDS

Electricity is a convenient form of energy. The deployment of electromedical devices in health care has advanced patient care, improved diagnosis, and expanded the treatment of diseases. However, improper use of electricity may lead to electrical shock, fire, or even explosion, which may lead to patient and staff injuries. The heating and arcing from electricity may cause patient burn or ignite flammable materials such as drapes, alcohol prep solutions, or even the body hair of patients. Together with enriched oxygen content in the surrounding atmosphere, fire and explosion hazards are eminent.

When an electrical current passes through a patient, it creates different effects on tissue. Tissue effects due to electrical current depend on the following factors:

- the magnitude and frequency of the current
- the current path
- the length of time that the current flows through the body
- the overall physical condition of the person

Skin is a natural defense against electrical shock because the outermost layer of skin (the epithelium) has very low conductivity. The skin is a good insulator (relatively high resistance) surrounding the more susceptible internal organs. The resistance of 1 cm^2 of skin is about 15 kΩ to 1 MΩ (note that the resistance decreases with increasing contact area). However, skin conductivity can increase 100 to 1,000 times (e.g., become 150 Ω) when it is wet.

Due to the nature of medical evaluations and treatments, patients are more susceptible to electrical shocks. Some reasons of the increased electrical hazards are listed below:

- In hospitals, skin resistance is often bypassed by conductive objects such as hypodermic needles, and fluid-filled catheters introduced through the skin.
- ECG/EEG electrodes use electrolyte gel to reduce skin resistance.
- Fluid inside the body is a good conductor to current flow.
- Patients are often in a compromised situation (e.g., under anesthesia). They may not be sensitive to or able to react to heat, pain, or other discomfort.
- Clinicians do not necessary have knowledge of electricity and maintaining a safe electrical environment.

As an example, a patient in an intensive care unit may have several fluid-filled catheters connected to his or her heart to allow pressure measurements in the heart chambers. This same patient could be in an electrical bed; be connected with ECG electrodes, temperature probes, respiration sensors, and intravenous lines; be covered by a hypothermic blanket; and be connected to a ventilator. All of these connections have the potential to conduct a hazardous current to the patient.

An electrical current can produce reversible or irreversible damage to tissue as well as stimulate muscle and nerve conduction. Table 12–1 shows

Table 12–1.
Potential Hazards from Electrical Current (External Contact).

Current Level	Physiological and Tissue Effect
1 mA	Threshold of perception. The person begins to sense the presence of the current.
5 mA	Maximum accepted safe current.
10 mA	Maximum current before involuntary muscle contraction. May cause the person's finger to clamp onto the current source. ("let go" current).
50 mA	Perception of pain. Possible fainting, exhaustion, mechanical injury.
100–300 mA	Possible ventricular fibrillation.
6A	Sustained myocardial contraction; temporary respiratory paralysis; may sustain tissue burns.
≥ 10 A	All of the above plus severe thermal burns.

the human physiological and tissue effects of a one-second external contact with a 60 Hz electrical current.

Example 1

A patient is touching a medical device with one hand and grabbing the handrail of a grounded bed. If the ground wire of the medical device is broken and there is a fault in the medical device that shorted the chassis of the device to the live power conductor (120V), what is the risk current passing through the patient? Assume that each skin contact has a resistance of 25 kΩ and the internal body resistance is 500 Ω.

Solution

If the ground wire of the medical device is intact, a large fault current will flow to ground and blow the fuse of the device or trip the circuit breaker of the power distribution circuit. If the ground of the device is open, a current will flow through the patient to ground. The total resistance of the current path is 25 + 25 + 0.5 kΩ = 50.5 kΩ.

The current passing through the patient is therefore $= \dfrac{120 \text{ V}}{50.5 \text{ k}\Omega} = 2.4$ mA.

According to Table 12–1, the patient should feel the presence of the current. Although this amount of current is not large enough to blow the fuse or trip the circuit breaker, the level is not high enough to endanger the patient

Experimental work on dogs had shown that ventricular fibrillation could be onset by a current as small as 20 microamperes (50–60 Hz) applied directly to the heart. Note that this current is 5,000 times below the "possible ventricular fibrillation" current (100 mA according to Table 12–1) applied externally. In addition, it was shown that the threshold current triggering these physiological effects increases with increasing frequency. For example, the "let go" current increases from 10 mA to 90 mA when the frequency is increased from 60 Hz to 10 kHz. Very high frequency current (e.g., 500 kHz) used in electrosurgical procedures will not cause muscle or nerve stimulation, and therefore will not cause ventricular fibrillation. Moreover, skin burn and tissue damage can still occur at high current.

MACROSHOCK AND MICROSHOCK

The physiological effects described in Table 12–1 are often referred to as macroshocks, whereas shocks that arise from current directly flowing through the heart are referred to as micro shocks. Figure 12–1a and Figure 12–1b show the differences between macro and microshocks. In a macroshock, the electrical contacts are at the skin surface. The risk current is distributed through a large area of the patient's body. As shown in Figure 12–1a, only a portion of the risk current flows through the heart. In a microshock, the entire risk current is directed through the heart by an indwelling catheter or conductor.

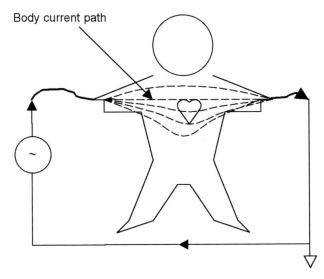

Figure 12–1a. Macroshock.

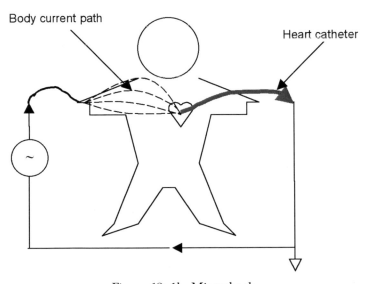

Figure 12–1b. Microshock.

Example 2

If the patient in Example 1 has a heart catheter (a conductor connected directly to the heart) and it is connected to ground, calculate the risk current.

Solution

Since the catheter bypassed one skin-to-ground contact, the resistance of the current path is now reduced to $25 + 0.5$ kΩ = 25.5 kΩ. The risk current therefore is equal to $\dfrac{120 \text{ V}}{25.5 \text{ k}\Omega} = 4.7$ mA.

Although this current level is still considered safe for external contact (Table 12–1), this amount of current under this situation (directly flowing through the heart) will trigger ventricular fibrillation (>20 μA).

Table 12–2 shows the physiological effect of such current through the heart. Note that this level of current is below the threshold of perception (listed in Table 12–1), which suggests that the person will not be able to feel the risk current even when it is sufficient to cause a microshock. Both macroshock and microshock can injure patients or cause death. Table 12–3 summarizes the characteristics of macroshock and microshock.

Table 12–2.
Potential Hazards from Electrical Current (Cardiac Contact).

Current Level	Physiological Effect
0–10 μA	Safe for a normal heart
10–20 μA	Ventricular fibrillation may occur
20–800 μA	Ventricular fibrillation

Table 12-3.
Characteristics of Macroshock and Microshock.

Macroshock	Microshock
Requires two contact points with the electrical circuit at different potentials	Requires two contact points with electrical circuit at different potentials
High current passing through the body	Low current passing directly through the heart
Skin resistance is usually not bypassed, i.e., external skin contact	Skin resistance is bypassed
Usually due to equipment fault such as breakdown of insulation, exposure of live conductors, short circuit of hot line to case	Usually due to leakage current from stray capacitors

The term *leakage current* is mentioned frequently in articles on patient safety. Leakage current is not a result of a fault. It flows between any energized parts of an electrical circuit and its grounded parts. Leakage current generally has two components—one capacitive and the other resistive. Capacitive leakage current exists because any two conductors separated in space have a certain amount of capacitance between the conductors. This undesired capacitance is called stray capacitance. When an alternating voltage is applied between two conductors, a measurable amount of current will flow (e.g., between the primary winding and the metal case of a power transformer, or between power conductors and the grounded chassis). The resistive component of leakage current is primarily due to imperfect insulation between conductors. Since no substance is a perfect insulator, some small amount of current will flow between a live conductor and ground. However, because of its relatively small magnitude compared to the capacitive leakage current, resistive leakage current is often ignored.

In addition to electrical shocks and fire hazards described above, the loss of electricity in health care settings can also create problems and compromise the safety of patients. Table 12–4 summarizes different electrical hazards in the health care environment.

Example 3

The total stray capacitance between the live conductors and ground of a medical device powered by a 120 V, 60 Hz power supply is 0.22 pF. Find the total capacitive leakage current flowing to ground.

Solution

Impedance due to the stray capacitance is

$$\frac{1}{2\pi f C} = \frac{1}{2\pi 60 \times 0.22 \times 10^{-9}} \Omega = 12 \text{ M}\Omega.$$

Therefore, magnitude of the capacitive leakage current is $\dfrac{120 \text{ V}}{12 \text{ M}\Omega} = 10 \text{ }\mu\text{A}.$

PREVENTION OF ELECTRICAL SAFETY HAZARD

Risk current is defined as any undesired current, including leakage current that passes through the body of a patient. Although it cannot be avoided, it can be minimized by appropriate equipment deployment and proper

Table 12–4.
Summary of Electrical Hazards.

Type of Hazard	Nature of Hazard
Macroshock	• Burns–including external (skin), internal, and cellular • Pain and muscle contraction–may cause physical injury • Ventricular fibrillation
Microshock	• Ventricular fibrillation
Fire and Explosion	• Damage and burn caused by heat or sparks from electrical short circuit, overload in the presence of fuel, and enriched oxygen environment
Electrical Failure	• Lost of function of life-supporting equipment • Disruption of service and treatment • Panic

utilization. Some simple user precautions that medical personnel can take to ensure patient and staff safety are:

1. Medical personnel should ensure that all equipment is appropriate for the desired application. Medical equipment usually has an approval label on it that informs the operator of the risk level of the equipment. One example of such classification and its meaning is shown in Table 12–5. A patient leakage current is a current flowing from the patient applied part through the patient to ground or from the patient through the applied part to ground.
2. Ensure that the medical equipment is properly connected to an electrical outlet that is part of a grounded electrical system. The power ground will provide a low-resistance path for the leakage current.
3. Users of medical devices should be cautioned about any damage to the equipment, including signs of physical damage, frayed power

Table 12–5.
Classification of Medical Electrical Equipment
(CAN/CSA C22.2 No. 601-1 M90)

Equipment Type	Intended Application	Maximum Allowable Patient Leakage Current (µA) under	
		Normal Conditions	Single Fault Conditions
B	Equipment with causal patient contact, usually have no patient applied parts	100	500
BF	Equipment with patient applied parts	100	500
CF	Equipment with cardiac applied parts, i.e., connected to the heart or to great vessels leading to the heart	10	50

cords, et cetera.

4. Ensure that there is an equipment management program in place so that periodic inspections and quality assurance measures are performed by qualified individuals to ensure equipment performance and safety.

In addition to these user precautions, electrical systems and medical devices can incorporate designs to lower the risk of electrical hazards. The remainder of this chapter describes such designs.

GROUNDED AND ISOLATED POWER SYSTEMS

Figure 12–2 shows the line diagram of a common grounded electrical system. In a grounded system, there are three conductors: the hot, the neutral, and the ground (these wires are colored black, white, and green, respectively, in a single phase 120 V North American power distribution system). The neutral wire is connected to the ground wire at the incoming substation or at the main distribution panel. In a 3-wire grounded system, the voltages between the hot and neutral wires and between the hot and ground wires are both 120 V. Under normal conditions, there is no voltage between the neutral and ground conductors.

An isolated power system is shown in Figure 12–3. In this distribution system, a line isolation transformer is placed between the power supply transformer and the power outlets. In an isolated power system, there is no neutral wire as both lines connected to the secondary of the transformer are not tied to ground; they are floating with respect to ground (has no conduction path to ground). The voltage between the lines is 120 V. The color coding for the line 1, line 2, and ground conductor of an isolated power system is brown, orange, and green, respectively. Both line conductors are protected by circuit breakers that are mechanically linked together.

In a grounded power distribution system, a short circuit between the hot conductor to ground creates a large current to flow from the hot conductor to ground. The spark and heat produced can create a fire. In an enriched oxygen environment, an explosion may occur if flammable gas is present. However, in an isolated power system, a short circuit to ground will not produce any significant current as none of the line conductors are connected to ground (no return path exists for the fault current). As a result, fire and explosion hazards due to ground faults are eliminated. Line isolation transformers were required by building codes in operating rooms to prevent explosion hazard when flammable anesthetic agents were used. Some jurisdictions have dropped these requirements as flammable anesthetic agents are no longer used in health care facilities.

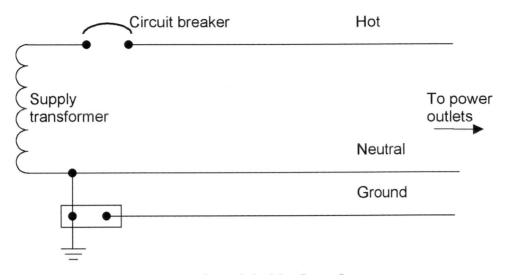

Figure 12–2. Grounded 3-Wire Power System.

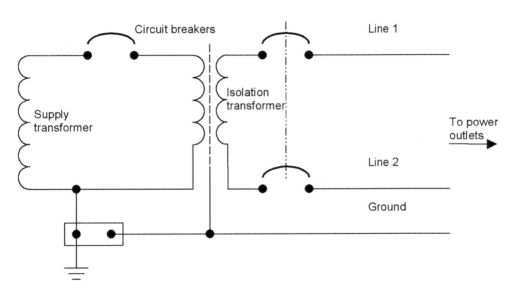

Figure 12–3. Isolated Power System.

Consider a ground fault (a hot conductor is connected to the grounded chassis) occurring on a medical device plugged into a grounded power system (Figure 12–4). If the ground conductor is intact, very little current will flow through the patient; all current will be diverted through the ground conductor to ground even when the patient is touching the chassis. The circuit breaker in the hot wire will detect this excessive current and disconnect (or

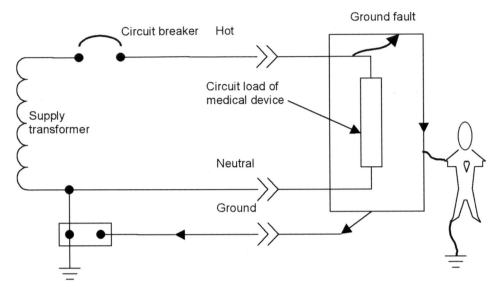

Figure 12–4. Ground Fault on 3-Wire Power System.

trip) the circuit. An intact ground connection is an effective first line of defense against electrical shock.

Example 4

Consider the situation in which the chassis of the medical device in Figure 12–4 is not solidly grounded, if the ground fault current creates a 20 V potential difference between the chassis of the medical device to ground, calculate the risk current when

   i) The patient is touching the chassis and also touching a grounded object.
   ii) The patient with a grounded heart catheter is touching the chassis.

Solution

   i) Assuming the resistance of the current path is 50 kΩ, the risk current is 20 V/50 kΩ = 0.4 mA. This current is harmless and is not even noticeable by the patient.
   ii) Assuming the resistance of the current path is 25 kΩ when one skin contact resistance is bypassed by the catheter, the risk current is 20 V/25 kΩ = 0.8 mA. The microshock current will trigger ventricular fibrillation in the patient.

Normally, the circuit breaker will disconnect the device from power in a fraction of a second to minimize patient injury. A grounded system with a protective circuit breaker or fuse is relatively safe to prevent electrical shock to the patient when a ground fault happens. However, a spark may jump between the hot and ground conductor at the fault location. Sparks may create a fire or an explosion under the right situation.

Example 5

The ground connection of a medical device has a resistance of 1.0 Ω. If the leakage current is 100 μA and a patient touching the grounded chassis has a resistance to ground = 25 kΩ, find the risk current flowing through the patient.

Solution

The patient resistance is parallel to the ground connection resistance, the current flowing through the patient resistance is $\left| \dfrac{100 \ \mu A \times 1 \ \Omega}{(25 \ k\Omega + 1 \ \Omega)} \right| = 4.0$ nA. When the ground is intact, only 4 nA of current flows through the patient; with a broken ground, the full leakage current (100 μA) will flow through the patient.

For an isolated power system, a single ground fault between the line conductors and ground will not produce a noticeable fault current as there is no conduction path to complete the electrical circuit. However, if the fault is a short circuit between one of the line conductors to the chassis of the medical device, the chassis will become hot and therefore create a potential shock hazard to the patient. A line isolation monitor (LIM) is used in an isolated power system to detect this fault condition. A LIM is a device that monitors the impedance of the line conductors to ground by periodically (several times per second) connecting each of the line conductors to ground and measuring the ground current (Figure 12–5). A LIM is usually set to sound an alarm when the ground current exceeds 5 mA. Some alarms can be set from 1 to 10 mA. A LIM can detect a ground fault in an isolated power system as well as deterioration of the insulation between line conductors and ground. However, it cannot detect a broken ground conductor nor can it eliminate microshock hazards.

Example 6

An isolated power system with a LIM set to sound an alarm at 5 mA is supplying power to a patient location. The patient has a grounded heart catheter

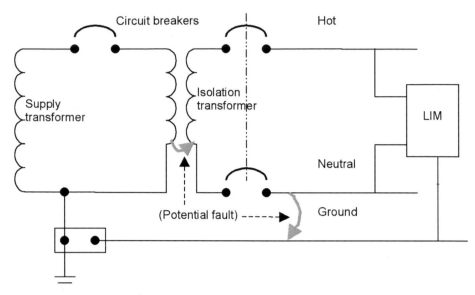

Figure 12–5. Isolated Power System with Line Isolation Transformer.

and is touching another medical device. If the leakage impedance due to capacitive coupling of the windings of the line isolation transformer is 25 kΩ and there is an insulation failure between a line conductor and the chassis of the medical device (line shorted to metal chassis), what is the risk current to the patient assuming the patient impedance is 30 kΩ resistive?

Solution

The current flowing through the patient is equal to the line voltage divided by the total impedance of the current path.

$$\text{The magnitude of the risk current} = \left| \frac{120 \text{ V}}{(30 \text{ k}\Omega - \text{j}25 \text{ k}\Omega)} \right| = 3.0 \text{ mA}.$$

The low level leakage current will not trigger the alarm of the LIM. However, this will be a fatal current if it is allowed to flow directly through the heart of the patient. In either case, the risk current would have been prevented to flow through the patient if the equipment enclosure is properly grounded.

SIGNAL ISOLATION

Example 6 shows that an isolated power system with a line isolation transformer is not sufficient to prevent microshock. In order to reduce microshock hazard, medical equipment with patient applied parts in contact with the heart or major blood vessels (F-type applied parts) are designed such that the applied parts are electrically isolated from the power ground. Isolation is achieved by using an isolation barrier with electrical impedance of over 10 MΩ (such that the leakage current is lower than 10 µA). Figure 12–6 shows the block diagram of such a signal isolated device. The components enclosed by the dotted line are electrically isolated from the power ground. Note that in order to achieve total isolation, the power supplies to the components before the signal isolation barrier will also need to be isolated. There are two different ground references in an isolated patient applied part medical device. The ground reference for the nonisolated part of the circuit are connected to the power ground, while the ground reference for the isolated components are connected to the ground reference of the isolated power supply. These two grounding references are not connected together and are differentiated by two different grounding symbols (Figure 12–6).

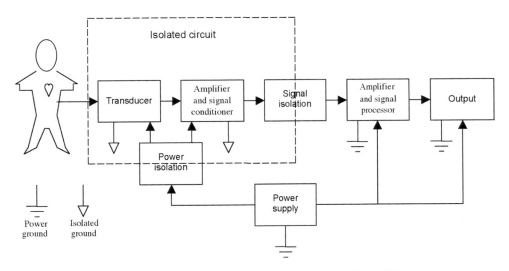

Figure 12–6. Block Diagram of Medical Device with Signal Isolation.

Signal isolation is achieved by an isolation barrier. Common isolation barriers used in medical instrumentation are isolation transformers or optical isolators (Figure 12–7). Isolation transformers used in signal isolation are much smaller in size than those used in power system isolation as they do not need to transform high power. Furthermore, they have much higher isolation impedances. Optical isolators break the electrical conduction path by using light to transmit the signal through an optical path. Figure 12–7a shows a simple optical isolator using a light-emitting diode (LED) and a phototransistor. The signal applied to the LED turns the LED on at high voltage level and off at low voltage level. The phototransistor is turned on and off according to the light coming from the LED. Since low-frequency signals often suffer from distortion when passing through isolation barriers, a physiological signal is first modulated with a high-frequency carrier (e.g., 50 kHz) before being sent through the isolation barrier. A demodulator removes the carrier and restores the signal to its original form on the other side of the isolation barrier. The signal at the output of the isolation circuit should be the same as the signal at the input.

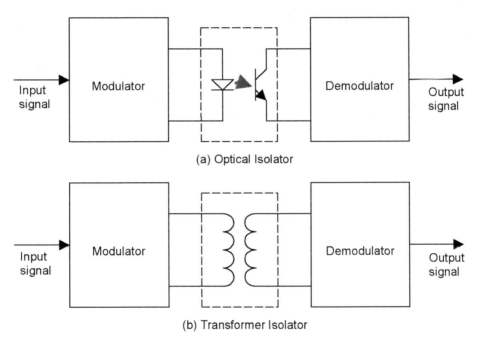

Figure 12–7. Optical and Transformer Signal Isolation.

OTHER METHODS TO REDUCE ELECTRICAL HAZARD

Equipotential Grounding

For a patient with the skin impedance bypassed, a tiny voltage can create a microshock hazard. For example, with a current path impedance of 2 kΩ, a voltage difference of 20 mV is sufficient to cause a 10 μA patient risk current. For this reason, it is desirable to protect electrically susceptible patients by keeping all exposed conductive surfaces and receptacle grounds in the patient's environment at the same potential. It is achieved by connecting all ground conductors (equipment cases, bed rail, water pipes, medical gas outlets, etc.) in the patient's immediate environment together and making common ground distribution points in close proximity to patients.

Ground Fault Circuit Interrupters

For an electrical device, the current flowing into the hot conductor should be equal to the current in the neutral conductor. When there is a current flowing from the hot conductor to ground, such as the existence of leakage current or a ground fault, the current in the hot conductor is different from that in the neutral conductor. A ground fault circuit interrupter (GFCI) senses the difference between these two currents and interrupts the power when this difference, which must be flowing to ground, exceeds a fixed value (e.g., 6 mA). Figure 12–8 shows the principle of a GFCI. Under normal conditions, there is no magnetic flux in the sensing coil as the hot and neutral current are equal. When there is a large enough hot to ground current, the

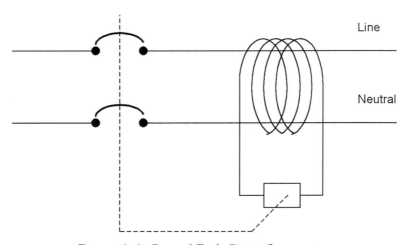

Figure 12–8. Ground Fault Circuit Interrupter.

net magnetic flux will trip the circuit breaker.

If a person is touching a hot conductor with one hand and a grounded object with the other, a risk current will flow from the hot conductor through the patient to ground. The GFCI detects the current difference in the hot and neutral conductors and interrupts the power before it becomes a problem. This protects the person from macroshock. GFCIs are commonly used in wet locations where water increases the electrical shock hazard. However, a GFCI is not used in critical patient care areas (OR, ICU, CCU) where life support equipment may be in use as it may be too sensitive to cause unnecessary power interruption.

Double Insulation

A device with double insulation has an additional protective layer of insulation to ensure that the outside casing has a very high value of resistance or impedance from ground. This separate layer of insulation prevents contact of any person with any exposed conductive surface. Usually the outside casing of the equipment is made of nonconductive material such as plastic. Any exposed metal parts are separated from the conductive main body by the addition of a protective, reinforcing layer of insulation. All switch levers and control shafts must also be double insulated (e.g., using plastic knobs). In order to be acceptable for medical equipment, the outer casing must be waterproof, that is, both layers of insulation should remain effective, even when there are spillages of conductive fluids. Double insulated equipment need not be grounded, so its supply cord does not have a ground pin.

Batteries and Extra-Low-Voltage Power Supply

The higher the power supply voltage, the higher the current that will flow through a person in an electrical accident. To reduce the voltage, one can use a step-down transformer or a low-voltage battery. In general, a voltage not exceeding 30 V_{rms} is considered as extra-low voltage. Such voltage is safe to touch for a healthy person. However, excessive heat from a direct short circuit (e.g., a battery short circuit), can create burn or explosion hazards. Battery-powered equipment is very common in health care settings because in addition to its lower electrical risk, it provides mobility to the equipment as well as the patient. A common type of equipment using a battery as the main source of power is the infusion pump.

Table 12–6 summarizes the effectiveness of different electrical safety protection measures discussed above toward microshock and macroshock.

Table 12–6.
Summary of Shock Prevention Methods

	Macroshock	*Microshock*
Proper Grounding	Yes	Yes
Double Insulation	Yes	Yes
Isolated Power System	Yes	No
Isolated Power with LIM	Yes	No
Isolated Patient Applied Parts	Yes	Yes
Equipotential Grounding	N/A	Yes
Ground Fault Circuit Interrupter	Yes	No
Battery Powered	Yes	Yes
Extra-Low Voltage (AC)	Yes	No

MEASUREMENT OF LEAKAGE CURRENT

It was mentioned earlier that the levels of electrical shock threshold current increase with increasing frequency. Figure 12–9 shows the approximate relationships between the threshold current and the power frequency. The higher the frequency, the higher the risk current to trigger physiological effects. To take into account the frequency-dependent characteristics of the human body's response to risk current, a measurement device to measure device leakage current is specified in the International Electrotechnical Commission standard (IEC601-1) on electrical safety testing of medical devices and systems. The measurement device consists of a passive network

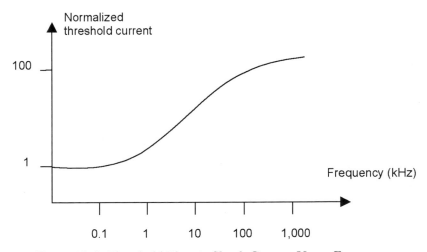

Figure 12–9. Threshold Electric Shock Current Versus Frequency.

with a true RMS millivoltmeter, which essentially simulates the impedance of the human body as well as the frequency-dependent characteristics of the body to risk current. Figure 12–10 shows the IEC601-1 leakage current mea-

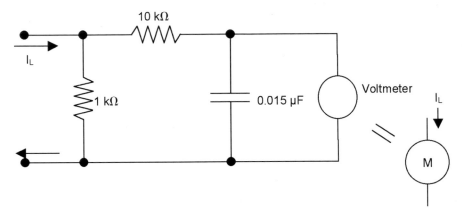

Figure 12–10. IEC601-1 Leakage Current Measurement Device.

surement device.

If the leakage current flowing into the measurement device is I_L, the current flowing through the capacitor I_1 is equal to

$$I_1 = I_L \left(\frac{1 \times 10^3}{1 \times 10^3 + 10 \times 10^3 + X_C} \right)$$

where $X_C = \dfrac{1}{j2\pi f \times 0.015 \times 10^{-6}}$ Ω.

The voltage across the capacitance as measured by the voltmeter is equal to

$$V_m = I_1 X_C = I_L \left(\frac{1 \times 10^3}{1 \times 10^3 + 10 \times 10^3 + X_C} \right) X_C = I_L \left(\frac{1 \times 10^3}{11 \times 10^3 + X_C} \right) X_C$$

For a direct current, $f = 0$ and $X_C = \infty$, therefore, $V_m = 10^3 \, I_L$.

From this relationship, if the voltmeter is measuring 1 mV, the leakage current is equal to 1 μA. Therefore, if the voltmeter is set to read in mV, the value displayed is the leakage current in μA.

For low-frequency current such as 60 Hz power frequency, $X_C = -j177 \times 10^3 \, \Omega$, therefore

$$V_m = \left| \frac{1 \times 10^3 \times (-j177) \times 10^3}{11 \times 10^3 + (-j177) \times 10^3} \right| I_L = \frac{10^3 \times 177}{177.3} I_L \approx 10^3 \, I_L$$

However, when *f* is very large, $X_C \rightarrow 0$, therefore,

$$V_m = I_L \left(\frac{1 \times 10^3}{11 \times 10^3 + X_C} \right) X_C = 0$$

This analysis illustrates that the IEC601-1 leakage current measurement device has an inverse characteristic to the threshold electrical shock response (Figure 12–9). Instead of having different threshold current levels for different leakage current frequencies (e.g., 10 μA at 60 Hz and 90 μA at 10 kHz), one can fix the threshold current limits and use the IEC601-1 measurement device to compensate for the frequency response (e.g., 10 μA maximum allowable leakage current for all frequencies). Figure 12–11 shows how the

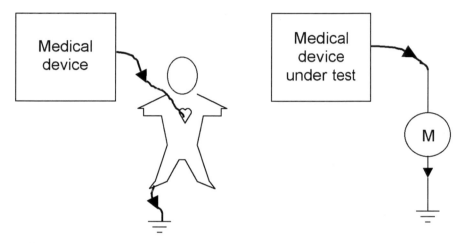

Figure 12–11. Use of IEC601-1 Measurement Device for Leakage Current.

measurement device is used to measure the patient leakage current flowing from the device through a patient applied parts to ground.

Interested readers should refer to the Standards (e.g., IEC60601) for the leakage current limits and the details of how and what to measure.

Chapter 13

MEDICAL WAVEFORM DISPLAY SYSTEMS

OBJECTIVES

- State the functions and characteristics of medical chart recorders and displays.
- Identify the basic building blocks of a paper chart recorder.
- Explain the construction of mechanical stylus and thermal dot array recorders.
- Explain the principles of operation of laser printers and ink-jet printers.
- Explain the terms *non-fade*, *waveform parade*, and *erase bar* in medical displays.
- Compare and explain the principles of different types of medical displays.
- Analyze the performance characteristics of medical display systems.

CHAPTER CONTENTS

1. Introduction
2. Paper Chart Recorders
3. Visual Display Monitors
4. Performance Characteristics of Display Systems

INTRODUCTION

For a medical device, the output device is the interface between the device and its users. Some common output devices found in medical equipment are listed in Table 1–3 of Chapter 1. They include paper records, audible alarms, visual displays, et cetera. A video monitor that displays a medical waveform such as an electrocardiogram is a typical medical output device. The principles of paper chart recorders and video display monitors are discussed in this chapter.

PAPER CHART RECORDERS

The function of a paper chart recorder in a medical device system is to produce records of physiological waveforms and parameters. These records can be used:

- as a snapshot of the patient's physiological condition for future reference, or
- to record an alarm condition so that it can be reviewed later by a medical professional.

Charts are often considered as medical records and therefore are required to be stored for a long period of time (e.g., 7 years for an adult patient in Canada). A paper chart recorder may use ink (e.g., ink stylus, ink-jet) or heat (e.g., thermal stylus, thermal dot array) to produce the waveform on a piece of paper. In an ink recorder, ink from an ink reservoir is supplied to a writing mechanism to produce the waveform on a piece of paper. Recorders using thermal styli or thermal dot array print heads require the use of heat-sensitive or thermal papers. Unlike ordinary paper, thermal paper is coated with a special chemical that turns dark when heat is applied. Thermal paper is more expensive than ordinary paper. However, the design and maintenance of thermal writers are simpler than those of ink writers.

Paper chart recorders can be divided into two categories: continuous paper feed recorders and single page recorders. Thermal dot array print heads are commonly used in continuous paper feed recorders. Lasers printers are in general the recorder of choice for single page recorders. Examples of paper chart recorders are listed in Table 13–1.

Table 13–1.
Paper Chart Recorders.

Continuous Paper Feed	Mechanical stylus recorder; thermal dot array recorder
Single Page Feed	Ink-jet printer; laser printer

Continuous Paper Feed Recorders

A continuous feed paper recorder draws paper from a paper roll or a stack of fanfolded paper. It can continuously record a waveform for an extended period of time. Two types of continuous paper feed chart recorders are found in medical devices: the mechanical stylus recorders and the thermal dot array recorders.

Mechanical Stylus Recorders

A mechanical stylus recorder consists of an electromechanical transducer to convert the analog electrical signal (e.g., amplified biopotential signal) to a mechanical motion. This motion is mechanically linked to a writing device such as an ink pen or a thermal stylus. The writing device leaves a trace on the chart paper as it moves across the paper. The paper is fed from a paper chart assembly that includes a paper supply mechanism and a writing table. The paper supply is driven by a motorized paper driving mechanism. Figure 13–1 shows a paper chart recorder setup using a galvanometer as the electromechanical transducer. A servomotor drive can replace the galvanometer to drive the mechanical stylus.

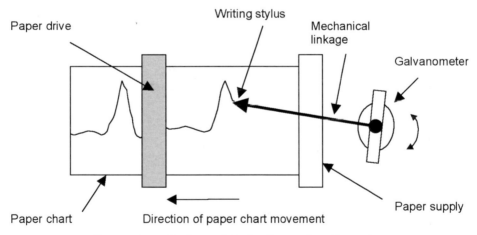

Figure 13–1. Mechanical Stylus Paper chart Recorder.

Thermal Dot Array Recorders

In a thermal dot array recorder, the electromechanical transducer is replaced by a thermal dot array printhead. The printhead of a thermal dot array recorder consists of a row of heater elements placed on top of the moving thermal paper as shown in Figure 13–2. Each of these heater elements can be independently activated to leave a black dot on the heat-sensitive paper. The analog electrical signal is first converted to a digital signal and then processed to heat the appropriate dots in the printhead. The paper supply and drive assembly is similar to that of the mechanical stylus recorder. Movement of the paper in conjunction with the appropriate addressing of the thermal elements on the printhead produces the image on the paper. As there are only a finite number of thermal elements on the printhead, the trace recorded on the paper is not continuous like the trace produced by a mechanical stylus writer. The vertical resolution of the recorder is limited by the number of thermal elements in the printhead. Paper chart recorders used in physiological monitors usually have resolution better than 200 dots per inch (dpi). Table 13–2 lists the major functional components of the mechanical stylus recorder and the thermal dot array recorder.

Mechanical stylus chart recorders are being replaced by thermal dot array recorders in medical devices as they have fewer mechanical moving parts. Mechanical stylus recorders require a higher level of maintenance due to wear and tear and misalignment problems.

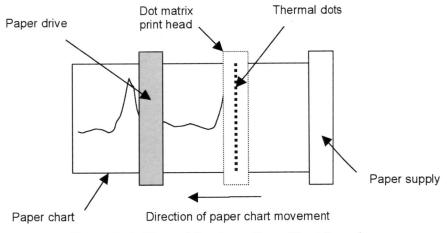

Figure 13–2. Thermal Dot Array Paper Chart Recorder.

Single Page Feed Recorders

Single page feed recorders use standard size paper (such as 8.5" by 11" paper) and therefore can record only a finite duration of the waveform on a single sheet of paper. Off-the-shelf laser printers or ink-jet printers are commonly used. Figure 13–3 shows the construction of a laser printer.

Table 13–2.
Main Building Blocks of Continuous Paper Feed Chart Recorders.

Mechanical Stylus Recorder	*Thermal Dot Array (Dot Matrix) Recorders*
An electromechanical device (galvanometric or servomotor drive) to convert electrical input signal to mechanical movement.	The analog electrical signal is converted to digital signal via an A/D converter.
An arm to transmit the mechanical movement to the stylus.	The digital signal is being processed to heat the appropriate dots in the dot matrix printhead.
A stylus to leave a record of the signal on the chart paper as it moves across the paper. It can be an ink stylus or a thermal stylus.	The activated dot in the print head will leave a black dot on the heat-sensitive paper.
A chart paper assembly consisting of a paper supply mechanism and a paper writing table.	
A paper drive mechanism to move the chart paper across the table.	

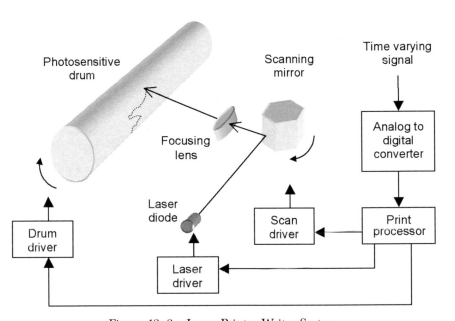

Figure 13–3a. Laser Printer Writer System.

Laser Printers

For a laser printer, the time varying signal such as an ECG is first converted to digital signal by an analog to digital converter. A photosensitive drum in the printer rotates at a constant speed. The speed of rotation of the drum determines the paper speed of the chart. The rotational motion of the scanning mirror reflects the laser beam to move across the surface of the

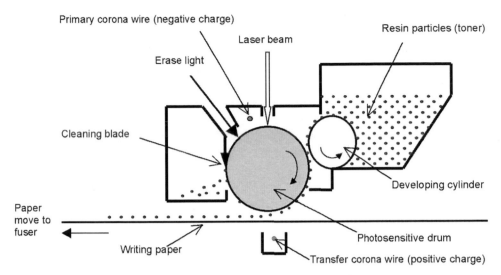

Figure 13–3b. Laser Printer Printing System.

drum (Figure 13–3a). The laser diode is switched on and off by the print processor according to the ECG signal and the position of the scanning mirror. The section of the rotating photosensitive drum acquires a negative charge when it passes by the primary corona wire (Figure 13–3b). When the laser beam reflected by the scanning mirror strikes the spots on the drum where dots are to be printed, the spots on the surface of the negatively charged drum become electrically neutral. As the drum rotates, new rows of neutral spots form in response to the laser pulses.

The surface of the developing cylinder contains a weak magnet field. As the developing cylinder rotates, it attracts a coating of dark resin particles (toner) that contain bits of negatively charged ferrite. As the resin particles on the developing cylinder move closer to the photosensitive drum, these particles, due to their negative charge, are repelled by the negative charged area on the drum and moved to the neutral spots that were created earlier by the laser beam.

As the resin particles on the drum move toward the paper, they are being attracted to the paper by the positive charge on the paper created by the transfer corona wire. The image on the drum is therefore transferred onto the paper.

As the drum continues to rotate, a cleaning blade removes all residue resin particles on the drum surface and an erase lamp introduces a fresh negative charge uniformly on the entire surface of the drum. This prepares the drum to receive the next part of the page information.

To fix the image on the paper, the resin particles are heat-fused onto the paper and the charge on the paper is neutralized by passing the paper over a grounded wire brush. Laser printers have resolution of 600 dpi or higher.

Ink-Jet Printers

An ink-jet printer has a printhead with multiple print elements as shown in Figure 13–4a. Each element consists of a tiny aperture with a heat transducer behind it. When activated, the heater boils the ink and forms a vapor bubble behind the aperture. The vapor pressure forces a minute drop of ink out toward the printing surface to create a single image dot.

The printhead is coupled to an ink reservoir to form the print cartridge. The print cartridge is driven by a servomotor to move back and forth across the paper. Together with the translational motion of the paper, a time varying waveform can be recorded on the paper (Figure 13–4b). Instead of using heat to create the ink-jet, some printers use the mechanical vibration force created by a piezoelectric crystal to eject the ink onto the paper.

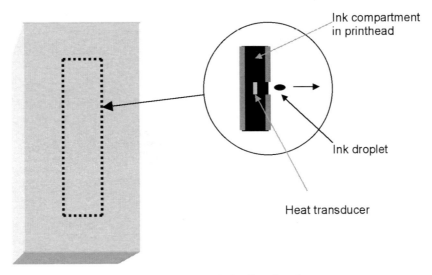

Figure 13–4a. Ink-Jet Printhead.

VISUAL DISPLAY MONITORS

In a physiological monitoring system, a visual display monitor provides real-time visual information for the medical professional to assess the condition of the patient. Some common monitors used in medical applications are:

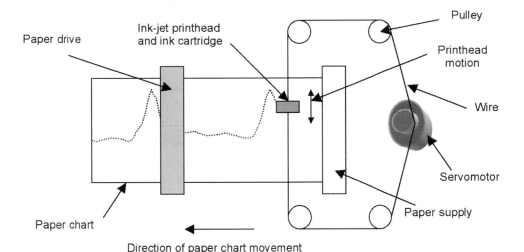

Figure 13–4b. Ink-Jet Paper Chart Recorder.

- Cathode ray tube (CRT)
- Liquid crystal display (LCD)
- Plasma display
- Electroluminescent display

Cathode Ray Tube Displays

The cathode ray tube has been used for a long time as an efficient and reliable visual display monitor for medical devices. Figure 13–5a shows the main components of a CRT. It is also called an oscilloscope.

The electron gun provides a continuous supply of electrons by heating the cathode filament (thermal ionic effect). These electrons are attracted and accelerated toward the screen due to the high voltage (several kV) applied across the anode and cathode. When the high-velocity electron beam hits the phosphor screen, it emits visible light photons at the location of impact. To deflect the beam to a desired location on the screen, a voltage is applied across two pairs of deflection plates located above, below, and on each side of the electron beam. In normal time-base operations, a saw-tooth waveform voltage is applied across the horizontal deflection plates. If no signal is applied across the vertical deflection plates, this saw-tooth voltage moves the electron beam horizontally back and forth across the tube. When the time varying waveform to be displayed is amplified and applied across the vertical deflection plates, it causes the electron beam to move in the vertical direction according to the voltage level of the signal. When the signal frequency

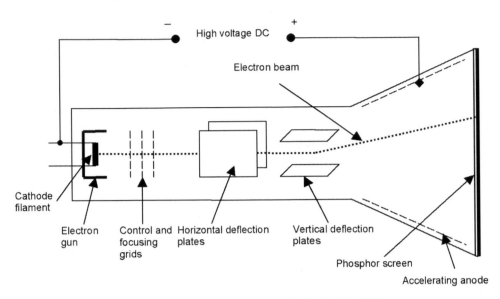

Figure 13–5a. Basic Structure of Cathode Ray Tube.

is a multiple of the frequency of the saw tooth waveform, a steady waveform of the signal is displayed on the screen of the CRT (Figure 13–5b).

Adjusting the frequency of the saw-tooth waveform so that a steady signal is displayed on the CRT screen is called triggering. Automatic triggering is done by feeding the signal to be displayed to a frequency detector and using this frequency to generate the frequency of the saw-tooth horizontal

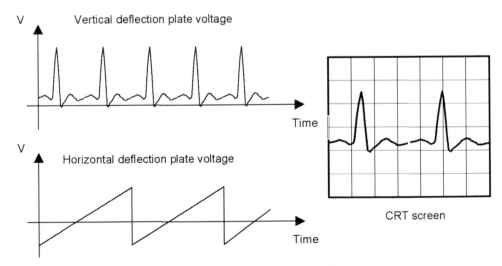

Figure 13–5b. Cathode Ray Tube Display.

deflection signal. The amplitude of the signal displayed on the screen can be adjusted by changing the amplification factor (sensitivity control) of the amplifier feeding the vertical deflection plates.

In order to control the brightness of the display and the convergence of the electron beam to a small dot when it reaches the phosphor screen, control voltages are applied to a set of control and focusing grids in front of the electron gun. Instead of using electrostatic deflection plates, some oscilloscopes use electromagnetic coils to provide horizontal and vertical deflections to the electron beam.

For a fast-moving repetitive waveform, the persistence of the phosphor and the response time of the human eye will make a triggered waveform appear to be continuous and stationary on the screen. For nonperiodic waveforms, as each sweep (one cycle of the saw-tooth waveform) produces a different trace of waveform on the screen, no stationary waveform will be seen. For slow time varying signals, since the phosphor can scintillate only for a fraction of a second, the trace will appear as a dot moving up and down across the screen (this is why old physiological monitors were referred to as bouncing ball oscilloscopes). To produce a steady display even from nonperiodic and slow varying signals, a storage oscilloscope is required. Figure 13–6 shows the block diagram of a storage oscilloscope. Instead of sending the signal to be displayed directly to the vertical deflection plates, the signal is first converted to digital format by an analog to digital converter (ADC) and stored in the memory. This slow varying signal is then reconstructed and swept across the screen many times faster than its original frequency so that it can be seen as a solid trace on the screen. This category of display is called non-fade displays.

There are two types of non-fade displays: one is "waveform parade" and the other is "erase bar." In a waveform parade non-fade display, the wave-

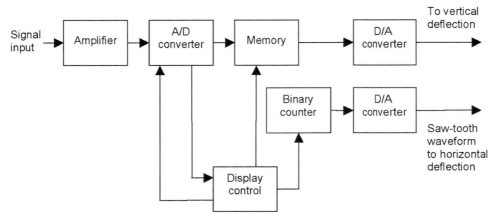

Figure 13–6. Storage Oscilloscope.

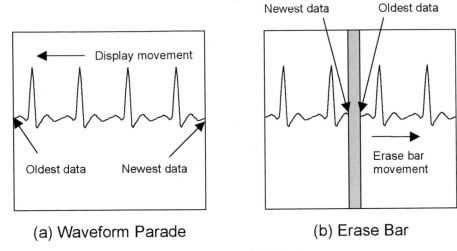

(a) Waveform Parade   (b) Erase Bar

Figure 13–7. Non-fade Display.

form appears to be moving across the screen with the newest data coming out from the right-hand side of the screen and the oldest data disappearing into the left-hand side (Figure 13–7a). In an "erase bar" non-fade display, the data appear to be stationary. A cursor (or a line) sweeps across the screen from left to right (Figure 13–7b). The newest data emerges from the left-hand side of the cursor while the oldest data are erased as the cursor moves over them. When the cursor has reached the right edge of the screen, it disappears and then reappears from the left edge of the screen.

CRT displays are bright, have good contrast ratio (ratio of output light intensity between total bright and dark), high resolution, and high refreshing rate. However, they are heavy, bulky, and may have uneven resolution across the screen.

Liquid Crystal Displays

Liquid crystal displays (LCDs) have gained popularity to replace CRTs as the display of choice for medical devices in recent years. LCDs are lightweight, compact, and robust compared to CRTs. LCDs operate under the principle of light polarization. A typical liquid crystal cell is shown in Figure 13–8. Liquid crystal, which has the ability to rotate polarized light, is sandwiched between two transparent electrodes and two polarizers with axes aligned in the same direction to each other. The light from a light source at the back of the cell is polarized by the first polarizer before it passes through the liquid crystal and then to the other polarizer. When no voltage is applied across the electrodes, the axis of the polarized light is rotated (or twisted) 90°

by the liquid crystals. As the axis of the analyzing polarizer is in line with that of the polarizing polarizer, the polarized light is blocked and therefore no light will exit from the other end. When a voltage (about 5 to 20 V) is applied across the electrodes, the twisting effect of the liquid crystal disappears. Since the axis of the polarized light is in line with the axis of the analyzing polarizer, the polarized light can exit through the other end with little attenuation. By switching the voltage across the electrodes, the liquid crystal cell can be turned on (bright) or off (dark). This is called a twisted nematic (TN) LCD.

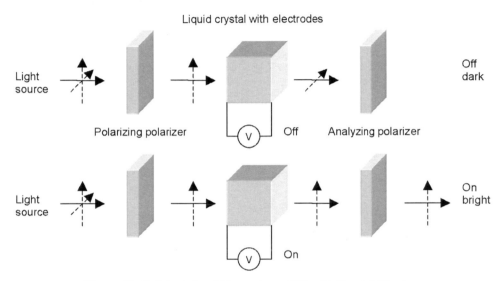

Figure 13–8. Principle of Operation of Liquid Crystal Display.

To illustrate the operation of a two-dimensional display, a 5 pixel × 5 pixel LCD panel with column electrodes and a polarizer on one side plus row electrodes and a polarizer on the other side of the LCD crystal is shown in Figure 13–9. Each of the 25 pixels sandwiched between the horizontal and vertical addressing electrodes can be turned on and off by applying appropriate voltages to the rows and column electrodes. For example, if we want to turn on the pixel B-3, the column electrode B will be connected to a positive voltage and the row electrode 3 will be connected to a negative voltage. To display a time varying signal, a display driver converts the input signal to be displayed into column and row addressing sequences to turn the pixels on and off.

The brightness of a pixel is controlled by adjusting the "on" time or the applied voltage across the liquid crystal. The longer the duty cycle of the

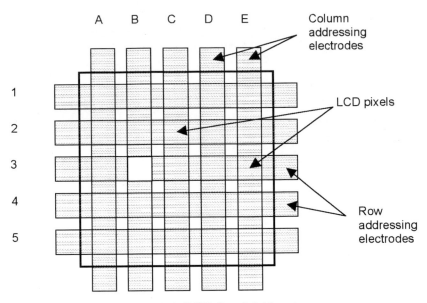

Figure 13–9. LCD Panel Addressing.

applied voltage, the brighter the pixel appears to be. To add color to the display, primary color filters (red, green, and blue) are overlaid on top of the pixel elements. Multiple colors are created by combining different intensities of these primary colors. As it requires three pixels to form one color pixel, a color LCD display will require three times as much pixel to achieve the same resolution as a monochromatic monitor. A 640 × 480 color LCD panel requires 920,000 LCD pixel elements.

For this type of LCD display, the addressing frequency and hence the screen refreshing rate is limited by the capacitance formed by the addressing electrodes and the LCD crystal (two conductors separated by an insulator). Earlier LCD panels using passive addressing electrodes suffered from slow refreshing rate and often showed a "tail" following a fast-moving object. Employing thin film transistors (TFT) to form an active matrix (AM) has substantially increased the screen refreshing rate in modern LCD displays. However, since each pixel element requires one TFT, AMLCD panels are more expensive than passive LCD panels. Figure 13–10 shows the schematic diagram of a single pixel element of an AMLCD. For a 640 × 480 color display, 920,000 TFT are required to be fabricated on a single substrate.

A LCD does not emit light photons. An external light source is therefore required to display images on a LCD. A back-lit LCD has a light source located at the back of the LCD (Figure 13–8). A reflective LCD uses a mirror at the back to reflect light coming from the front, such as daylight or ambient light. Other than its slower screen refreshing rate, a LCD has lower

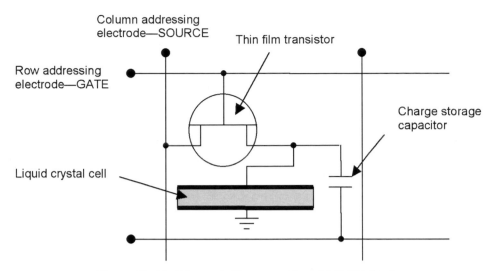

Figure 13–10. Schematic Diagram of an AMLCD Pixel.

contrast ratio and narrower viewing angle (brightness of the LCD is lower when viewing from the sides and above or below the display) than a CRT.

Plasma Panel Displays

Plasma panels used in low-resolution and alphanumeric displays are established technology and have been proven to be rugged and reliable. In recent years, high-resolution large flat panel plasma displays are used in consumer products such as televisions as well as medical applications. Plasma is a gas made up of free-flowing ions and electrons. When an electrical current is running through plasma, it creates a rapid flow of charged particles colliding with each other. These collisions excite the gas atoms, causing them to release energy in the form of photons. In xenon-neon plasma, most of these photons are in the ultraviolet region, which is invisible to the human eye. However, these ultraviolet photons can interact with a phosphor material to produce visible light.

The cross-sectional view of a plasma display cell is shown in Figure 13–11. The cell is sandwiched between two glass plates. The addressing electrodes are surrounded by a dielectric insulating material covered by a magnesium oxide protective layer. The plasma is trapped in an enclosure coated with phosphor.

In a plasma flat panel display, each pixel is made up of three separate plasma cells or sub-pixels with phosphors chosen to produce red, green, and blue light. Different colors can be produced by combining different intensities of these primary colors by varying the current pulses flowing through each of the three sub-pixels. Similar to a LCD, row and column addressing electrodes are used to produce the image. Plasma panels are less bulky than a CRT, and they have a higher contrast ratio and higher response rate than a LCD. However, they require higher driving voltage than a LCD (150–200 V).

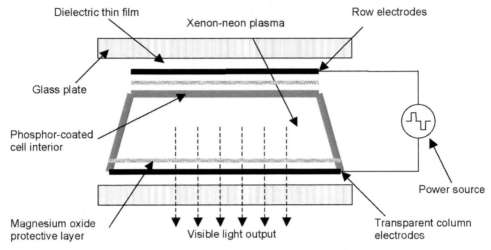

Figure 13–11. Basic Construction of a Plasma Display Cell.

Electroluminescent Displays

Electroluminescent (EL) displays contain a substance (such as doped zinc sulfide) that produces visible light when an electric field is applied across it. Figure 13–12 shows an electroluminescent panel with the electroluminescent material between rows and columns of addressing electrodes. Electroluminescent displays are thin and compact, with high response rate, and acceptable brightness. However, they are not as popular than LCD in medical applications as they require relatively high driving voltage (170–200 V) and have lower power efficiency.

Table 13–3 shows a general comparison of the three common display technologies.

PERFORMANCE CHARACTERISTICS OF DISPLAY SYSTEMS

The output of a display system is often used in diagnosis or to monitor the condition of a patient during medical treatment. The accuracy of the dis-

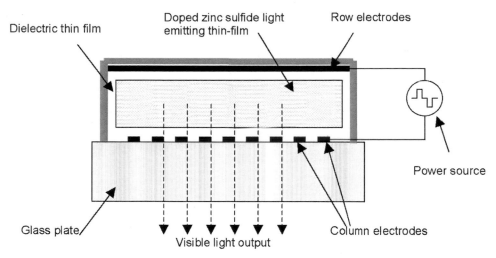

Figure 13–12. Basic Construction of Electroluminescent Display.

Table 13–3.
Comparison Chart on Display Technologies

	CRT	*LCD*	*Plasma*	*EL*
BRIGHTNESS	High	Need light source	High	High
CONTRAST RATIO	High	Low	High	High
READABILITY UNDER BRIGHT DAYLIGHT	Washout	Yes	Washout	Washout
RESOLUTION	Good	Good but expensive	Good but expensive	Good but expensive
VIEWING ANGLE	Wide	Narrow	Wide	Wide
REFRESHING RATE	High	Low	High	High
WEIGHT	Heavy	Light	Medium	Medium
SIZE	Bulky	Thin	Thin	Thin
DRIVING VOLTAGE	High	Low	Medium	Medium
COST	Low	High (for AMLCD)	High	High

play can therefore affect the medical outcome. This section studies the performance characteristics of the paper chart recorders and the video display monitors discussed earlier in this chapter. Most of the medical device performance characteristics and parameters discussed in Chapter 2 apply to the display systems. Some of them are discussed below.

Sensitivity

The function of a paper chart recorder as well as a video display monitor is to convert the electrical input signal (usually a voltage signal) to a vertical deflection (distance). The sensitivity therefore is usually measured in distance per unit voltage. For example, the vertical sensitivity of an electrocardiograph (ECG) may be 5 mm/mV, 10 mm/mV, or 20 mm/mV. Many medical devices with an output display have an internal calibration signal to enable users to quickly verify the accuracy of the sensitivity. An example is the 1 mV internal calibration square pulse of an electrocardiograph. When invoked, the size of the square pulse will be shown according to the sensitivity setting. For example, when set at 10 mm/mV, a square pulse with 10 mm amplitude will be recorded or displayed. An external calibration signal can also be applied to the input to verify the accuracy of the display.

Paper/Sweep Speed

A physiological signal is often a time varying signal. The distance on the horizontal axis of the display represents the elapsed time of the signal. For an ECG monitor, a common paper speed of the recorder and sweep speed of the monitor is 25 mm/sec. To check the accuracy of the paper speed or sweep speed, a repetitive signal of known frequency is applied to the input of the display device. The horizontal distance of one cycle of the output signal is measured. The sweep speed of the display is equal to this distance divided by the period of the applied signal.

Resolution

Resolution of a display is a measure of the smallest distinguishable dimension of an image on the display. For a paper chart recorder using a thermal dot array, the resolution may be 8 dots/mm in the vertical direction and 32 dots in the horizontal direction. For a video monitor, the resolution may be expressed as 1,280 × 800 pixels. If the dimensions of this monitor are 40 cm × 22.5 cm, the display resolution is 32 pixels/cm horizontally and 20 pixels/cm vertically.

Frequency Response

Like any transducers and functional components, a display of a medical device has limited bandwidth. A typical frequency response of a display system is shown in Figure 13–13. An ideal display system should have a transfer function with the lower cutoff frequency (f_L) lower than that of the signal that is going to be displayed and an upper cutoff frequency (f_U) higher than that of the signal. The regions of the transfer function between the upper and lower cutoff frequency should be constant or flat.

Example 1

An electrocardiogram is shown. If the sensitivity and paper speed settings are 10 mm/mV and 25 mm/sec, respectively, find the amplitude of the ECG signal and the patient's heart rate. (Note: One small square on the chart equals 1 mm).

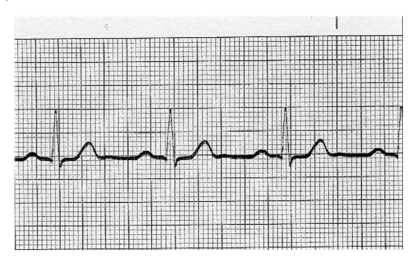

Solution

The amplitude of the R wave is 10 mm. As the sensitivity setting is 10 mm/mV, the input ECG signal amplitude is 1 mV.

The distance between two QRS complexes is 25 mm (one cycle). With a paper speed of 25 mm/sec, this represents a period of 1 second. Therefore, the heart rate is 60 beats per minute.

The frequency response transfer function of the display system can be obtained by inputting a sinusoidal signal of known amplitude and frequency and measuring the amplitude of the output. By changing the input frequency and repeating the measurement, the frequency response transfer function can be plotted. Using this method to obtain the lower cutoff frequencies of a low-frequency signal such as an electrocardiograph ($f_L = 0.01$ Hz) can be difficult and time-consuming. In practice, the lower cutoff frequency of the display (or any system) can quickly be estimated by assuming that the display

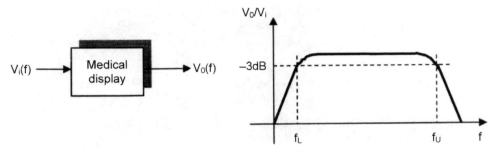

Figure 13–13. Frequency Response of a Medical Display System.

behaves like a first-order high pass filter. To find the cutoff frequency of the high pass RC filter as shown in Figure 13–14, a step function is applied to the input to produce the step response from the output. From the step response, f_L can be obtained from the equation:

$$f_L = \frac{1}{2\pi RC}$$

where the exponential decay time constant RC can be obtained by using the equation:

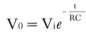

$$V_0 = V_i e^{-\frac{t}{RC}}$$

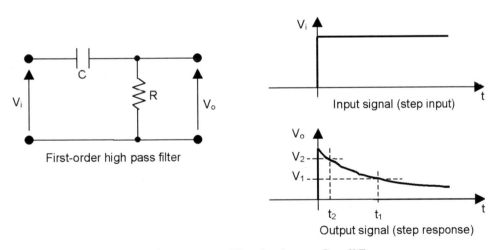

First-order high pass filter

Input signal (step input)

Output signal (step response)

Figure 13–14. Estimation of Display Lower Cutoff Frequency.

Example 2

Find the lower cutoff frequency of a paper chart recorder if the step response is as shown in Figure 13–14.

Solution

Using the exponential decay equation $V_0 = V_i e^{-\frac{t}{RC}}$, at time t_1 and t_2,

$V_1 = V_i e^{-\frac{t_1}{RC}}$, and $V_2 = V_i e^{-\frac{t_2}{RC}}$, dividing the first equation by the second gives

$\dfrac{V_2}{V} = e^{-\frac{(t_2 - t_1)}{RC}} \Rightarrow RC = \dfrac{t_1 - t_2}{\ln \dfrac{V_2}{V_1}}$. But $f_L = \dfrac{1}{2\pi RC}$, so the lower cutoff frequency

of the chart recorder can be calculated by looking up the voltage V_1 and V_2 at time t_1 and t_2 from step response.

Alternatively, if we pick t_2 as the start of the step input and t_1 is the time when the step response dropped to 50% of the initial value, from the above-derived equation

$RC = \dfrac{t_1 - t_2}{\ln \dfrac{V_2}{V_1}}, f_L = \dfrac{1}{2\pi RC} \Rightarrow f_L = \dfrac{1}{2\pi} \dfrac{\ln \dfrac{V_2}{V_1}}{t_1 - t_2} = \dfrac{1}{2\pi} \dfrac{\ln 2}{t_1} = \dfrac{0.11}{t_1}$, where

t_1 is the time elapsed when the output decreases to 50% of the initial value.

Example 3

The following chart paper recording was made by an electrocardiograph in response to a step input. Estimate the lower cutoff frequency f_L of the unit if the paper speed is 25 mm/s. The vertical axis of the chart is 1 mV/div. and the horizontal axis is 5 mm/div.

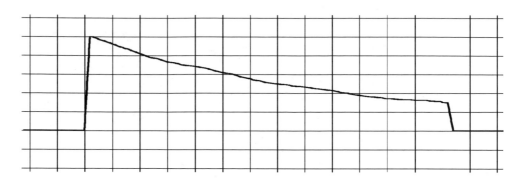

Solution

The 50% amplitude of the output is seven divisions from the beginning of the step input. Assuming the response is a first-order high pass filter. Using the equation

$f_L = \dfrac{0.11}{t_1}$ derived above, $t_1 = \dfrac{7 \times 5 \text{ mm}}{25 \text{ mm/s}} = 1.4 \text{ s}$

Therefore, $f_L = \dfrac{0.11}{t_1} = \dfrac{0.11}{1.4} = 0.079 \text{ Hz}$

Chapter 14

PHYSIOLOGICAL MONITORING SYSTEMS

OBJECTIVES

- State the functions of a physiological monitor.
- Sketch the functional block diagram of a typical multiparameter patient monitor.
- List the common physiological parameters being monitored.
- Identify the common features of a bedside, ambulatory, and central monitor.
- Explain the advantages and shortcomings of a telemetry patient monitoring system.
- Explain the two algorithms of ECG arrhythmia detection.
- List the desirable characteristics of a patient monitoring network.
- Differentiate ring, bus, and star network topologies.
- Differentiate host-terminal, client-server, and peer-to-peer networks.
- Describe the characteristics of Ethernet and Token Ring network protocols.
- State the characteristics of different types of network connections.
- List the functions of a network interface card, repeater, bridge, and router.

CHAPTER CONTENTS

INTRODUCTION

Since the early 1960s, it has been recognized that some patients with myocardial infarction or those suffering from serious illnesses or recovering from major surgery benefit from treatment in a specialized intensive care unit (ICU). In such units, cardiac patients thought to be susceptible to life-threatening arrhythmia could have their cardiovascular function continuously monitored and interpreted by specially trained clinicians.

Technological advances led to the ability to monitor other physiological parameters. Temperature transducers such as thermistors made it possible to continuously record patient temperature. Through impedance plethysmography, respiration could be monitored using ECG electrodes. The development of accurate, sensitive pressure transducers gave clinicians the ability to continuously monitor venous and arterial blood pressures; improved catheters made it possible to monitor intracardiac pressures and provide relatively easy and safe methods of measuring cardiac output. Noninvasive means were developed to monitor parameters such as oxygen saturation level in blood.

As clinical knowledge continues to advance and become more sophisticated, special cardiac care units (CCUs) evolved to centralize cardiovascular monitoring. When patients in danger of cardiac arrest are grouped together with trained staff, resuscitation equipment, vigilance, and combined with prompt responses to cardiac emergencies, lives can be saved. The concept of intensive specialized care assisted by continuous electronic monitoring of physiological parameters has been applied to specialties other than cardiology, resulting in the formation of other special care units such as pulmonary ICUs, neonatal ICUs, trauma ICUs, and burn units.

FUNCTIONS OF PHYSIOLOGICAL MONITORS

Patient monitors continuously or at prescribed intervals measure physiological parameters and store them for later review, and thus can free up some clinicians' time from performing other tasks. In addition, monitors with built-in diagnostic capabilities can alert clinicians when abnormalities such as tachycardia (abnormally high heart rate) occur. Most physiological monitors carry out the following basic functions:

- **Sense**–pick up and transform the physiological signal into a more machine friendly format (e.g., a pressure transducer to convert blood pressure waveform to an electrical signal)
- **Condition**–amplify, filter, level shift, etc.
- **Analyze**–make measurements and interpretations of the signal (e.g., extract heart rates from ECG waveform)
- **Display**–show the output in visual (e.g., waveforms, numerical values) or audio formats
- **Alarm**–provide visual and audio warning when some limits are exceeded
- **Record**–store information on paper or electronic media

In a modern patient care ward such as an ICU, several physiological parameters of a patient are usually being monitored. Instead of having multiple single-parameter monitors clustered around a patient, a multiparameter monitor is used. A multiparameter monitor has the capability to capture several physiological parameters simultaneously. In addition to saving space, a multiparameter monitor is more economical as the modalities may share some common fundamental components. Figure 14-1 shows a three-parameter monitor capable of measuring ECG, blood pressure, and temperature.

Each of the three modules captures (senses and conditions) a physiological signal from the patient. As the modules are sharing the remainder of the

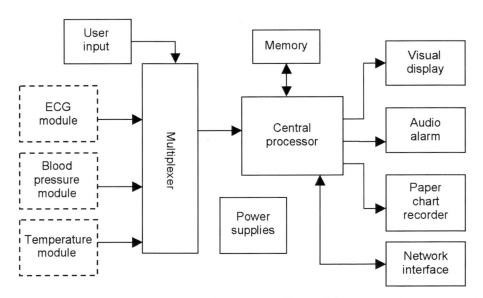

Figure 14–1. A multiparameter Patient Monitor.

device components, the signals from the modules are multiplexed and sent to the central processor. The processor analyzes the signals and extracts necessary information from them (such as heart rate from the ECG, systolic and diastolic values from the blood pressure waveform). Such information is then compared with preset parameters to trigger audio or visual alarms. The physiological waveforms as well as numerical information are displayed in the video monitor and hard copies are created by the paper chart recorder. The monitor may also be connected to a central monitor or to the hospital information system through a computer network.

METHODS OF MONITORING

The simplest form of patient monitoring is shown in Figure 14–2a, where the patient's physiological parameters are displayed at bedside only. This assumes either a one-to-one nurse–patient ratio or a physical grouping of patients that permits viewing of the monitor by the nursing staff. Since alarms must be at the bedside in this type of system, nursing response must be immediate to prevent unnecessary psychological stress accompanying an alarm.

The need for patient privacy in the confines of a single room and the need to economize on nursing staff led to the use of both bedside and a remote monitoring station (commonly refers to central monitoring station). Extending the patient–nurse ratio from 1:1 to 2:1 or even 3:1 permits a more economical approach of surveillance (Figure 14–2b). Under such an arrangement, it is also possible to remove alarms from the patient's range of hearing. Furthermore, the central monitoring and physical layout allows nurses to maintain visual contact with patients and displayed parameters while still able to engage in other nursing duties in the work area.

The grouping of monitors permits the economical addition of components that can be selectively applied to any bed. For example, through suitable grouping, a single chart recorder to provide hard copy rhythm strips can be configured to serve multiple (e.g., four to six) patient beds. Such a central recorder can be programmed to print either on demand by the user or automatically in the event of an alarm.

MONITORED PARAMETERS

Some examples of physiological parameters being monitored are:
• Electrocardiograph–heart rate, arrhythmia, ST segment level

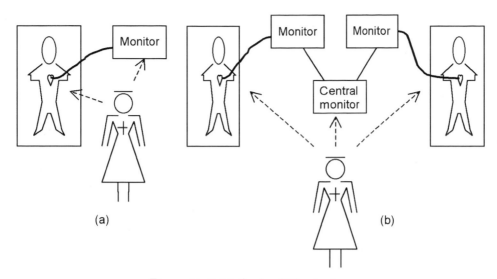

Figure 14-2. Methods of Monitoring.

* Hemodynamics–systolic, diastolic, and mean blood pressure; cardiac output
* Respiration
* Temperature
* End-tidal carbon dioxide level (EtCO$_2$)
* Percentage oxygen saturation (%SaO$_2$)
* Blood gas (PO$_2$, PCO$_2$)

While surface ECG, noninvasive blood pressure, and S$_p$O$_2$ are basic parameters being monitored in most specialty areas, additional monitoring needs are required in different areas of care. For example, end tidal carbon dioxide (EtCO$_2$) and bispectral index (level of consciousness) monitoring on patients under general anesthesia are often required in the operating room.

CHARACTERISTICS OF PATIENT MONITORING SYSTEMS

The purpose of a patient monitoring system is to monitor vital physiological parameters so that clinicians can be alerted to adverse changes in the patient's condition and provide appropriate interventions. A typical system often consists of a number of bedside monitors, a few ambulatory monitors, a central station, and sometimes a telemetry system. In a modern patient monitoring systems, all of the above are connected via a patient monitoring network.

Bedside Monitors

A bedside monitor is positioned beside the patient bed location to acquire physiological signals from the patient. The monitor is either mounted on the wall or placed on a shelf beside the patient's bed. Catheters and leads physically connect the transducers or electrodes on the patient to the input modules of the monitor. Some of the common features of a bedside monitor are:

- Multiple traces display–able to display more than one trace of the same or different physiological parameters. For example, a four-channel monitor can be configured to display two channels of cascaded ECG, one arterial blood pressure, and a $\%S_aO_2$ waveforms.
- Alarms–provide visual and/or audio alerts when physiological variables are outside certain preset values. Usually have silencing feature and are able to automatically reset into "ready" mode after powered OFF and ON.
- Freeze capability–able to freeze the waveform displaying on the screen for more detailed analysis.
- Trending capability–receive input from any number of slowly changing physiological variables and plot a continuous record of this variable over a long period of time. For example, plotting the number of ectopic beats, heart rate, respiration rate, temperature, and blood pressure over time (1, 8, and 24 hour basis).
- Recording–able to record a physiological waveform on a printing device. The printing device may be integrated with or networked to the beside monitor.

A bedside monitor can be preconfigured or modular. For a preconfigured monitor, all physiological parameters are built in as an integral part of the monitor at the factory (e.g., a monitor comes with one ECG, one temperature channel, and two blood pressure channels). For a modular bedside monitor, each physiological parameter is an individual module. A bedside monitor can be custom-configured by the clinician at the bedside by selecting the modules to meet the monitoring needs of the patient. Modules can be inserted and removed easily by the user. Although the cost of a modular monitor is usually higher than that of a preconfigured monitor with the same features, a modular designed monitoring system is more economical and provides greater flexibility than that of a preconfigured design. For example, instead of having cardiac output measurement capability in all the monitors in a 12-bed ICU, three cardiac output modules can be shared among 12 modular monitors as cardiac output measurements are done on an intermittent basis and not on all patients.

Ambulatory Monitors

Very often, a patient staying in a hospital has to be transported from one patient location to another or to another hospital. For example, a patient in the Emergency Department may need to be moved to Radiology to have a CT scan. To facilitate patients who require uninterrupted monitoring, a smaller, battery-powered monitor that can be brought along with the patient is necessary. Ambulatory monitors are special monitors that can be transported with the patient. Some manufacturers have ambulatory monitors that use the same bedside monitor modules. Such a system can avoid having to disconnect the patient cables and catheters from the bedside monitor and reconnect to the ambulatory monitor. To prepare for transport, a user simply removes the modules from the bedside monitor (while still connected to the patient) and inserts them into the ambulatory monitor.

Central Station

The location relationship between the patient bed areas and the nursing work areas should be one where the nurse is never far from his/her patients when he/she is carrying out his/her routine tasks away from the patient, and where he/she can maintain visual observation of the patients. Similarly, the patient, frequently anxious, gains much reassurance by being able to keep the staff in view and by knowing that they are never far away should he/she need help. Therefore, a properly designed central station should maintain two-way visibility between the nurses on duty and each of his/her patients.

In practice, the central station is an extension of the bedside monitor and provides information from all patients at one location. Typically, one or more large multitrace central monitors and one or more chart recorders are located at the central station. By observing the central monitor, all patient activities can be observed at a glance. In addition, a chart can be printed automatically or manually from the central recorder at the central station.

The central monitor is usually a large multitrace instrument capable of displaying several waveform traces at the same time. A basic central monitor has the following capabilities:

- Display multiple traces per monitor
- Waveform selection and position controls for each of the traces on the central display
- Waveform freeze capability on all traces
- Display digital values indicated at the bedside along with alarm limit settings
- Selective trending of parameters

It may also include the following capabilities:

- Arrhythmia detection and ST segment analysis
- Record keeping (e.g., medication and drug interaction)
- Connection to the hospital information system (HIS) for patient information downloading, retrieval, and billing

The central chart recorder is interfaced with the monitoring alarm system to instantly record the signal if an alarm occurs. It is usually a multi-channel recorder capable of simultaneously printing a number of traces from the bedside monitors. The recorder can also be used manually to produce a printout of selected traces from any beside monitors upon demand or, when so equipped, can automatically provide a printout at predetermined time intervals.

TELEMETRY

A conventional ECG patient cable confines the patient to the bedside monitor and limits his/her mobility. Exercise is considered beneficial to coronary patients; increase in mobility often increases the rate of recovery. This limitation can be removed by an ECG telemetry system. A telemetry system removes hardwired connections by replacing it with radio frequency links. ECG telemetry was developed in the 1950s for stress testing. It now replaces or supplements hardwired monitors in acute care units. A typical ECG telemetry system consists of:

- A radio transmitter, about the size of a deck of cards, carried by the patient on a belt or in a pocket
- Surface (or skin) electrodes attached to the patient, which, through lead wires, feed the ECG signal into the transmitter
- A bedside or central station receiver that detects the radio wave and reconstructs the ECG waveform

An ECG telemetry systems can be found in progressive care and coronary (or cardiac) care (CCU) units. It allows continuous monitoring of patients who require less care and need mobility. Typically, a CCU patient whose ECG rhythm has satisfactorily stabilized will be put on telemetry where ECG monitoring continues to detect dangerous arrhythmia. However, ECG telemetry has the following shortcomings:

- Increased system's complexity and cost
- ECG artifacts associated with increased mobility
- Decreased reliability (loss of signal, range limit, electrical interference)
- Delays in locating patients because the freedom afforded by telemetry encourages wandering

In a typical ECG telemetry system, the patient wears a transmitter, which is connected to three or more skin electrodes that detect the ECG signal (Figure 14–3). The ECG signal is modulated and transmitted into the free space. The receiver at the receiving station decodes the signal and displays the waveform and heart rate on the monitor. Telemetry is also available for other physiological parameters.

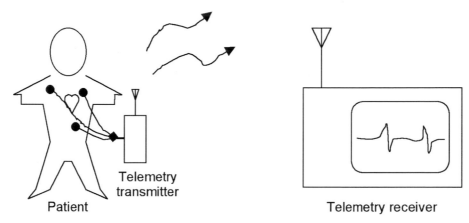

Figure 14–3. ECG Telemetry System.

ARRHYTHMIA DETECTION

ECG is an important physiological parameter in patient monitoring. When a patient has a heart problem such as myocardial infarction, the ECG waveform is different from that of a healthy individual. A computerized arrhythmia detection system continuously analyzes the ECG waveforms and attempts to recognize arrhythmias and to alarm on certain ones. Most patient monitors with arrhythmia detection capability specifically identify and count different types of arrhythmia. The computer in the monitor measures QRS complexes, compares beat intervals, follows some algorithm to classify individual beats, and recognizes arrhythmias. The computer may use additional criteria, such as width, prematurity, heart rate, and compensatory pause, to further classify the type of arrhythmia. In general, there are two types of algorithms in arrhythmia detection:

1. Waveform feature extraction
2. Template (matching or cross-correlation variety)

Waveform feature extraction measures several QRS characteristics (e.g., width, prematurity, height, and area). This is often used in combination with a compression (data reduction) technique such as AZTEC (Amplitude-Zone-Time-Epoch-Coding). AZTEC converts the sample ECG signal to a series of constant-amplitude or sloped line segments for more efficient input to the computer (see Figure 14–4). The computer then identifies the QRS complex and makes the required measurements.

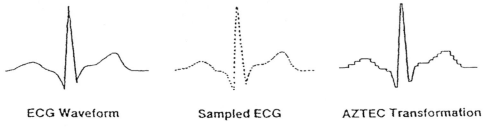

ECG Waveform   Sampled ECG   AZTEC Transformation

Figure 14–4. AZTEC ECG Compression.

These measurements are then compared to criteria stored in the computer system to differentiate between normal and abnormal beats. As the computer reviews each beat, it groups those with similar features (e.g., height, weight). In most systems, the computer then classifies the beats as normal, paced, premature, et cetera.

In template matching, the computer samples each beat at approximately 16–40 points. These values are then mathematically matched with the values from previously stored beats or a general set of templates. In template matching, the beat is classified as normal, abnormal, or questionable based on the number of points on the sampled beat that violate the template boundaries (see diagram below).

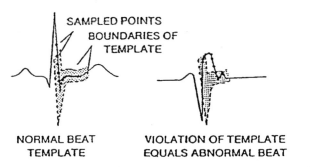

SAMPLED POINTS
BOUNDARIES OF
TEMPLATE

NORMAL BEAT   VIOLATION OF TEMPLATE
TEMPLATE   EQUALS ABNORMAL BEAT

Figure 14–5. Template Matching Arrhythmia Detection Algorithm.

Template cross-correlation algorithm uses a calculated correlation coefficient (a number from –1 to +1) to mathematically determine how closely the beat matches one of a set of stored templates. A correlation coefficient greater than or equal to some criterion (e.g., ≥ 0.9) constitutes a match between the sampled beat and the template.

With both template algorithms, questionable beats are usually classified as noise or artifact if similar beats are not detected within a specified time period (generally under 1 minute) or within a certain number of beats (e.g., 500). Those that are seen again are classified as abnormal beats.

All algorithms are subject to error, resulting in misclassification of noise and artifact as arrhythmia and incorrect categorization of arrhythmia. Since the "normal" QRS complex of a patient may change with time and condition, the system must "relearn" the patient's normal QRS from time to time to minimize false alarms.

PATIENT MONITORING NETWORKS

To connect the central and bedside monitors, a "Patient Monitoring Network" is required. A "network" is a group of computerized devices connected by one or more transmission media for communication or sharing of resources and data. The transmission links can be wired or wireless. Resources to be shared in a network can be hardware (such as hard disks, printers), software, or human resources (such as accessing remote clinical experts for consultation). Data to be shared can be any information such as medical images, physiological waveform, or patient information. A network can be a local area network (LAN), which operates in a small area, or a wide area network (WAN), which connects a number of LANs over a large geographic area.

Some desirable characteristics of a patient monitoring network in health care applications are:

- Easily adaptable and configurable to all site-specific requirements (i.e., different number of monitored bedside system, distances, etc.)
- Easy and fast to move information throughout the network
- Allow modifications or changes to system without loss of required function of the rest of the system
- Disconnect and reconnect equipment to system without disruption
- Scalable and allow variability of monitoring parameters
- Compatible with other network equipment and system (i.e., adheres to industry standards)

Network Topologies

Components in a network can be physically connected in different ways. The following diagrams show some possible network topologies (physical ways of connections) for a patient physiological monitoring network system.

In a ring topology, data passes through each instrument on the way around the circle. In a bus (or tree) topology, the main data are on pipeline or bus. Each computer receives the same information. In a star topology, the central controller connects to other computers like branches radiating out from the center. It may include satellites.

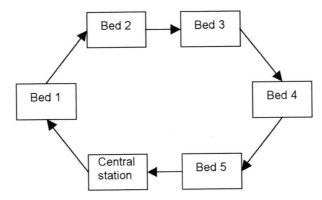

Figure 14–6a. Ring Network Topology.

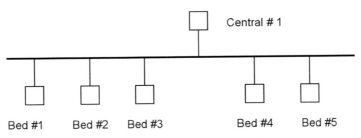

Figure 14–6b. Bus Network Topology.

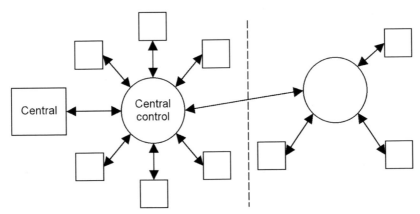

Figure 14–6c. Star Network Topology.

Network Protocols

The ARCnet network protocol, developed in the 1970s by Datapoint, was once a significant industrial standard to handle data link in networking. However, due to its low transmission rate (2.5 Mbps), it was slowly taken over by the Ethernet and Token Ring in the 1980s. Today, Ethernet is the dominant data link protocol used in computer networking, including physiological monitoring. The characteristics of the ethernet and token ring protocols are:

Ethernet

- Ethernet LANs were first developed by Xerox in the 1970s
- Adhere to the IEEE 802.3 Standard
- 10 Mbps (10 Base-2 Thinnet) to 100 Mbps (Cat. 5 UTP fast Ethernet) to Gbps bandwidth
- Access methodology is CSMA/CD (carrier sensed with multiple access and collision detection)
- All stations share the same bus
- A station ready to transmit will listen to make sure that the bus is not in use
- Upon a collision (two or more stations were transmitting simultaneously), each will wait for a random period of time and then retransmit
- Quite efficient for low traffic LANs
- BUS–10 Base-2 (Thinnet) or 10 Base-5 (Thick Ethernet)
- STAR–10 Base-T (UTP), center of the STAR is a HUB or concentrator

Token Ring

- Token Ring LANs were created by IBM and introduced as the IEEE 802.5 Standard
- Called a logical ring, physical star
- 4 or 16 MBps bandwidth
- Uses Token-passing access methodology
- Guarantees no data collisions and ensures data delivery
- Sequential message delivery as opposed to Ethernet's broadcast delivery
- Contention is handled through a TOKEN that circulates past all stations
- Token Ring LANs can be set up in a physical ring or a physical star
- The center of the STAR is called a multistation access unit (MAU)

To handle networking and transportation of information, the TCP/IP (transport control protocol and internet protocol) is by far the most commonly used network protocol today to resolve addresses, route information, and ensure reliable data delivery.

Networks Models

There are three main network models, each of which is characterized by how it handles traffic and data.

Host-terminal

- A host computer connected to dump terminals
- The central host handles processing
- Terminals provide display and keyboard input

Client-server

- Intelligent client workstations connected to a server computer
- Application can be customized and processed at the workstation
- Considered as a distributed processing network
- The server provides services such as file and printer access to the workstations
- Can have more than one server, e.g., a file server and a printer server in a network

Peer-to-peer

- Two or more computers connected and running the same network software
- Each can do its own processing
- Good for small networks to share resources such as printers, storage, application software, etc.

Network Operating Systems

Most modern commercial network operating systems (NOS) can work with Ethernet and Token Ring. Examples are the Novell Netware, Microsoft Windows NT and 2000 Servers, UNIX, et cetera.

Network Connection Components

Transmission Links

The network hardware and software will determine the data transfer rates between networks and the components within a network. In LANs or WANs, the cables connecting the components are often one of the major factors affecting the data transfer rate. The type of connection and the distance will limit the maximum data transfer rate. Hardwired systems can use twisted copper wires, coaxial cables, shielded cables, or fiber-optic cables. Wireless links can use infrared, radio frequency, or microwave for data transmission. For rapid transmission of a large amount of data (e.g., for video conferencing), high-speed links are available through telephone or cable companies. Many organizations have installed such high-speed links as the backbone of their WAN. Examples of high-speed links are Integrated Services Digital Network (ISDN), which has a transmission rate of 64 to 128 Kbps; T–1 lines with a rate of 1.44 Mbps; and Fiber Distributed Data Interface (FDDI) with a rate of 100 Mbps.

Network Interconnection Devices

A number of interconnection devices can be found in a computer network system. Some of the common devices are:

Network interface card (NIC)

- The interface between the computer and the physical network connection
- Responsible for sending and receiving binary signals according to the network standards
- Each NIC has a unique physical address

Hubs

- A device to connect several computers
- Signals sent to the hub are broadcasted to all ports (where computers or network devices are connected) of the hub

Switches

- A device to connect several computers
- Signals sent to the switch are broadcast to selected ports

Repeaters

- A device to extend network cabling segments over longer distances
- Basic functions are to receive, amplify, and transmit signal

Bridges

- An internetworking device to connect small number of LANs together
- When a bridge receives a packet or a message, it reads the address and forward the message if it is not local
- Reduce traffic congestion because it will not pass local packets to other LANs

Routers

- An internetworking device to direct traffic across multiple LANs or WANs

- Communicate to each other using a routing protocol that includes a routing table
- The routing table stores information about network accessibility and optimal routing routes

Health Care Network Standards

With the need to share information, LANs and WANs are installed in hospitals, clinics, and communities. To allow data transfer between terminal units connecting to these networks, standards are developed to enhance the connectivity of different medical devices and systems. Examples of standards for the exchange of patient and clinical data are HL7 (Health Level 7) for electronic data exchange in health; and DICOM (Digital Imaging and Communications in Medicine) for vendor-independent digital medical images transfers between equipment.

DICOM standard sets the basis for interoperability between imaging devices that claim to support DICOM features. It facilitates equipment from different manufacturers to communicate to each other. DICOM 3 supports a subset of the OSI upper level service and is implemented in software.

HL7 is a standard for the exchange, management, and integration of data that supports clinical patient care and the management, delivery, and evaluation of health care services. Level 7 refers to the highest level of the ISO-OSI communication model–the application level. This level addresses definition of the data to be exchanged, the timing of interchange, and the communication of certain errors to the application. It supports such functions as security checks, participant identification, availability checks, exchange mechanism negotiations, and, most importantly, data exchange structuring.

Chapter 15

ELECTROCARDIOGRAPHS

OBJECTIVES

- Explain the origin of ECG signal and the relationships between the waveform and cardiac activities.
- Explain projection of the three-dimensional cardiac vector and analyze the relationships between the ECG leads.
- Define 12-lead ECG, the electrode placements, connections, and their relationships.
- Differentiate between diagnostic and monitoring ECG and explain the effects of changing bandwidth on the display waveform.
- Identify and analyze the functional building blocks of an ECG machine.
- Study typical specifications of an electrocardiograph.
- Evaluate causes of poor ECG signal quality and suggest corrective solution.

CHAPTER CONTENTS

INTRODUCTION

The class of medical instrumentation to acquire and analyze physiological parameters is called diagnostic devices. This chapter introduces an important diagnostic medical device to monitor and analyze the heart condition through collecting and evaluating electrical potential generated from cardiac activities. This medical device is called electrocardiograph, and the record of the electrical cardiac potential as a function of time is called the electrocardiogram. The first ECG came into clinical use in the 1920s using electron vacuum tube amplification, an oscilloscope for display, and a string galvanometer for recording. ECG has since evolved into a group of highly sophisticated devices to acquire cardiac potentials, perform diagnostic analysis and interpretation, as well as provide information storage and communication.

ORIGIN OF THE CARDIAC POTENTIAL

The natural pacemaker of the heart is a small mass of specialized heart muscle cells called the sinoatrial (SA) node. The SA node generates electrical impulses that travel through specialized conduction pathways in the atrium (Figure 15–1). As a result of this electrical activation, the atrial muscle contracts to pump blood from the atria through the two atrioventricular valves into the ventricles.

While causing the atrial muscle to contract, this electrical impulse continues to travel and eventually reaches another specialized group of cells called the atrioventricular (AV) node. In the AV node, the electrical impulse is delayed by about 100 ms before it arrives at the Bundle of His and its two major divisions, the right and left bundle branches. These branches then break into the Purkinje system, which conducts the electrical impulse to the inner wall of the ventricles, causing the ventricles to contract and pump blood from the right ventricle into the lung and from the left ventricle to the rest of the body. The time delay of the electrical impulse in the AV node allows blood to be emptied from the atria to the ventricles before the ventricular contraction. This coordinated contraction of the atria and ventricles maximizes the throughput of the cardiac contraction. Figure 15–2 shows the time delay of the electrical stimulation reaching different locations of the heart conduction pathway.

The contraction and relaxation of the heart due to synchronized polarization and depolarization of the cells in the cardiac muscles produce an electric current that spreads from the heart to all parts of the body. The spread-

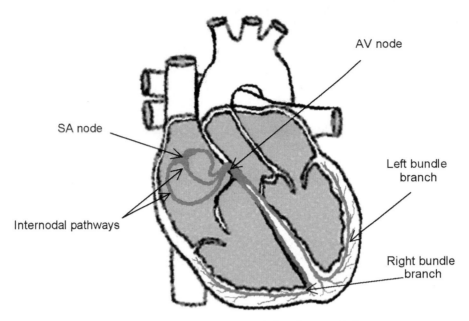

Figure 15–1. The Heart's Electrical Conduction Pathways.

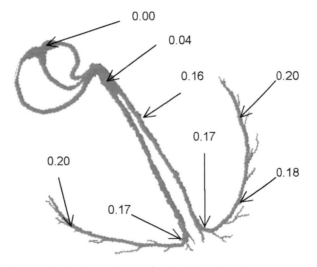

Figure 15–2. Time Delay (sec) of Cardiac Conduction.

ing of this current creates differences in potential at various locations on the body. Figure 15–3a shows a typical action potential plotted against time obtained from a pair of electrodes placed on a ventricular muscle fiber bundle under normal cardiac activity. It shows rapid depolarization (contraction) and then slow repolarization (relaxation) of the muscle fiber. As there are many fiber bundles contracting and relaxing at slightly different times in a cardiac cycle, the result of these electrical potential forms a cardiac vector of changing magnitude moving in three dimensions with time. The potential difference measured using a pair of electrodes placed on the surface of the body is the projection of the cardiac vector to the line joining the two electrodes. The waveform obtained by plotting this potential difference between a pair of electrodes placed on opposite sides of the heart as a function of time is called the electrocardiogram (or ECG).

THE ELECTROCARDIOGRAM

An ECG obtained from electrodes placed on the surface of the body (or skin) is called a surface ECG. A typical surface ECG is shown in Figure 15–3b. It consists of a series of waves (P, Q, R, S, and T) corresponding to different phases of the cardiac cycle. Roughly speaking, the P wave corresponds to the contraction of the atria, the QRS complex marks the beginning of the contraction of the ventricles, and the T wave corresponds to the relaxation of the ventricles. In a normal heart, relaxation of the atria occurs at the same time as the contraction of the ventricles. The voltage variation due to atrial relaxation is not visible because of the large amplitude of the QRS complex. The amplitude of the R wave for surface ECG is about 0.4 to 4 mV. Typical amplitude is 1 mV with a cycle time of 1 second (60 beats per minute). Figure 15–4 shows the relationship between the surface ECG and the depolarization of the heart. In a normal cardiac cycle:

- The P wave precedes the depolarization of the atria.
- The PQ (or PR) interval is a measure of the elapsed time from the onset of atrial depolarization to the beginning of ventricular depolarization.
- The QRS complex marks the start of the depolarization of the ventricles.
- The QT interval marks the period of depolarization of the ventricle.
- The T wave reflects ventricular repolarization.

Delay due to total interruption or nonresponsiveness of some part of the pathway causes changes in the ECG. For example, if a large nonconductive area develops in the wall of the ventricle, the shape or duration of QRS will be altered. Any marked cardiac abnormality such as problems with the SA or AV nodes or in the ventricular conduction pathways will be reflected by changes in amplitude and shape of the ECG waveform. Surface ECG is an important diagnostic tool for clinicians to gain insight into different abnor-

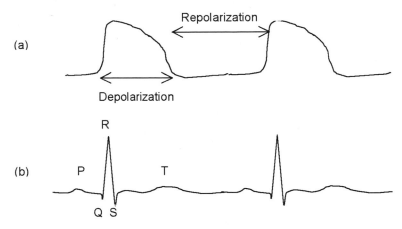

Figure 15–3. (a) Action Potential of a Cardiac Fiber Bundle and (b) Surface ECG.

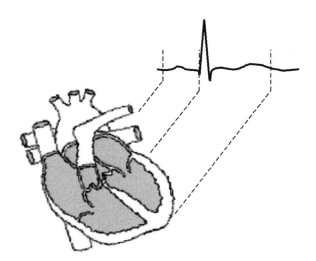

Figure 15–4. Surface ECG and the Cardiac Cycle.

mal heart conditions. Examples of some cardiac arrhythmias (abnormal heart rhythms) revealed in diagnostic ECG are shown in Figure 15–5.

An electrocardiogram can be used to diagnose physiological conditions of the heart (e.g., to track heart rhythm and heart rate). Figure 15–5b reviews a premature ventricular contraction caused by an ectopic focus from the ventricles. Figure 15–5c is the most severe consequence of ventricular condition, which occurs when each muscle fiber within the myocardium contracts and relaxes at its own pace with no coordination. In ventricular fibrillation, the heart loses its ability to pump blood into the circulatory system.

ECG is an important diagnostic tool of the heart. An ECG stress test

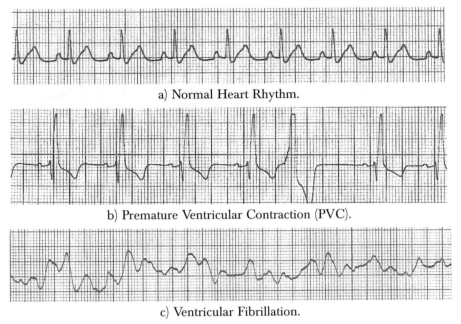

a) Normal Heart Rhythm.

b) Premature Ventricular Contraction (PVC).

c) Ventricular Fibrillation.

Figure 15–5. Normal and Arrhythmic ECG.

(ECG taken when the patient is exercising) is an example of a diagnostic ECG. When a patient's heart rhythm is monitored while staying in a hospital, it is called monitoring ECG. In general, diagnostic ECG contains more information than monitoring ECG due to two major factors:

1. The bandwidth of diagnostic ECG (e.g., 0.05 Hz to 120 Hz) is wider than that of monitoring ECG (e.g., 0.5 Hz to 40 Hz).
2. There are more leads (projection of the cardiac vector) taken simultaneously in diagnostic ECG than monitoring ECG.

The effects of machine bandwidth and lead configurations on ECG will be discussed in more detail later in this chapter.

In a critical care area in a hospital, monitoring of a patient's ECG provides the following information:

- Early warning signs of more major arrhythmias that may follow
- Immediate detection of potentially fatal arrhythmia by means of alarms
- Feedback on the effectiveness of a treatment intervention
- Correlation between cardiac rhythm and treatment variables
- Permanent record of ECG waveform on a routine basis

When an out-patient's ECG must be monitored over an extended period of time, an ambulatory ECG (or sometimes called Holter ECG) is used.

An ambulatory ECG can record the patient's heart rhythm continuously during normal daily activities, say, 24 hours. During monitoring, the patient wears a small ECG machine with a built-in magnetic tape recorder or a semiconductor memory. ECG is acquired from skin electrodes attached to the patient and stored in the memory. After the acquisition period, the memory is downloaded to a reader terminal by a cardiology technologist and the ECG is read and interpreted by a cardiologist.

ECG LEAD CONFIGURATIONS

In earlier discussion, we learned that the cardiac vector has a varying magnitude and pointing to different directions with time; also, an ECG is the potential difference measured against time from the projection of the cardiac vector into a direction according to the placement of the pair of electrodes. If ECG electrodes are connected to the right arm (RA), left arm (LA), and left leg (LL) of the patient, one projection of the cardiac vector can be obtained by connecting the electrodes attached to the left leg and right arm to the input terminals of a biopotential amplifier. A different projection of the same cardiac vector can be measured between the left arm and the right arm electrodes and similarly another projection between the left leg and right arm. These projections (or lead vectors) in the patient's frontal plane can be approximated by an equilateral triangle called the Einthoven's triangle. Figure 15–6 shows the projections of the cardiac vector at a certain time instant on the Einthoven's triangle.

The ECG obtained between the limb electrodes LA (+) and RA (–) is called lead I (Figure 15–7), between LL and RA is called lead II, and

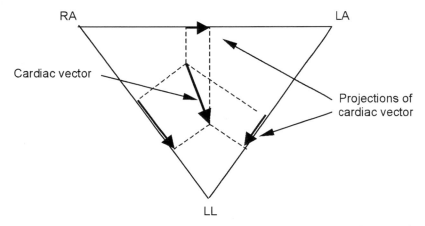

Figure 15–6. Projection of Cardiac Vector in the Frontal Plane.

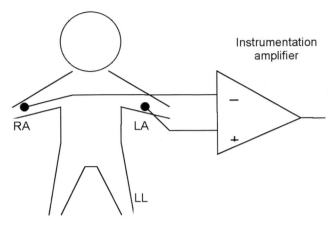

Figure 15–7. ECG Lead I Measurement.

between LL and LA is called lead III. Figure 15–8 shows the configurations of these limb leads. Note the polarities of the electrodes.

If the potential is measured across a limb electrode and the average of two other limb electrodes, the ECG obtained is called an augmented limb lead. Figure 15–9 shows the connections of the augmented limb leads aVR,

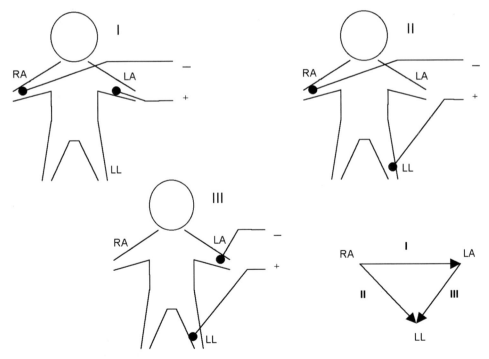

Figure 15–8. ECG Limb Leads.

aVL, and aVF (note that R stands for right, L stands for left, and F stands for foot). The average of the limb potentials is obtained by connecting two identical value resistors to the limb electrodes and then connected to the inverting input of the instrumentation amplifier. The limb leads (I, II, and III) and the augmented limb leads (aVR, aVL, and aVF) together are called the frontal plane leads.

The frontal plane leads represent the projection of the three-dimensional cardiac vector onto the two-dimensional frontal plane. In order to reconstruct the entire cardiac vector, the cardiac potential projected onto another plane is required. Figure 15–10 shows the position of the electrode placements on the chest of the patient to obtain the precordial leads (or the chest leads). The precordial leads represent the projection of the cardiac vector on the transverse plane of the patient. To measure the precordial leads, potential of each of the chest electrodes is referenced to the average of the three limb electrodes (that is why they are sometimes referred to as unipolar leads). Figure 15–11 shows the connections to obtain the chest leads. Note that all resistors to the limb electrodes are of equal value. Which precordial lead is being measured depends on the position of the electrode on the chest of the patient (Figure 15–10). The six frontal plane leads and the six precordial leads form the standard 12-lead ECG configuration. A summary of the electrode positions for the standard 12-lead ECG is shown in Table 15–1.

Note that altogether nine electrodes (three on the frontal plane and six on the transverse plane) are necessary to obtain the 12-ECG leads simultaneously. In practice, a tenth electrode attached to the patient's right leg is used either as the reference (grounded) or connected to the right-leg-driven circuit for common mode noise reduction (see Chapter 11). Figure 15–12 shows the characteristic ECG waveform from a standard 12-lead measurement.

Table 15-1.
Standard 12-Lead ECG Electrode Placement.

Lead	Positive Polarity	Negative Polarity
	Electrode Placement	
I	left arm (LA)	right arm (RA)
II	left leg (LL)	right arm (RA)
III	left leg (LL)	left arm (LA)
aVR	right arm (RA)	$\frac{1}{2}$ (LA + LL)
aVL	left arm (LA)	$\frac{1}{2}$ (RA + LL)
aVF	left leg (LL)	$\frac{1}{2}$ (RA + LA)
V1 through V6	chest positions	$\frac{1}{3}$ (LA + RA + LL)

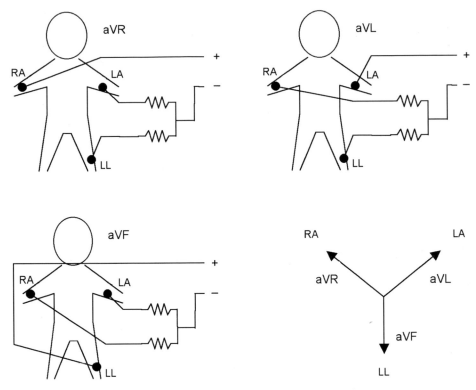

Figure 15–9. ECG Augmented Limb Leads.

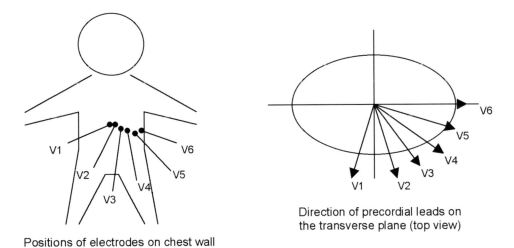

Positions of electrodes on chest wall

Direction of precordial leads on
the transverse plane (top view)

Figure 15–10. ECG Precordial Leads.

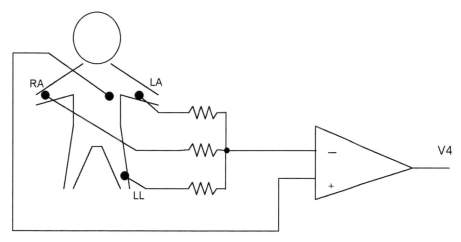

Figure 15–11. Connections for the Chest Leads.

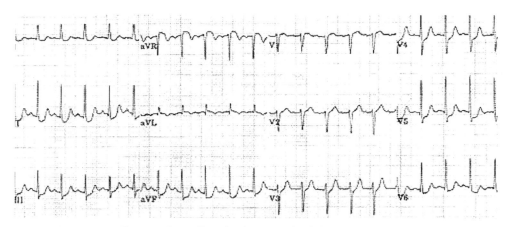

Figure 15–12. Standard 12-Lead ECG Waveform.

STANDARD 12-LEAD ECG AND VECTORCARDIOGRAM

From the definition of the limb leads, lead I is the difference in potential between the electrodes attached to the left arm and the right arm. That is: lead I = E_{LA} – E_{RA}, similarly lead II = E_{LL} – E_{RA}, and lead III = E_{LL} – E_{LA}.

The sum of Lead I and Lead III equals to Lead II:

Lead I + Lead III = (E_{LA} – E_{RA}) + (E_{LL} – E_{LA}) = E_{LL} – E_{RA} = Lead II

This result agrees with the vector relationships between lead I, lead II, and lead III shown in Figure 15–8.

For the precordial lead V_n, where $n = 1$ to 6,

$$V_n = E_n - \frac{E_{RA} + E_{LA} + E_{LL}}{3}$$

For the augmented limb leads,

$$aVR = E_{RA} - \frac{E_{LA} + E_{LL}}{2} = \frac{2E_{RA} - E_{LA} - E_{LL}}{2} = -\frac{(E_{LL} - E_{RA}) + (E_{LA} - E_{RA})}{2}$$

Since lead I (or I) $= E_{LA} - E_{RA}$ and lead II (or II) $= E_{LL} - E_{RA}$,

$$aVR = -\frac{II + I}{2} \text{, similarly, one can show that}$$

$$aVL = E_{LA} - \frac{E_{RA} + E_{LL}}{2} = \frac{I - III}{2} \text{, and}$$

$$aVF = E_{LL} - \frac{E_{RA} + E_{LA}}{2} = \frac{II + III}{2}.$$

Furthermore, augmented leads can be obtained by subtracting the average potential of the three limb electrodes from one of the limb electrode potential:

$$E_{LL} - \frac{E_{RA} + E_{LA}' + E_{LL}}{3} = \frac{2E_{LL}}{3} - \left(\frac{E_{RA}}{3} + \frac{E_{LA}}{3}\right) = \frac{2}{3}\left(E_{LL} - \frac{E_{RA} + E_{LA}}{2}\right) = \frac{2}{3}aVF.$$

Similarly, one can show that

$$E_{LA} - \frac{E_{RA} + E_{LA} + E_{LL}}{3} = \frac{2}{3} aVL \text{, and}$$

$$E_{RA} - \frac{E_{RA} + E_{LA} + E_{LL}}{3} = \frac{2}{3} aVR.$$

Consider the Wilson network shown in Figure 15–13. If the corners of this triangular resistive network are connected to electrodes on the right arm, left arm, and the left leg of the patient, V-, V_{R}-, V_{L}-, and V_{F}- are equal to:

$$V_- = \frac{E_{RA} + E_{LA} + E_{LL}}{3}$$

$$V_{R-} = \frac{E_{LA} + E_{LL}}{2}$$

$$V_{L-} = \frac{E_{RA} + E_{LL}}{2}$$

$$V_{F-} - \frac{E_{RA} + E_{LA}}{2}.$$

These terminals on the network can therefore be used as the negative reference to measure the augmented and precordial ECG leads. The Wilson network allows using only one electrode connection at each location. It also avoids the need to remove and reconnect lead wires and electrodes during ECG measurement. Figure 15–14 shows the connections to obtain lead I, lead aVR, and a chest lead. Typical resistance values of R and R1 in the network (Figure 15–13) are 10 kΩ and 15 kΩ, respectively.

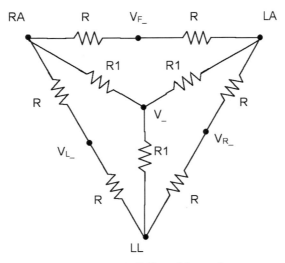

Figure 15–13. Wilson Network.

Figure 15–15 shows the acquisition block (or patient interface module) of a single channel 12-lead ECG machine. During operation, it uses a multiplexer or a number of mechanical switches to select which two input combinations of electrodes are connected to the instrumentation amplifier. Note that for this machine only one lead can be measured at a time. In a fully digital machine, the Wilson Resistor Network may be eliminated. The lead signals from such a digital system are derived mathematically from the electrical potentials from the individual electrodes using the lead relationships derived previously.

In order to simultaneously measure more than one ECG lead, more than one instrumentation amplifiers are usually required. Figure 15–14 shows a three-channel ECG machine measuring lead I, lead aVR, and one chest lead simultaneously. In general, to measure all 12 leads simultaneously, the electrocardiograph will need to have 12 sets of instrumentation amplifiers as well as 12 display channels. Some machines are using sampling and time-division multiplexing techniques.

Other than the standard 12-lead ECG, other lead systems or lead loca-

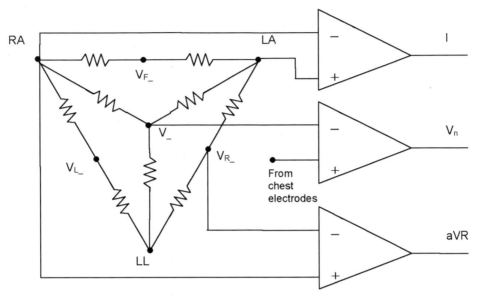

Figure 15–14. Use of Wilson Network in ECG Measurement.

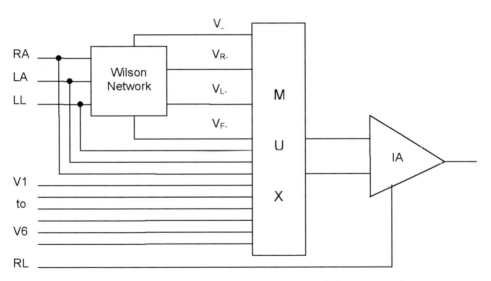

Figure 15–15. A Single Channel 12-Lead ECG Front End.

tions are used in diagnostic electrocardiography. One such commonly used lead is the esophageal lead, which is obtained by swallowing an electrode into the esophagus so that the electrode is directly behind and close to the heart of the patient. The esophageal electrode is often referenced to the average of the limb leads.

Another interpretation of the electrical cardiac activity is the vectorcardiogram. It was discussed earlier that the cardiac vector changes in both magnitude and direction (in three dimensions) as the electrical impulse spreads through the myocardium. A vectorcardiogram depicts these changes as a function of time during the cardiac cycle. Figure 15–16 show the magnitude and direction of the cardiac vector projected onto the frontal plane at five different time intervals during the QRS complex (i.e., ventricular contraction). The vector at t_1 is zero, which corresponds to the quiescent time before the ventricle starts to contract. When the current starts to flow toward the apex of the heart, causing the ventricle to contract, the cardiac vector starts to grow in magnitude as well as change in direction. The vectors at time intervals t_2 to t_5 are shown in Figure 15–16. The elliptical figure (or loop) traced by the cardiac vector during the QRS interval using the quiescent point as reference is called the QRS-vectorcardiogram. A smaller loop, referred to as the T-vectorcardiogram, is also produced by the T wave. As the magnitude of the T wave is about 0.2 to 0.3 mV and happens about 0.25 second after the QRS, it is a much smaller loop that appears about 0.25 second after the disappearance of the QRS-vectorcardiogram. A still smaller P-vectorcardiogram can be recorded during atrial depolarization. Like the conventional electrocardiogram, the vectorcardiogram can be used in the diagnosis of certain heart conditions.

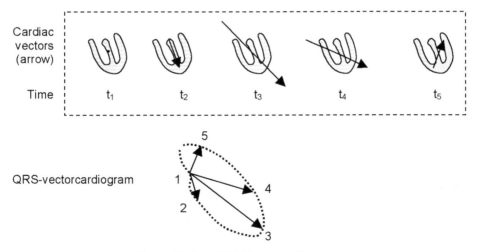

Figure 15–16. QRS-Vectorcardiogram.

FUNDAMENTAL BUILDING BLOCKS
OF AN ELECTROCARDIOGRAPH

Figure 15–17 shows the functional block diagram of a typical electrocardiograph. The function of each block is described below.

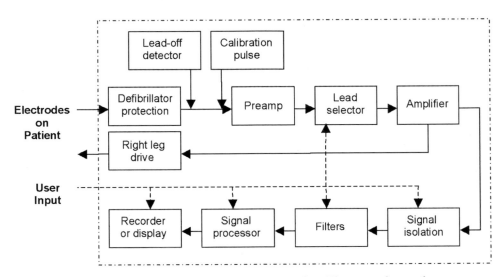

Figure 15–17. Functional Block Diagram of an Electrocardiograph.

Defibrillator Protection

As the ECG electrodes are connected to the patient's chest, they will pick up the high-voltage impulses during cardiac defibrillations. Gas discharge tubes and silicon diodes are used for defibrillator protection (see Chapter 11, Figs. 11–17 and 11–18) to prevent the high-voltage defibrillation discharge from damaging sensitive electronic components.

Lead-Off Detector

When an electrode or lead wire is disconnected, the output of the ECG may display a flat baseline with noise. This may be misinterpreted as asystole. A lead-off (or lead fault) detector can prevent such misinterpretation. A simple lead-off detector is shown in Figure 15–18. In this design, a very large value resistor (>100 MΩ) is connected between the positive power supply and a lead wire to allow a small DC current to flow via the electrode through the patient to ground. Under normal situation, due to the relatively small electrode/skin impedance, the DC voltages created at the input terminals of the operation amplifier are very small and almost of equal value. However, if an electrode or a lead wire comes off from the patient, the amplifier will be saturated since the voltage at one input of the amplifier will rise to the level of the power supply. In this case, the lead-off LED will turn on to alert the user to a lead fault.

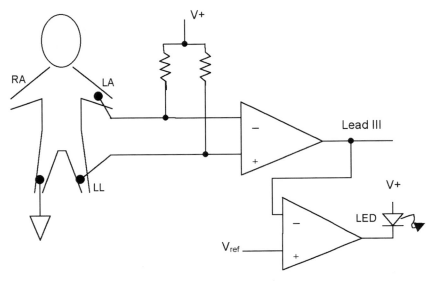

Figure 15–18. Lead-Off Detector.

Preamplifier

The magnitude of surface ECG is from 0.1 to 4 mV. A system, especially one with long unshielded lead wires, may pick up noise of up to several mV through electromagnetic coupling. Therefore, it is important to amplify this small signal as close to the source as possible before it is corrupted by noise. Most ECG machines amplify the potential signals picked up by the electrodes in a preamp module or patient interface module located near the patient.

Lead Selector

The lead selector selects the ECG lead to be displayed or recorded. In a multichannel machine, the lead selector also configures the sequence and format of the display or printout.

Amplifier

Typically the magnitude of the ECG at the surface of the body is about 1 mV, but this value may vary substantially from patient to patient. For example, the ECG of a critically ill patient may be as low as 0.1 mV or as high as 3 mV. The electrocardiography must have some means of controlling the size of the ECG waveform. This is also called SIZE, GAIN, or SENSITIVITY adjustment. Typical sensitivity settings are 5, 10, or 20 mm/mV.

Right-Leg-Driven Circuit

Electrical equipment and wiring near the electrocardiograph may induce common mode signal of several mV magnitude on the patient's body. The right-leg-driven circuit is to suppress this common mode signal so that it will not mask the ECG signal (see Chapter 11).

Calibration Pulse

A built-in reference voltage of 1 mV is applied to the input of the electrocardiograph. This reference signal is displayed on the screen and on the printout to inform the user that the machine is functioning properly and that it has the necessary gain to display the ECG signal coming from the patient.

Signal Isolation

The function of the signal isolation circuit is to reduce the leakage current to and from the patient through the electrode/lead connection for microshock prevention. A module consisting of a FM modulator, an opto-isolator, and a demodulator is commonly used to serve this purpose.

Filter

The frequency bandwidth for a diagnostic quality ECG is from 0.05 to 150 Hz. Such diagnostic mode bandwidth allows accurate presentation of the electrical activities of the patient's heart. Monitoring mode is used where a gross observation of the electrical activity of the patient's heart is necessary but requires little analysis or details. Interference and baseline drift can be reduced by a bandwidth less than that required for a diagnostic-quality ECG. For monitoring, a bandwidth of 1 to 40 Hz is reasonable and will allow recognition of common arrhythmias, while providing reasonable rejection of artifacts and power frequency (60 or 50 Hz) interference. However, some distortion of the ECG will occur. Most electrocardiographs have built-in upper and lower cutoff frequency selection to allow the user to choose the optimal bandwidth for the situation. A power frequency rejection filter (notch filter) can also be switched on or off by the user to minimize power frequency interference.

Signal Processor

Signal processing functions in ECG machines can range from simple heart rate detection to sophisticated arrhythmia analysis and classification. Some common features for signal processing are:

- Heart rate detection and alarm
- Pacemaker pulse detection
- Waveform measurement: PR interval, QRS duration, etc.
- Arrhythmia analysis and classification: e.g., occurrence and frequency of PVC
- Diagnosis and interpretation

Recorder or Display

The acquired waveform of diagnostic ECG can be displayed on a monitor (LCD or CRT) or printed out from a paper chart recorder. In either case, the speed of the waveform traveling across the screen of the monitor or the speed of the paper in the chart recorder can be adjusted. Typical speeds are 12.5, 25, and 50 mm/s. For a multichannel ECG machine, the display format can be selected to display a combination of ECG leads. For example, a "3 × 4 + 3R" print format from a six-channel paper chart recorder is shown in Figure 15–19. In this format, the 12 ECG leads are displayed in three rows of 4 ECG leads. Each of the leads is displayed for 2.5 seconds. In addition, three leads selected by the user are displayed for the entire 10 seconds.

TYPICAL SPECIFICATIONS OF ELECTROCARDIOGRAPHS

The specifications of a typical 12-lead electrocardiograph are:
- Input channels: simultaneous acquisition of up to 12 ECG leads
- Frequency response: –3dB @ 0.01 to 105 Hz
- CMRR: >110 dB
- Input impedance: >50 MΩ
- A/D conversion: 12 bits

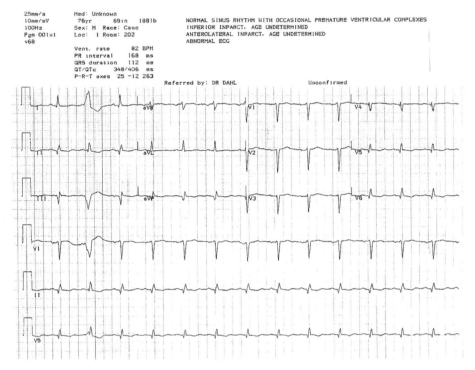

Figure 15–19. A "3 × 4 + 3R" Printout of a 12-Lead ECG.

- Sampling rate: 2,000 samples/sec per channel
- Writer type: thermal digital dot array with 200 dots per inch vertical resolution
- Writer speed: 1, 5, 25, and 50 mm/sec, user selectable
- Sensitivities: 2.5, 5, 10, and 20 mm/mV, user selectable
- Printout formats: 3, 4, 5, 6, and 12 channels, user selectable channel, and lead configurations
- Dimensions: 200 (H) × 40 (W) × 76 (D) cm
- Power requirements: 90 VAC to 260 VAC, 50 or 60 Hz
- Certifications: IEC 601

ECG DATA STORAGE, NETWORK, AND MANAGEMENT

With the advancement in electronic data storage and computer network technologies, modern ECG machines are capable of electronically stored and shared information through computer networks. In a hospital, wireless ECG telemetry, diagnostic review stations, ECG machines, and electronic storage can be integrated into an "ECG data management system" via a local area network (LAN). Multiple hospitals, through wide area network (WAN), can also be configured to communicate and share resources such as mass storage or archive. In a paperless cardiology, ECG data can be readily stored, retrieved, transferred, and viewed at any designated location.

COMMON PROBLEMS

Abnormality in ECG waveform may be grouped into the following three categories:

1. Artifacts due to electrode problems may be caused by

- Improper positioning of electrodes on the patient
- Loose contact between the electrode and the patient
- Dried-out electrode gel
- Bad connection between the lead wire and the electrode
- Failure to properly prepare (clean, shave, and abrade) the patient site for electrode attachment

2. Artifacts due to physiological interference may be caused by

- Skeletal muscle contraction
- Breathing action
- Patient movement
- Involuntary muscle contraction (e.g., tremor)

3. Artifacts due to external interference may be caused by

- Power frequency interference coupled to the lead wires or as common mode voltage on the patient (60 Hz interference in North America)
- Radiated electromagnetic interference from other equipment (e.g., 500 kHz interference from an electrosurgical unit)
- Conductive interference from the power line or ground conductor (e.g. high-frequency noise from switching power supplies)
- Interfering signals from other equipment connected to the patient (e.g., pacemaker or neural stimulator pulses)
- Power interruption and supply voltage fluctuation

Figure 15-20 shows some common artifacts in ECG acquisitions. Figure 15-20a shows a typical ECG waveform with power frequency interference. One can see 60 even, regular spikes in a 1-second interval if the timescale is expanded. Severe 60 Hz interference is often caused by improper patient or equipment grounding. It may also occur when the ECG lead wires are placed too close to power cables or improperly grounded electrical equip-

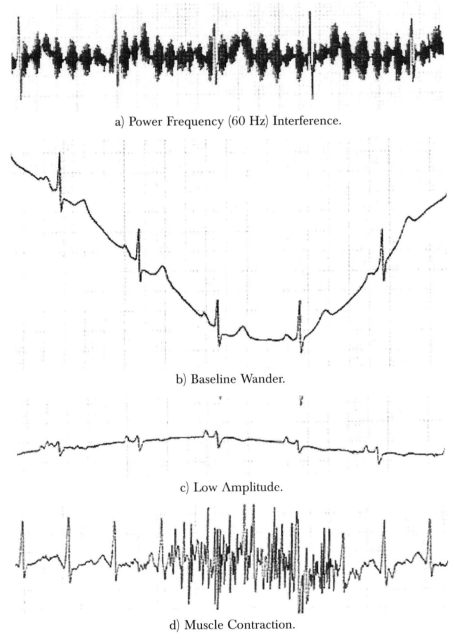

a) Power Frequency (60 Hz) Interference.

b) Baseline Wander.

c) Low Amplitude.

d) Muscle Contraction.

Figure 15–20. Common ECG Artifacts.

ment. Turning on the built-in 60 Hz notch filter (if available) can eliminate such interference. Grouping the lead wires may reduce the interference amplitude. Figure 15–20b shows an ECG with wandering baseline. This can be caused by poor skin preparation, bad electrode contact, dried-out or expired electrode, patient movement, or patient's respiratory action. Figure 15–20c shows an ECG waveform with abnormally small amplitude. Poor skin contact, improperly prepared skin, or dried-out electrode may be the cause. Figure 15-20d shows ECG artifacts due to skeletal muscle contraction. Muscle artifacts will usually disappear when the patient is relaxed and calmed down.

Chapter 16

ELECTROENCEPHALOGRAPHS

OBJECTIVES

- Explain electroneurophysiology and the sources of signals.
- Outline the signal characteristics and clinical applications of EEG.
- Describe different types of EEG electrodes and their applications.
- Explain the 10–20 electrode placements and montages.
- Identify the characteristics of EEG waveform.
- Sketch and explain the functional block diagram of an EEG machine.
- Identify causes of poor EEG signal quality and suggest corrective solutions.

CHAPTER CONTENTS

INTRODUCTION

Electroneurophysiology refers to the study of electrical signals from the central and peripheral nervous systems for functional analysis and diagnosis. These signals are recorded using extremely sensitive instruments to pick up tiny electrical signals produced by the system. Electroencephalography was developed by the German psychiatrist Hans Berger in the mid 1920s, evolved in the 1930s for clinical use, and expanded quickly in the 1940s. It includes the field of electrocorticography–multichannel recordings from the exposed brain cortex. Today, there are four main areas in electroneurophysiology: electroencephalography (EEG), evoked potential (EP) studies, polysomnography (PSG), and electromyography (EMG).

Electroencepholography is a procedure in which small electrical signals produced by the brain are recorded. These signals are generated by the inhibitory and excitatory postsynaptic potentials of the cortical nerve cells. An electroencephalograph is a machine that captures these brain signals. The electrical potential measured due to these signals plotted against time is called an electroencephalogram (EEG). EEG may be used to diagnose conditions such as epilepsy and cerebral tumors. In EEG measurements, electrodes are generally placed on the skull of the patient, although some clinicians may use electrodes that penetrate the skin surface or electrodes that are placed directly on the surface of the cerebral cortex. EEG signals measured directly at the surface of the brain or by needle that penetrated the brain are typically of amplitude from 10 µV to 3 mV, whereas signals acquired on the surface of the skull are typically from 1 to 500 µV. Figure 16–1 shows a general configuration of EEG recording.

Evoked potentials (EP) are performed to analyze the various nerve conduction pathways in the body. Stimulation such as a sound or flashing light is imposed on the subject to initiate a nerve signal transmission. If the signal is not getting through, a lesion in the particular nerve pathway may be pre-

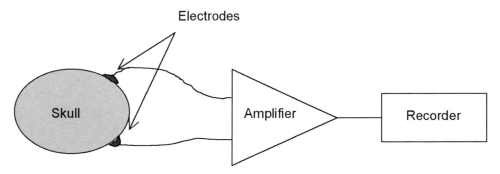

Figure 16–1. General Configuration of EEG Recording.

sent. EP studies, for example, are useful in diagnosing problems in the visual and auditory pathways.

Polysomnography (PSG) is the study of sleep disorders by recording EEG, physiological parameters, and various muscle movements. PSG can be used in diagnosing and treating sleep disorders such as insomnia and sleep apnea.

Electromyography (EMG) is the study of the electrical activities of muscles and their peripheral nerves. It may be used to determine whether the muscles are functioning properly or if the nerve conduction pathway is healthy.

This chapter focuses on EEG, EMG and EP studies are discussed in Chapter 17.

ANATOMY OF THE BRAIN

The brain is the enlarged portion and also the major part of the central nervous system (CNS), protected by three protective membranes (the meninges) and enclosed in the cranial cavity of the skull. The brain and spinal cord are bathed in a special extracellular fluid called cerebral spinal fluid (CSF). The CNS consists of ascending sensory nerve tracts carrying information to the brain from different sensory transducers throughout the body. Information such as temperature, pain, fine touch, pressure, et cetera is picked up by these sensors, and delivered via the nerve tracts to be processed in the brain. The CNS also consists of descending motor nerve tracts, originating from the cerebrum and cerebellum, and terminating on motor neurons in the ventral horn of the spinal column.

The three main parts of the brain are the cerebrum, the brainstem, and the cerebellum. The cerebrum consists of the right and left cerebral hemispheres, controlling the opposite side of the body. The surface layer of the hemisphere is called the cortex and is marked by ridges (gyri) and valleys (sulci); deeper sulci are known as fissures. The cortex receives sensory information from the skin, eyes, ears, et cetera. The outer layer of the cerebrum, approximately 1.5–4.0 mm thick, is called the cerebral cortex. The layers beneath consist of axon and collections of cell bodies, which are called nuclei. The cerebrum is divided by the lateral fissure, central fissure (or central sulcus), and other landmarks into the temporal lobe (responsible for hearing), the occipital lobe (responsible for vision), the parietal lobe (containing the somatosensory cortex responsible for general sense receptors), and the frontal lobe (containing the primary motor and premotor cortex responsible for motor control).

The brainstem is an extension of the spinal cord, which serves three purposes:

1. Connecting link between the cerebral cortex, the spinal cord, and the cerebellum
2. Integration center for several visceral functions (e.g., heart and respiratory rates)
3. Integration center for various motor reflexes

The cerebellum receives information from the spinal cord regarding the position of the trunk and limbs in space, compares this with information received from the cortex, and sends out information to the spinal motor neurons

APPLICATIONS OF EEG

EEG can be used as a clinical tool in diagnosing sleep disorders, epilepsy, and multiple sclerosis. It can also be used in bispectral index monitoring as an indicator of the depth of anesthesia in surgery. It is an effective tool in ascertaining a patient's recovery from brain damage or to confirm brain damage.

A normal EEG usually consists of a range of possible waveforms from low-frequency, nearly periodic waves with large delta components in deep sleep, to high-frequency, noncoherent beta waves measured on the frontal lobe channels during vigorous mental activity. Under a relaxed state, the EEG is characterized by alpha waves from the occipital lobe channels. Opening and closing the eyes results in an evoked response. Examples of the characteristics of some common EEG applications follow.

Brain Death

Absence of EEG signals is a definition of clinical brain death.

Epilepsy and Partial Epilepsy

Epilepsy may be classified into the following categories:

• Generalized epilepsy–affects the entire brain
• Grand mal seizures–large electrical discharges from entire brain that last from a few seconds to several minutes. It is apparent on all EEG channels and may also be accompanied by skeletal muscle twitches and jerks

- Petit mal seizures–this is a less severe form of epilepsy with strong delta waves that last from 1 to 20 seconds in only part of the brain, and therefore appears in only a few EEG channels

Diagnosing Sleep Disorders

In normal sleep, the alpha rhythms are replaced by slower, larger delta waves. EEG monitoring can also determine if and when a subject is dreaming due to the presence of rapid, low-voltage interruptions, indicating paradoxical sleep, or rapid-eye-movement (REM) sleep.

CHALLENGES IN EEG ACQUISITION

Measurement of EEG signals using surface electrodes in general is more difficult than measuring ECG signals because:

- The electrical potentials are conducted through a number of nonhomogeneous media before reaching the scalp. Table 16–1 lists the values of resistivity of different body tissues.
- Since tissues have higher resistivity than the cerebral spinal fluid (CSF) that overlies the brain, the CSF is acting as a region of high conductivity, having a shunting effect on electrical currents.
- Muscles over the temporal region and above the base of the skull provide pathways of high conductivity, allowing the shunting of local voltages well beneath the skin.
- Because of this spatial conductivity arrangement, the electrical potential difference measured actually shows the resultant field potential at a boundary of a large conducting medium surrounding an array of active elements (i.e., activities of the nuclei and some axons).
- In addition, utilization of any nervous functions would cause or inhibit electrical activities of related parts of the brain, leading to a change

Table 16–1.
Tissue's Electrical Resistivity.

Body Part	Resistivity (Ω-cm)
Blood	100–150
Heart muscle	300
Thoracic wall	400
Lung	1,500
Dry skin	6,800,000

in the electrical potentials on the scalp. Electrical activities will also be a function of age, state of consciousness, disease, drugs, and whether external stimulation is used.

EEG is then, in general, the scalp surface measurements of the total effects of all the electrical activities in the brain. It is assessed in conjunction with patient records, clinical symptoms, and other physiological parameters.

EEG ELECTRODES AND PLACEMENT

Types of EEG Electrodes

Depending on the nature of EEG studies, different types of electrodes are used. Surface electrodes, due to their noninvasive application, are the most commonly used electrodes. Needle, cortical, subdural, and depth electrodes are examples of invasive electrodes. Common materials for EEG electrodes are Ag/AgCl, Au-plated Ag, stainless steel, and platinum. The constructions and placements of some are described next.

In an EEG measurement using surface (or scalp) electrodes, the electrodes are made to be in contact with the scalp of the patient. Electrodes may be in the form of a flat disk (1 to 3 mm in diameter) or a small cup with a hole at the center for injection of electrolyte gel. Materials such as platinum, gold, silver, or silver/silver chloride are used for EEG surface electrodes. Earlobe electrodes and nasopharyngeal electrodes are some of the other noninvasive electrodes. In order to minimize noise and artifact problems, surface electrodes must be affixed to the scalp. One of two methods can be used:

1. Using collodion (a viscous fluid) to attach the electrode to the scalp. It is applied to the electrode site and dried using a jet of air. Electrolyte gel is then injected into the electrode through a hole in the center. Low-melting-point paraffin may be used as a substitute for collodion.
2. Adhesive conductive paste is placed directly on the desired location with the electrode pressed into the center of the paste.

Needle electrodes are sharp wires usually made of steel or platinum. There are inserted into the capillary bed between the skin and the skull bone. They can be applied quickly and provide slightly better signal quality than scalp electrodes. Although it is relatively safe, EEG measurement using needle electrodes is an invasive procedure.

Cortical electrodes are used during neurosurgical procedures such as excision of epileptogenic foci. They are applied directly onto the surface of the exposed cortex. These electrodes consist of metal balls or saline-soaked wicks that may be held in place by swivel joints mounted on a bracket of a head frame for easy three-dimensional positioning. Figure 16–2 shows an example of the setup.

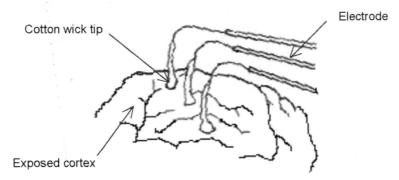

Figure 16–2. Cortical Electrodes.

Subdural electrodes are used to localize epileptiform activity and to map cortical function. They consist of a number of disk electrodes mounted on a thin sheet of flexible translucent Silastic™ rubber. The electrodes are made of platinum or stainless steel. Subdural electrodes are often configured as linear strips or rectangular grids with a number of electrode contact points.

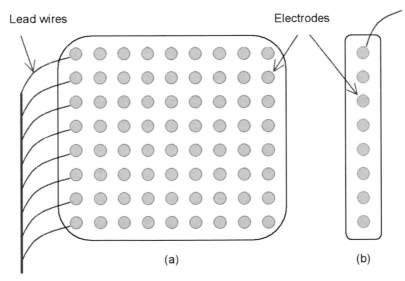

Figure 16–3. Subdural Electrodes (a) Grid, (b) Single Column Strip.

They are designed to be placed on the surface of the cortex. A single column strip can also be inserted into the intracranial cavity through a small burr hole opening. Subdural grids are placed over the cortical convexity in open cranial procedures to cover a large surface area. Figure 16–3 shows such electrodes.

Depth electrodes are fine, flexible plastic electrodes attached to wires that carry currents from deep and superficial brain structures. These currents are recorded through contact points mounted on the walls of the electrodes. Fine wires extending through the bores of the electrodes are inserted with stylets placed in the bores. Stereotactic depth electrodes are useful, for example, in determining the site of origin in temporal lobe epilepsy and as stimulating electrodes for the treatment of movement disorders. Either local or general anesthesia is applied when the electrodes are being inserted into the brain.

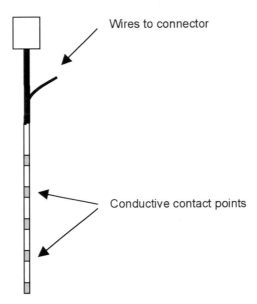

Figure 16–4. Depth Electrodes.

Risks of Implanted EEG Electrodes

Infection is considered the major risk of implanted EEG electrodes. Recent studies reported an infection rate of about 2–3%. Meticulous surgical techniques and procedures to prevent cerebrospinal fluid leakage keep the risk of infection low.

Another risk from electrode placement is hemorrhage. Significant intracerebral hemorrhages have been reported, but the incidence is 1% or less. Direct brain injury due to passing of the depth electrodes has not been demonstrated because the electrodes are so thin that they normally dissect neural tissue without imposing much injury.

Surface (or Scalp) Electrode Placement

The international 10–20 system of electrode placement provides uniform coverage of the entire scalp. Based on the proven relationship between a measured electrode site and the underlying cortical structures and areas, electrodes are symmetrically spaced on the scalp, using identifiable skull anatomical landmarks as reference points. It is termed "10–20" because electrodes are spaced either 10% or 20% of the total distance between a given pair of skull landmarks. These landmarks are:

*   Nasion—the root of the nose
*   Inion—ossification or bump on the occipital lobe
*   Right auricular point—right ear
*   Left auricular point—left ear

Figure 16–5 shows the locations of the electrodes in the 10–20 system and Table 16–2 lists the names of the electrode positions.

Table 16–2.
Nomenclature for the 10–20 System.

Scalp Leads

Brain Area	Left Hemisphere	Midline	Right Hemisphere
Frontal Pole	Fp1		Fp2
Frontal	F3		F4
Inferior Frontal	F7		F8
Mid-Frontal		Fz	
Mid-Temporal	T3		T4
Posterior Temporal	T5		T6
Central	C3		C4
Vertex or Mid-Central		Cz	
Parietal	P3		P4
Mid-Parietal		Pz	
Occipital	O1		O2

Non Scalp Leads (reference)

Auricular	A1		A2
Nasopharyngeal*	Pg1		Pg2

Note: * optional leads

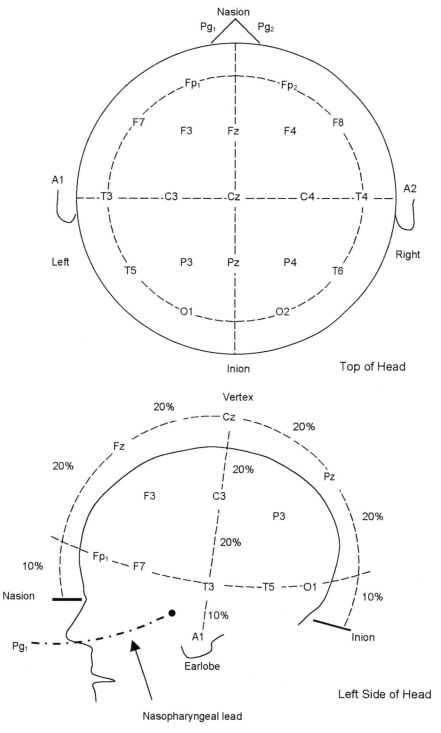

Figure 16–5. International 10–20 System Electrode Placement.

The use of the 10–20 system ensures reproducible electrode placement to allow more reliable comparison of EEGs from the same patient or different patients. Additional electrodes may be placed between a pair of adjacent electrodes to more accurately localize an event or abnormality.

Scalp-Electrode Impedance

As the EEG signal is of such low amplitude, the impedance of each electrode should be measured before every EEG recording. The impedance of each electrode should be between 100 Ω and 5 kΩ. Impedance below 100 Ω indicates short circuit set up by conductive gel between two electrodes. Impedance above 5 kΩ signals poor electrode skin contact. In practice, electrode impedance is usually measured using an ohmmeter by passing a small alternating current from one electrode through the scalp to all other connected electrodes. An alternating current of approximately 10 Hz is used to avoid electrode polarization and prevent measurement error due to DC offset potential. If only one pair electrodes are used, the impedance should be between 200 Ω and 10 kΩ. In addition, minimizing the differences in impedance at the different electrode sites can reduce EEG signal size variations.

EEG WAVEFORM CHARACTERISTICS

The peak to peak amplitude of EEG waveforms measured using scalp electrodes lies between 0 and 500 µV. A wide variety of EEG patterns can be seen in different persons of the same age. An even greater variation can be found in different age groups. An EEG is considered normal if there is no abnormal pattern known to be associated with clinical disorders. An EEG with no abnormal pattern does not guarantee the absence of problems as not all abnormalities of the brain produce abnormal EEG. Figure 16–6 shows an EEG recording with normal rhythm followed by a run of epileptic events.

The frequency of EEG waveforms can be divided into four frequency ranges–beta, alpha, theta, and delta. The frequency bandwidths, locations, and conditions of acquisitions of these four bands are listed in Table 16–3.

FUNCTIONAL BUILDING BLOCKS OF EEG MACHINES

A very basic single channel electroencephalograph is shown in Figure 16–7. In practice, an EEG machine for use in a diagnostic laboratory contains

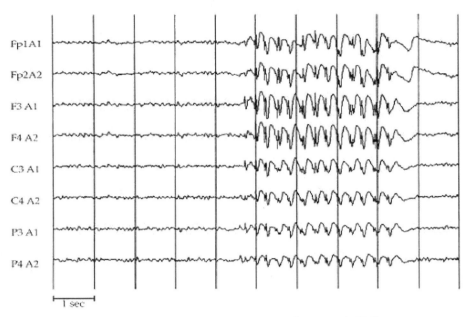

Figure 16–6. Normal and Abnormal (Epileptic) EEG.

Table 16–3.
Frequency of EEG Waves.

Waveform	Frequency (Hz)	Remarks
Beta Rhythm	13–30	Frontal-parietal leads Best when no alpha Prominent during mental activity
Alpha Rhythm	8–13	Parietal-occipital Awake and relaxed subject Prominent with eyes closed Disappear completely in sleep
Theta Rhythm	4–8	Parietal-temporal Children 2–5 years old Adults during stress or emotion
Delta Rhythm	0.5–4	Normal and deep sleep Children less than 1 year old Organic brain disease

more functions and options. Figure 16–7 shows the functional block diagram of a typical EEG machine. Their functions are discussed in this section.

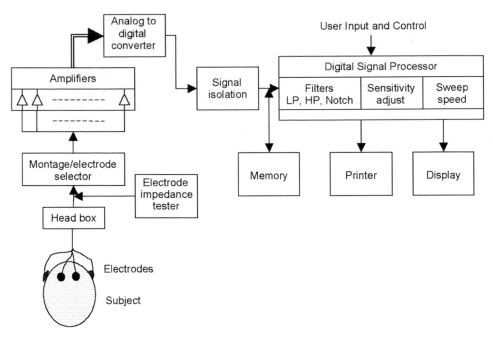

Figure 16–7. Functional Building Block of an EEG Machine.

Electrode Connections and Head Box

A head box is used to interface electrodes from the skull to the switching system. Each lead wire from the electrode applied to the skull is plugged into the corresponding location on the head box. An EEG referential head box for standard EEG application accepts 23 electrodes plus a few spares. The head box contains the first level of signal buffering and amplification to increase the signal level and provide a high input impedance to minimize common mode noise. Input impedance of a modern EEG machine is on the order of tens of MΩ.

Montage and Electrode Selector

Multichannel recordings are used to determine the distribution of electrical potential over the scalp. In order to gain insight into the activity at a given location, multiple differential signals from different combinations of electrode pairs are required. A montage consists of a distinct combination of differential signals of such multiple channel recordings.

Electrodes are attached in groups of 8 (or 10) in a montage. Because of this, EEG machines usually have 8 or 16 (or 10 or 20) differential amplifiers. There are two types of amplifier input connections:

1. Bipolar connection–measurements taken between two electrodes
2. Unipolar connection–all measurements have a common reference point

Figure 16–8 shows a unipolar connection. A common reference electrode for unipolar connection is the auricular or nasopharyngeal electrode. To facilitate grouping of electrodes, an electrode selection circuit is available at the front end of the EEG machine. Figure 16–9 is a diagrammatic representation of a multichannel electrode selector matrix. Any two electrodes can be switched to the input of any of the differential amplifiers. To facilitate diagnosis, certain electrode combinations are grouped together to form standard montages. Depending on the design, montage selection can be done digitally instead of using analog switches. Standard montages are usually built into EEG electrode selection function and can be programmed or modified by the user. Figure 16–10 shows the standard "referential" and "transverse bipolar" montages.

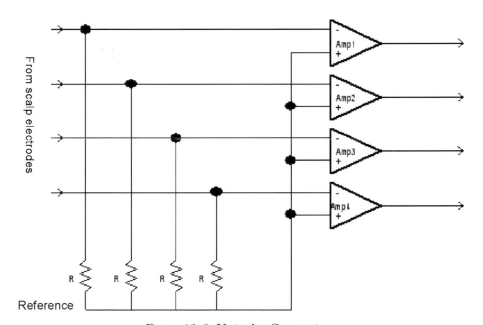

Figure 16–8. Unipolar Connection.

Amplifiers

The amplifier increases the signal level to the desired amplitude for the analog to digital converter and the display. Together with the digital processing circuit, it allows the operator to select a different level of sensitivities;

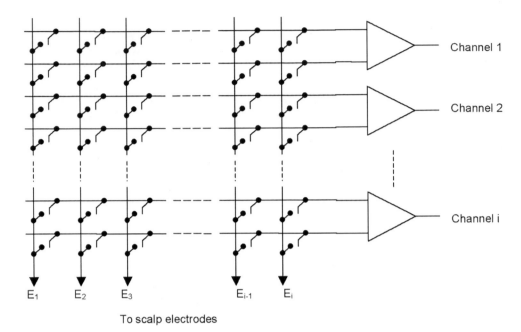

To scalp electrodes

Figure 16–9. Electrode Selection Matrix.

most EEG machines have two ranges of sensitivities: mV/cm or μV/mm. A common sensitivity setting for general applications is 7 μV/mm. Each channel of an EEG machine consists of a high gain differential amplifier with a gain of approximately 10,000. Depending on the number of channels, an EEG machine typically has 8, 10, 16, or 20 differential amplifiers.

Analog to Digital Converter

The ADC samples and converts the analog EEG signals to digital format so that they can be processed by the digital computer. Typical sampling rates is 1,000 samples/second with 12 bits (4,096 vertical steps) resolution.

Signal Isolation

The patient-connected parts are isolated from the power ground via optical isolators. Signal isolation prevents electric shocks (micro- and macroshocks) by reducing the amount of leakage current flowing to and from the patient.

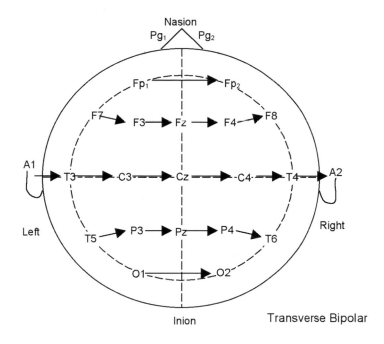

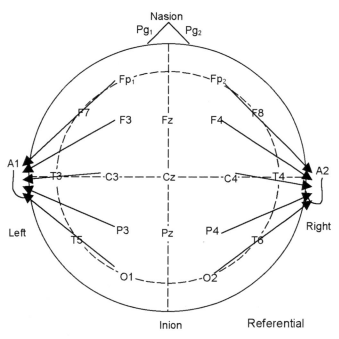

Figure 16–10. Transverse Bipolar and Referential Montages.

Filters

The signal bandwidths are individually selectable through software (older machines use analog filters). The high pass filter (low filter) is usually adjustable in steps from 0.1 to 30 Hz and the low pass filter (high filter) from 15 to 100 Hz. In addition, a notch filter (60 Hz in North America and 50 Hz in Europe and Asia) can be selected to reduce power frequency noise from line interference.

Sensitivity Control

Sensitivity of each channel can be adjusted individually to match the input signal amplitude and the output display. Typical sensitivity range is 2 to 150 µV/mm or 2 to 150 mV/cm. A sensitivity equalizer control allows verification of the accuracy of all channel sensitivities for the same input calibration signal.

Memory, Chart Speed, Display, and Recorder

Chart speeds of 10, 15, 30, and 60 mm/sec are supported in most machines. A mechanical paper chart recorder with ink styli on 11 × 17 inch fanfolded paper was used in older EEG machines. The huge volume of paper EEG records generated from each study used to create storage problems in EEG departments. With digital technology in the newer generation of machines, the EEG signals are stored in electronic memories and displayed on CRT or flat panel displays instead of written on paper. To further reduce the storage requirement, the neurologist may choose to remove nonpertinent EEG records and save only waveforms containing useful diagnostic information as patient records. To produce paper copies, laser printers are commonly used for digital EEG machines.

Electrode Impedance Tester

A small 10 Hz alternating current is used to measure the impedance of the electrode skin contacts. Electrode impedance testing is available on-demand in real-time modes on individual or all-channel basis. As discussed earlier, the impedance of a pair of electrodes should be between 200 Ω and 10 kΩ.

ERRORS AND PROBLEMS IN EEG RECORDING

EEG Artifacts

In EEG measurements, recorded signals that are noncerebral in origin are considered as artifacts. Artifacts can be either physiological or nonphysiological. Physiological artifacts arise from normal biopotential activities or movement activities of the patient. The primary sources of nonphysiological EEG artifacts include external electromagnetic interference and problems with the recording electrodes. While device hardware malfunction may cause problems, it is not a common source of EEG artifacts. Common sources of EEG artifacts are:

Artifacts due to physiological interference may result from:

- The heart potential results from either patient touching metal and creating second ground or pulsatile blood flow in brain
- Tongue and facial movement
- Eye movement
- Skeletal muscle movement (uncooperative patient or fine body tremors)
- Breathing
- High scalp impedance

Possible Solution:

- Must ensure that patient is calm; try to get him or her to relax

Artifacts due to electrode problems may result from:

- Improper electrode positioning
- Poor contact causing sharp irregular spikes, or the pickup of 60 Hz noise
- Electrodes not secured properly
- Dried-out electrode gel
- Oozing of tissue fluids in needle electrodes
- Frayed connections
- Sweat resulting in changing skin resistance

Possible Solution:

- Replace electrodes on scalp; ensure that electrode impedances are good (less than 10 kΩ between electrode pairs)

Artifacts due to electromagnetic interference (EMI) may result from:

- 60 Hz common-mode interference
- Radio frequency interference due to presence of electrical devices (e.g., an ESU)

- Defibrillation
- Presence of pacemakers and neural stimulators

Possible Solution:

- Look for proper grounding (no grounding or multiple ground loops) as well as shielding
- Remove sources of EMI
- Perform procedure in special EMI shielded room

Troubleshooting an EEG Problem

Troubleshooting EEG problems is similar to other troubleshooting scenarios having surface electrodes. Some common areas to look into are:

- Common-mode problems
- Problems compounded due to small signal levels (thousand times smaller than ECG)
- Problems with electrodes and leads (multiple)
- Use internal calibration control to check internal electronics and distinguish them from electrode problems
- Isolate problem to one channel, use internal calibration–if output is healthy, then electronics after calibration must be working properly
- For problems that happen with one channel only, can rule out common components such as power supply

Chapter 17

ELECTROMYOGRAPHY AND EVOKED POTENTIAL STUDIES

OBJECTIVES

- Explain EMG and EP studies.
- State clinical applications of EMG and EP studies.
- Sketch and explain a typical functional block diagram of an EMG/EP machine.
- Describe the constructions and applications of different types of surface and needle electrodes.
- Explain the characteristics of electrical activities from needle electrode examinations.
- Differentiate between motor response and sensory nerve action potential.
- Name common signal procession functions used in EMG/EP studies.
- Explain the purpose of signal averaging and how it can reduce noise level in EP studies.

CHAPTER CONTENTS

INTRODUCTION

In the previous chapter, the applications, signal acquisition, and functional building blocks of EEG were discussed. This chapter introduces electromyography (EMG) and evoked potential (EP) studies, which are other areas in electroneurophysiology. EMG studies the muscles and the nerves that innervate the muscles; EP studies look at the relationships between nerve stimulations and their responses.

CLINICAL APPLICATIONS OF EMG AND EP STUDIES

An EMG study may be used to establish the relationships between the signal morphology to the biomechanical variables. An example is comparing the biopotential signal frequency to muscle tension. In an EP study, a nerve may be stimulated by an electrical signal at one end and the reaction measured somewhere along the nerve itself to determine the time-location relationship between the stimulus and the response. Parameters such as nerve conduction velocity can also be determined.

There are two main areas of applications of EMG and EP studies: one is in kinesiology and the other in diagnostic.

In kinesiology, the main areas of interest are:

• Functional anatomy
• Force development
• Reflex connection of muscles

In electrodiagnostic, areas of analysis may involve:

• Creation of strength-duration curves to assess nerve and muscle integrity
• Determination of nerve conduction velocity to test for nerve damage or compression
• Analyzing firing characteristics of motor neurons and motor units, including analysis of motor unit action potentials (MUAPs) to detect signs of pathology such as fibrillation potentials and positive sharp waves

Figure 17–1 shows a typical configuration of an EMG/EP study. The EMG or EP is picked up by a pair of electrodes, one being the sensing electrode and the other acting as the reference. The signal is amplified, processed, and sent to a chart recorder. Depending on the type of studies, a stimulation signal may be applied.

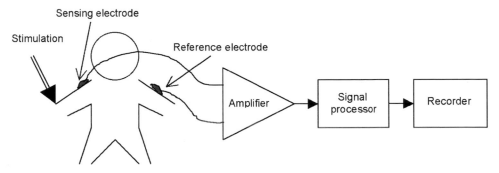

Figure 17–1. General Configuration of EMG/EP Recording.

ELECTRODES

A number of different electrodes may be used in EMG/EP measurements. The basic electrodes, including grounding, stimulating, and recording, are described next.

Grounding Electrode

As with all work involving electrical equipment, a ground electrode must be used. Grounding is essential for obtaining a response that is relatively free of artifact. In general, the ground electrode should be placed on the same extremity that is being investigated. The ground electrode in EP studies should be placed, if possible, halfway between the stimulating electrode and the active recording electrode. Usually the ground is a metal plate that is much larger than the recording electrodes and provides a large surface area of contact with the patient. Some clinicians may use a noninsulated needle inserted under the patient's skin. One should be careful not to apply more than one ground to the patient at any time. The presence of multiple grounds from different electrically powered devices can form "ground loops," which may create noise in the measurement.

Stimulating Electrode

In most cases, a peripheral nerve can be easily stimulated by applying the stimulus near the nerve. Therefore, most nerve stimulation is done to segments of nerve that lie close to the skin surface. Because of the need for proximity, the number of nerves accessible to the stimulation and the locations of the stimulation of that nerve are limited.

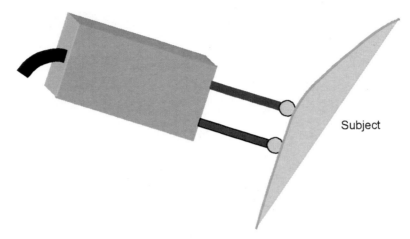

Figure 17–2. Stimulating Electrodes.

The stimulating electrodes are normally two metal or felt pads placed about 1 to 3 cm. apart (Figure 17–2). The electrodes are placed on the nerve with the cathode toward the direction in which the nerve is to conduct. The stimulation amplitude is adjusted until a maximal response is obtained and then by 25 to 50 percent more to ensure that the response is truly maximal. One may use a needle electrode to stimulate nerves deep beneath the skin. Other than electrical stimulation, visual or audible stimulations may be used in EP studies.

Recording Electrodes

Positioning of recording electrodes depends on the type of response being studied. In motor response recording, the active electrode is placed over the belly of the muscle being activated. This placement should be over the motor point to give an initial clear negative deflection (upward) in the response. In testing of sensory nerve, the active electrode is placed over the nerve itself to record the nerve action potential. The reference electrode is placed distal from the active electrode.

In motor response recording, surface electrodes may be used. Surface electrodes can be made of pure metal or Ag/AgCl in the shape of a circular disk of 0.5 to 1 cm in diameter. Surface electrodes such as flat buttons, spring clips, or rings are frequently used in sensory recording. However, bare-tip insulated needle electrodes placed close to the nerves are also used by many investigators. Some of the surface electrodes are shown below.

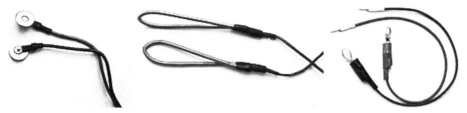

Figure 17–3. Surface Electrodes.

Needle Electrodes

Needle electrodes are commonly used in EMG/EP studies. They are used to evaluate individual motor units within a muscle to avoid picking up signals from other muscle units. The following paragraphs describe a few different types of needle electrodes.

A *monopolar needle electrode* has a very finely sharpened point and is covered with Teflon™ or other insulating material over its entire length, except for a tiny (e.g., 0.5 mm) exposure at the tip. The needle serves as the active electrode, and a surface electrode placed on the skin close to it serves as a reference. The main advantage of monopolar needle electrodes is that they are of small diameter and the Teflon™ covering allows them to easily insert into and withdraw from the muscle. Moving the needle causes less discomfort to the patient. However, repeated use of this electrode changes the size of the bare tip, thereby limiting the number of examinations for which it can be used. Because the active electrode tip and the surface electrode are separated by some distance, it is easier to pick up background noise from remote muscle contractions.

A *concentric needle electrode* consists of a cannula with an insulated wire inserted down the middle. The active electrode is the small tip of the center wire, and the reference electrode is the outside cannula. Concentric needles may have two central wires (bipolar), in which case the active and reference electrodes are at the tip and the outside cannula acts as the ground. Because the active and reference electrodes are closer together, only local motor unit

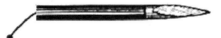

Figure 17–4. Monopolar Needle.

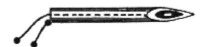

Figure 17–5. Concentric Needle.

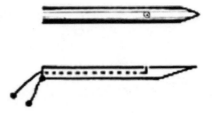

Figure 17–6. Single-Fiber Needle.

action potentials (MUAPs) are picked up by the electrode. Another advantage of this electrode is that no reference surface electrode is needed. The main disadvantage of the concentric electrode is that it has a larger diameter relative to other needle electrodes. Large diameter needle electrodes tend to cause more pain and are uncomfortable to move around.

Single-fiber needle electrodes are used for special studies. A single-fiber needle consists of a thin (e.g., 0.5 mm) stainless steel cannula with a fine (e.g., 25 µm) platinum wire inside its hollow shaft. The cut end of the platinum wire is exposed from a side opening near its tip.

SIGNAL CHARACTERISTICS

Most EMG signals have repetition frequencies in the range of 20 to 200 Hz. A single motor unit action potential (MUAP) has amplitude on the order of 100 µV and duration of 1 msec. The following paragraphs describe the electrical activities from needle electrode examinations.

The Muscle at Rest

Insertion Activity

Insertion activity is the response of the muscle fibers to needle electrode insertion. It consists of a brief series of muscle action potentials in the form of spikes. It is caused by mechanical stimulation or injury of muscle fibers, which may disappear immediately or shortly after (a few seconds) stopping needle movements.

Spontaneous Activity

Any activity beyond insertion constitutes spontaneous activity. It can be due the normal end plate noise, or to the presence of fasciculation (the ran-

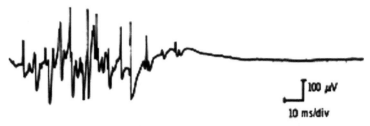

Figure 17–7. Needle Electrode Insertion Activity.

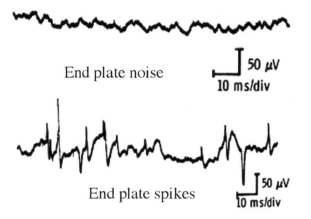

End plate noise

End plate spikes

Figure 17–8. Needle Electrode End Plate Noise.

dom, spontaneous twitching of a group of muscle fibers or a motor unit).

Spontaneous activity due to end plate noise when the needle is in the vicinity of a motor end plate can be monophasic (end plate noise) or biphasic (end plate spikes) potentials (a phase refers to the part of the wave between the departure and return to the baseline). The monophasic potentials are of low amplitude and short duration. The biphasic activity consists of irregular short duration biphasic spikes with amplitude of 100–300 µv.

The Muscle During Voluntary Effort

Voluntary activity can be divided into three stages of effort: mild, moderate, and full. Individual motor units can be studied with mild and moderate voluntary effort, while interference patterns are studied during full voluntary effort. Motor unit potentials are best studied with the same filter setting used for insertion and spontaneous activity (i.e., 16–32 Hz low cutoff and 8,000 Hz or more high cutoff frequency).

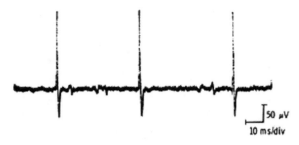

Figure 17–9. Mild Voluntary Effort.

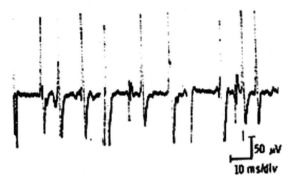

Figure 17–10. Moderate Voluntary Effort.

Mild Effort

Only a few motor units are observed at this stage. These are the smaller motor units as they are the ones to be recruited first. Amplitude, duration, and number of phases of individual motor units are measured.

Moderate Effort

The frequency and recruitment of motor units are best assessed during this stage. Motor units seen at this stage are larger than those seen with mild effort. As muscle effort increases, motor unit firing rates are increased and new motor units are recruited.

Full Effort

At maximum contraction, it is difficult to distinguish individual motor units as the firing rates are high and many motor units are recruited. When all the motor units are recruited a complete interference pattern is observed.

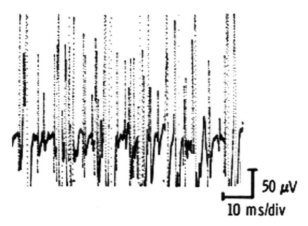

Figure 17–11. Full Voluntary Effort.

Motor Responses

A motor response is obtained by stimulating a nerve and recording from a muscle that it innervates. The muscle selected should have a fairly well-defined motor point and be isolated from other muscles innervated by the same nerve. The excitation of nearby muscles may alter the response and make it difficult to determine the exact onset of the desired motor response. A motor response may be characterized by its amplitude, duration, and wave form. The amplitude is measured from the baseline to the top of the negative peak (upward) of the motor response. The latency is measured from the onset of the stimulus to the point of takeoff from the baseline. In motor response studies, it is important to ensure maximal motor response by using supramaximal stimulation of the nerve (i.e., using 15 to 20 percent more than the minimum level of stimulation). The number and size of muscle fibers

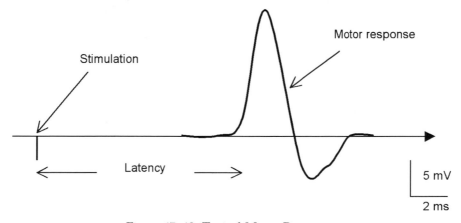

Figure 17–12. Typical Motor Response.

being activated determine the amplitude of the response. Decrease in the number of motor units or muscle fibers responding will affect the amplitude. The usual motor response has a fairly simple waveform. It may have one or two initial negative (up) peaks (the latter usually indicating two muscle being stimulated) and usually will be followed by a positive deflection (down) toward the end. If there is dispersion of the times when the motor units discharge, then the amplitude will be lowered and the response spread in time. The motor response also changes in relationship to the point of nerve stimulation. The more proximally the nerve is stimulated, the lower the amplitude and the longer the duration of responses.

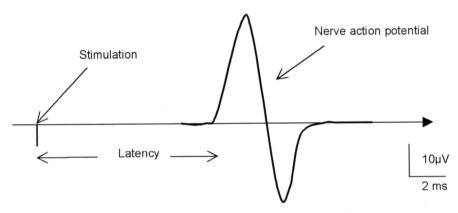

Figure 17–13. Typical Nerve Action Potential.

Sensory-Nerve Action Potentials

Sensory-nerve action potentials (NAPs) are obtained by stimulating a nerve and recording directly from it or one of its branches. The recording site must be remote from muscles innervated by that same nerve because muscle responses will obscure the much smaller NAP.

A NAP is characterized by its amplitude, duration, and wave form. The amplitude of the NAP is measured from the peak of the positive deflection to the peak of the negative deflection. The sensory distal latency is traditionally measured from the stimulus artifact to the takeoff or the peak of the negative deflection. When conduction velocities are calculated, the same takeoff of the proximal and distal responses should be used to determine the latency. The amplitude depends on the number of axons being stimulated and the synchrony with which they transmit their impulses. If the axons transmit impulses at comparable velocities, the response duration will be short and its amplitude high. However, if the axonal velocities are widely dispersed, the NAP duration will be longer and its amplitude lower.

Conduction Velocity

Conduction velocities can be determined by stimulating a nerve at two points and measuring the distance between those points. This method can eliminate the neuromuscular transmission time and is used for most motor nerves. In sensory studies, however, only one stimulation site is normally used. The conduction velocity (v) can be computed by measuring the distance (d) in millimeters (mm) between the two recording points and dividing it by the difference in latency (ms) between the proximal (t_p) and distal recording points (t_d), as indicated in this equation:

$$v = \frac{d}{t_d - t_p}, \text{ the result is expressed as meters per second (m/sec.).}$$

Conduction velocities are different in different nerves due to different anatomical conditions. However, several general principles apply to nerve conduction studies:

- The more proximal the segment of nerve being evaluated, the faster the velocity will be.
- If the extremity being tested is cold, the velocity will be slowed and the amplitude increased. This effect occurs especially in cold weather, and some provisions for warming the patient and using a fairly constant room temperature should be made.
- The shorter the segment between the two stimulation or recording points, the less reliable the calculated velocities will be, due to a greater effect on the margin of error by a shorter distance.
- Conduction velocities depend mostly on the integrity of the myelin sheath. In segmental demyelinating diseases, conduction velocities may drop to below 50% of normal values. Axonal loss will slow down the conduction velocity. Conduction velocity drop due to axonal loss is usually in the vicinity of 30% of normal values.

MACHINE SETTINGS

In studying sensory and motor responses, different filter, sweep speed, and sensitivity settings are used. Sensory studies are performed with the low frequency setting between 32 and 50 Hz and the high between 1.6 and 3 kHz. The sweep speed is set to 2 ms/div and the sensitivity at 10–20 µV/div. Motor studies are performed with the low frequency set to 16–32 Hz and the high frequencies to 8–10 kHz. Depending on the response's latency and duration, the sweep speed can be set to anywhere between 2 and 5 ms/div and the sensitivity between 2 and 10 mV/div.

SIGNAL PROCESSING

Signal processing plays an important role in EMG/EP studies. Described next are some signal processing functions commonly found in EMG/EP machines.

Filtering

Filters are used to eliminate unwanted signals such as electrical noise and movement artifact. The frequency spectrum of muscle action potentials lies between 2 Hz and 10 kHz. In practice, a band pass filter of 20 Hz to 8 kHz is often used because motion artifacts have frequencies less than 10 Hz and a high cutoff frequency is necessary to remove high-frequency noise.

Rectification and Integration

Because the raw signal is biphasic or polyphasic, a rectifier is sometime used to "flip" the signal's negative content across the zero axis, making the whole signal positive. Integration is used to calculate the area under the curve for quantization and comparison.

Amplification

A single MUAP has an amplitude of about 100 μV; signals detected by surface electrodes are in the range of 5 mV; signals detected by indwelling electrodes are in the range of 10 mV. All these signals must be amplified before they can be further processed. If a 1 V amplitude signal is required for the signal processor, an amplifier with a gain of 100 to 10,000 is necessary. Differential amplifiers with high common mode rejection ratio are used to minimize induced electrical noise, including 60 Hz power frequency noise, which is within the bandwidth of the signal. In addition, the impedance of the front-end amplifiers must be considerably higher than the impedance of the electrode/skin or electrode/muscle interfaces. Since indwelling electrodes have very high impedances (due to low surface area), very high amplifier input impedances (e.g., >100 MΩ) are necessary.

Spectral Analysis

Because EMG signal is actually a summation of MUAPs, some close and some at a distance from the recording electrodes, it is difficult to know which motor units contribute to the signal. In trying to differentiate normal from abnormal waveforms, some investigators, using spectral analysis, have tried to divide the signal's components into its constituent frequencies.

Signal Averaging

Signal averaging is a technique used in EP studies to extract the low amplitude evoked response from noise. The amplitude of the evoked nerve response is on the order of μV, while noise can be on the order of mV. This technique assumes that noise is random and that the evoked responses at the same location from identical stimulations are the same. Instead of recording the nerve response from a single stimulus, multiple nerve responses are recorded from repeating the same stimulation periodically over a period of time. The response from each stimulus is stored and the average is computed by an analog or digital computer. As all the nerve responses are the same, averaging will produce the same response. However, averaging random noise will reduce or eliminate the noise superimposing on the signal. In practice, an evoked potential is acquired from averaging 16 or more evoked responses.

Chapter 18

INVASIVE BLOOD PRESSURE MONITORS

OBJECTIVES

- Explain the origin of blood pressure waveform.
- Analyze the relationships between the blood pressure waveform and the cardiac cycle.
- Compare the magnitude and shape of the blood pressure waveform at different locations in the cardiovascular system.
- Describe the clinical setup for invasive blood pressure (IBP) monitoring.
- Sketch the block diagram of a typical IBP monitor.
- Explain the construction and characteristics of a resistive strain gauge blood pressure transducer.
- Define systolic, diastolic, and mean blood pressure and explain the principle of detecting these parameters.
- Identify common problems and potential sources of error in IBP measurement.

CHAPTER CONTENTS

1. Introduction
2. Origin of Blood Pressure
3. Blood Pressure Waveforms
4. Arterial Blood Pressure Monitoring Setup
5. Functional Building Blocks of an Invasive Blood Pressure Monitor
6. Common Problems and Causes of Errors

INTRODUCTION

The earliest attempt to record arterial blood pressure was performed in 1773 by Stephen Hales, a British scientist. Hales used an open-ended tube with one end inserted into an artery in the neck of a horse and the other end held at a high level (Figure 18–1). The blood from the horse rose to about 8 feet in the tube above the arterial insertion site and fluctuated by 2 to 3 inches between heartbeats. From the experiment, Hales was able to determine the blood pressure of the horse using the equation $P = \rho g h$ where ρ is the density of the blood, g the acceleration due to gravity, and h the height of the blood column. This chapter explores the principles and instrumentations of invasive blood pressure measurements in clinical settings. Although only blood pressure measurement is discussed, the same principle and, in fact, similar instrumentations are used in other physiological pressure measurements such as bladder pressure and intracranial pressure.

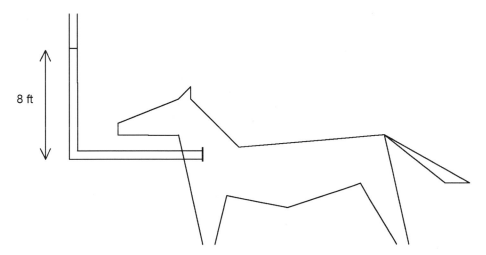

Figure 18–1. Hales's Experiment to Measure Arterial Blood.

ORIGIN OF BLOOD PRESSURE

In humans, circulation of blood is achieved by the pumping action of the heart. Atrial contraction pushes the blood from the right atrium through the tricuspid valve into the right ventricle and from the left atrium through the mitral valve into the left ventricle. The positive pressure created by the contraction of the ventricles forces blood to flow from the left ventricle through the aortic valve into the common aorta and from the right ventricle through the pulmonary valve into the pulmonary arteries (Figure 18–2). The blood from the aorta travels through the arteries and eventually reaches the capillaries, where oxygen and nutrients are delivered to the tissues and carbon dioxide and other metabolic wastes are diffused from the cells into the blood. This deoxygenated blood is collected by the veins and returned to the right atrium of the heart via the superior and inferior vena cavae. Contraction of the right atrium followed by the right ventricle delivers the deoxygenated blood to the lungs. Gaseous exchange takes place in the capillaries covering the alveoli of the lungs. Carbon dioxide is removed and oxygen is added to the blood. This oxygenated blood collected flows into the left atrium via the pulmonary veins and then into the left ventricle to start another round-trip in the cardiovascular system.

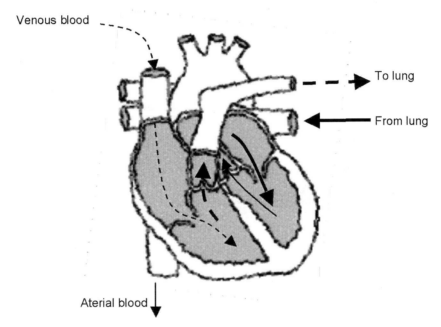

Figure 18–2. The Heart and Circulatory System.

The heart is the center of the cardiovascular system creating the pumping force. Every contraction of the heart produces an elevated pressure to push blood flow through the blood vessels. Relaxation of the heart allows blood to return to the heart chambers. Blood pressure within the cardiovascular system fluctuates in synchrony with the heart rhythm. The maximum pressure within a cardiac cycle is called systolic blood pressure, while the lowest is called the diastolic blood pressure. Blood pressure measured in an artery is called arterial pressure and pressure measured in a vein is called venous pressure. Although the S.I. unit of pressure is Pascal (Pa), the unit of blood pressure commonly used is still in millimeter mercury (mmHg). Figure 18–3 illustrates the timing of the cardiac cycle showing the blood pressures in the left ventricle, left atrium, and the common aorta. The pressure in the left ventricle starts to rise when the heart contracts (corresponding to the QRS complex of the ECG). When the blood pressure in the ventricle is above the pressure in the common aorta, the aortic valve opens, allowing blood to flow from the left ventricle into the aorta and then to the arteries. During the time when the aortic valve is open, the pressure in the common aorta is virtually the same as that in the ventricle. After the contraction, the heart relaxes, causing the ventricular pressure to drop rapidly. The pressure drop in the common aorta is slower than that in the ventricle due to the back-pressure from downstream and the elasticity of the blood vessels. As the pressure in the left ventricle falls below the pressure in the common aorta, the aortic valve (which is a one-way valve) closes, hence separating the left ventricle from the common aorta. The blood pressure in the common aorta fluctuates.

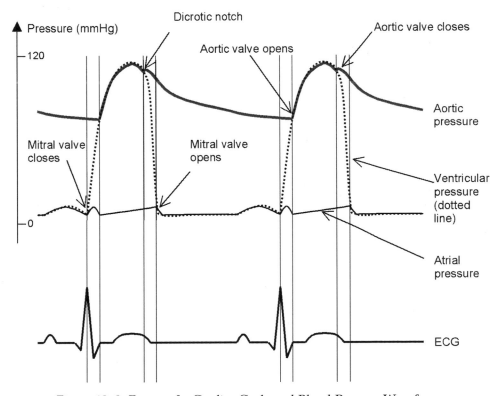

Figure 18–3. Events of a Cardiac Cycle and Blood Pressure Waveforms.

BLOOD PRESSURE WAVEFORMS

As the arterial blood flows into smaller blood vessels, the average (mean) pressure as well as the magnitude of fluctuations (difference between systolic and diastolic pressure) drop due to friction and viscosity. Arterial blood pressure eventually reaches its lowest level in the capillaries. Venus blood pressure is the lowest just before it enters the right atrium. Figure 18–4 shows the values of typical mean, systolic, and diastolic blood pressure measured at different locations in the cardiovascular system. Since the left ventricle is the primary pumping device in the cardiovascular system, the blood pressure is elevated from the lowest level at the inlet of the left atrium to almost the highest as it leaves the left ventricle.

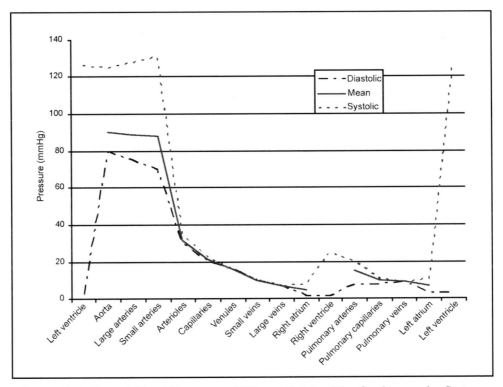

Figure 18–4. Typical Blood Pressure at Different Points of the Cardiovascular System.

Figure 18–5 shows a typical blood pressure waveform. Note that the blood pressure is referenced to the atmospheric pressure and does not go negative. Each cycle of fluctuation corresponds to one cardiac cycle. The characteristic dicrotic notch is a result of the momentum of blood flow and the elasticity of the blood vessels. When the pressure inside the ventricle is lower than that in the common aorta, the aortic valve closes and suddenly stops blood from flowing out of the left ventricle. The blood flow continues for a brief moment right after the valve closure due to the momentum of the blood velocity. This flow creates a transient pressure reduction in the aorta as well as in all arteries. The dicrotic notch is less noticeable in smaller arteries and disappears altogether in the capillaries. Within a cardiac cycle, the blood pressure goes from a minimum to a maximum. The maximum pressure is called the systolic pressure (P_S), while the minimum is the diastolic pressure (P_D). The mean blood pressure (P_M) is determined by integrating the blood pressure waveform over one cycle and dividing the integral by the period (T).

$$P_M = \frac{1}{T}\int_0^T P(t)dt.$$

In some older blood pressure monitors, the mean blood pressure is approximated by the equation:

$$P_M \approx P_D + \frac{1}{3}(P_S - P_D).$$

Figure 18–6 shows typical blood pressure waveforms at different locations of the cardiovascular system.

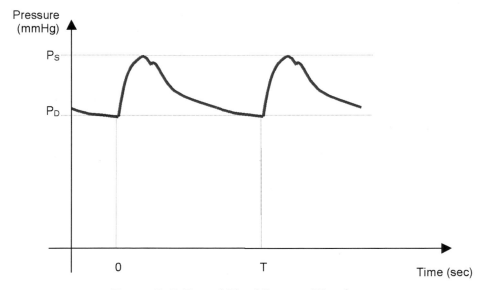

Figure 18–5. Typical Blood Pressure Waveform.

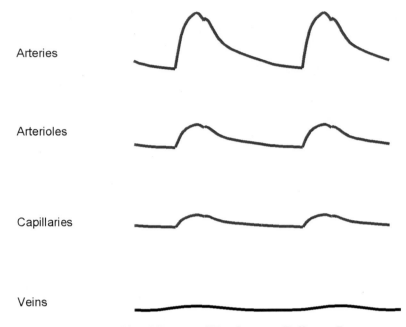

Figure 18–6. Blood Pressure Waveforms at Different Points
of the Cardiovascular System.

ARTERIAL BLOOD PRESSURE MONITORING SETUP

A typical arterial blood pressure monitoring setup is shown in Figure 18–7. Instead of inserting a pressure transducer into the blood vessel, it employs a less invasive approach by coupling a liquid column between an external pressure transducer and the blood in the vessel. In this commonly used invasive blood pressure monitoring setup, a catheter is inserted into an artery (or a vein if venous pressure is monitored), and an arterial pressure extension tube filled with saline is connected to the catheter. This setup is often referred to as the arterial line. The other end of the extension tube is connected to a pressure transducer. The transducer, which converts the pressure signal to an electrical signal, is connected to a pressure monitor to display the blood pressure waveform and the systolic, mean, and diastolic pressure values. To prevent blood clot at the tip of the catheter inside the blood vessel (blood clot will block the pressure signal from reaching the transducer), a bag of heparinized saline is connected to the extension tube. The bag is pressurized (to about 150 mmHg) to above the blood pressure in the vessel. Together with the continuous flush valve at the transducer set, this setup produces a slow continuous flow of heparinized saline flushing the catheter to prevent blood clot. The flow is very slow (less than 5 ml/hr) to avoid creating a pressure drop in the extension tube and catheter setup; otherwise it will affect the accuracy of blood pressure measurement. The rapid flush valve is used during initial setup to flush and fill the extension tube before it is connected to the indwelling catheter.

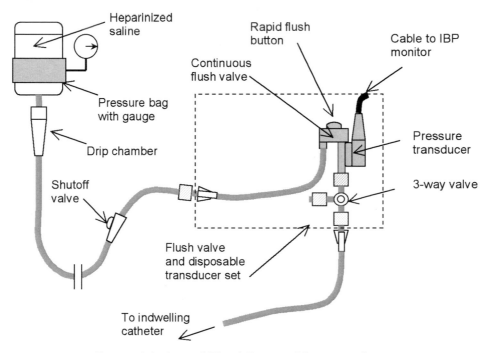

Figure 18–7. Arterial Blood Pressure Monitoring Setup.

The equivalent hydraulic circuit of the arterial line setup is shown in Figure 18–8a. In the setup, the patient port (which is the location of the catheter) is h meter above the transducer port (the point where the liquid in the extension tube interfaces with the pressure transducer). Therefore, the pressure P_x as seen by the transducer is the sum of the pressure due to the liquid column and the pressure P_P at the patient port (blood pressure of the patient), i.e.,

$$P_x = P_P + \rho gh, \tag{1}$$

where ρ is the density of the liquid in the extension tube and g is the acceleration due to gravity. This equation shows that the pressure as seen by the transducer is higher than the actual blood pressure by the product ρgh. Figure 18–8b shows the concept of introducing an offset P_0 to compensate for this overpressure phenomenon. The zeroing process performed during the initial setup is designed to allow the machine to determine the value of this offset.

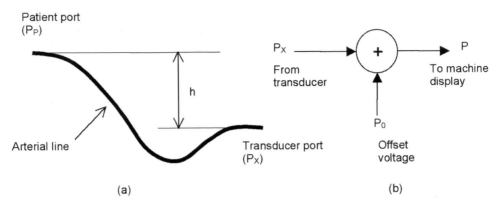

Figure 18–8. Zeroing of Blood Pressure Monitor.

From the compensation circuit and equation (1),

$$P = P_x + P_0 = P_P + \rho gh + P_0. \qquad (2)$$

During the initial zeroing process, the patient port is open to the atmosphere so that P_P becomes zero. Equation (2) therefore becomes

$$P = \rho gh + P_0. \qquad (3)$$

While the patient port is still exposed to atmospheric pressure, the operation invokes the zeroing sequence of the blood pressure monitor telling the monitor that this reading corresponds to zero pressure (i.e., P = atmospheric pressure = 0, or zero gauge pressure). Equation (3) now becomes

$$0 = \rho gh + P_0 \Rightarrow P_0 = -\rho gh.$$

The blood pressure monitor saves this value of P_0 in memory and exits the zeroing sequence. The operator then closes the patient port. The blood pressure monitor applies this offset to the transducer reading during subsequent pressure measurements. As long as the vertical height difference between the transducer port and patient port remains the same, the monitor will always display the true blood pressure of the patient. However, if the transducer is lowered (or the patient port is raised) after zeroing, the monitor will over-read the pressure (for every 2.5 cm decrease in the height difference, the pressure is over-read by 2 mmHg). The zeroing process will also compensate for any other constant offsets in the system, including offset from the pressure transducer.

Example

A patient is undergoing invasive blood pressure monitoring. the arterial line was zeroed at setup. The patient's systolic pressure and diastolic pressure were 125 and 80 mmHg, respectively. If the patient bed is raised by 4.0 inches (4.0 × 0.0254 = 0.10 m) while the level of the transducer remains the same, what will the pressure readings be?

Solution

Using the equation $P_0 = \rho gh$ and assuming the density of the saline in the extension tube has a density of 1,020 Kg/m^3, raising the patient by 4 inches (4.0 × 0.0254 = 0.10 m) will increase the offset pressure by

$$P_0 = 1{,}020 \text{ kg/m}^3 \times 9.8 \text{ m/s}^2 \times 0.10 \text{ m} = 1{,}000 \text{ Pa} = 7.5 \text{ mmHg.}$$

The blood pressure reading therefore becomes 132.5 and 87.5 mmHg.

In most prepackaged disposable transducers, the zero ports are attached to the transducers. In order to properly zero the system, the setup procedure requires that the zero port be located at the same level as the patient's heart. Instead of opening the patient port to the atmosphere during the zeroing process, the zero port attached to the transducer is open to the atmosphere. In this case, after correct zeroing, the monitor will display the blood pressure at the level of the patient's heart.

FUNCTIONAL BUILDING BLOCKS OF AN INVASIVE BLOOD PRESSURE MONITOR

Figure 18–9 shows a typical functional block diagram of an invasive blood pressure monitor. The following paragraphs describe the functions of each building block.

Transducer

The pressure transducer of an invasive blood pressure monitor converts the pressure signal to an electrical signal. Ideally, the transducer should have a linear characteristic with adequate frequency response to handle the rate of pressure fluctuations.

Figure 18–10a shows the cross-sectional view of a four-wired resistive strain gauge pressure transducer. The central floating block is connected to the four pretensioned strain wires with the other ends of the wires connect-

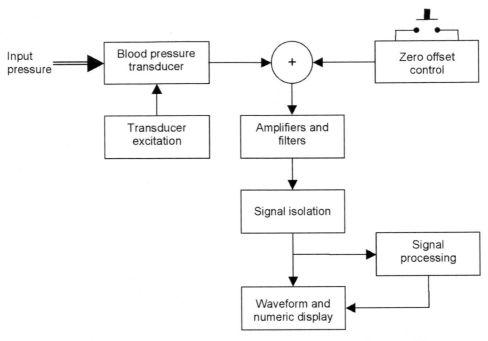

Figure 18–9. Functional Block Diagram of an Invasive Blood Pressure Monitor.

ed to the stationary frame of the transducer. The diaphragm in contact with the fluid chamber (or pressure dome) is mechanically connected to the central floating block by a rigid connecting rod. The blood pressure to be measured is transmitted via saline in the extension tube to the fluid chamber, forcing the diaphragm to move according to the pressure fluctuation. As the diaphragm moves, the strain wires will extend or retract according to the movement. The strain wires are connected in a bridge format with the electrical equivalent diagram as shown in Figure 18–10b.

For a higher applied pressure, strain wires 1 and 2 are stretched while 3 and 4 are relaxed. As a result, the resistance of the strain wires 1 and 2 (shown in the equivalent circuit) become higher while 3 and 4 become less. If an excitation voltage V_E is applied to the bridge, the output voltage V_o will vary according to the applied pressure. Although V_E is shown to be a DC voltage, AC excitation may be used. The sensitivity of a pressure transducer is often expressed in output voltage per unit pressure (e.g., 10 mV/mmHg) or in output voltage per unit excitation voltage per unit pressure (e.g., 2 mV/V/mmHg).

In older systems or systems using reusable transducers, resistive strain gauge or piezoelectric element transducers are used. Nowadays, disposable transducers using semiconductor piezoresistive strain gauges are commonly used. These transducers are mass-produced using semiconductor fabrication

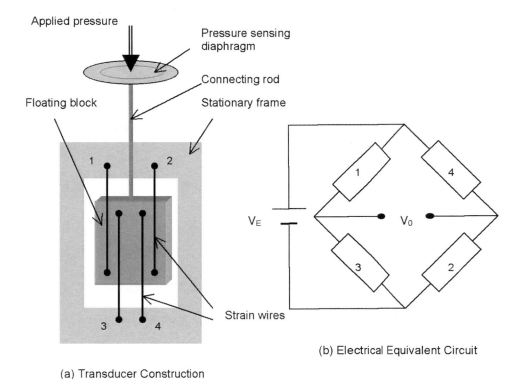

(a) Transducer Construction

Figure 18–10. Resistive Strain Gauge Pressure Transducer.

technology, which yields consistent performance at low cost. Disposable IBP transducers are prepackaged with the extension tube, flush valves, and connectors for single patient use.

The sensitivity of a disposable blood pressure transducer as specified in the AAMI Standards BP22 and BP23 is 5 µV/V/mmHg ± 1% when an excitation voltage of 4 to 8 V, DC to 5 kHz is used. This allows interchangeability of blood pressure transducers across different manufacturers of compatible blood pressure monitors.

Example

A special-purpose reusable pressure transducer has an output sensitivity of 2.0 mV/V/mmHg. If an applied pressure of $P = 200$ mmHg is applied and the excitation V_E is a 5.0 V peak to peak 100 Hz sinusoidal voltage source, what is the output voltage of the transducer?

Solution

Since

$$V_0 = \text{sensitivity} \times V_E \times P.$$

The transducer output voltage V_0 is calculated by:

$$V_0 = 2.0 \text{ mV/V/mmHg} \times 5.0 \text{ V}_{\text{p-p}} \times 100 \text{ mmHg} = 1{,}000 \text{ mV}_{\text{p-p}} \text{ or } 1.0 \text{ V}_{\text{p-p}}$$

The output voltage in this case is also 100 Hz sinusoid.

Zero Offset

The zero offset functional block is used during the zeroing procedure to determine and store the zero offset value. During blood pressure monitoring, this stored value is used to compensate for the offset due to the static pressure of the setup and the offset of the transducer circuit. For microprocessor-based machines, the zero offset value is stored digitally.

Amplifiers and Filters

For a systolic pressure of 120 mmHg, a standard disposable transducer (sensitivity = 5 μV/V/mmHg) with an excitation of 5 V produces an output of 3,000 μV or 3 mV; such small voltage must be amplified before it can be used by other parts of the monitor. Instrumentation amplifiers with high input impedance and high common mode rejection ratio are used for this purpose.

The fundamental frequency of the blood pressure waveform is the same as the heart rate (which is about 1 Hz). However, spectral analysis of a typical arterial blood pressure waveform (Figure 8–11b) shows a bandwidth from DC to about 10 Hz (Figure 8–11b). In order to reduce higher frequency artifacts and interferences, a low pass filter with a high cutoff frequency of 20 to 50 Hz is often built into the front-end analog circuit of the monitor.

Signal Isolation

Invasive blood pressure monitoring requires external access to major blood vessels. Both the saline solution in the arterial line and the blood in the artery conduct electricity. This setup forms a conduction path between the electromedical device and the patient's heart. The blood pressure monitor may become the source or sink of the risk current flowing through the heart. Signal isolation to break the conduction path is required to minimize the risk of electrical shock (both macro- and microshocks) to the patient.

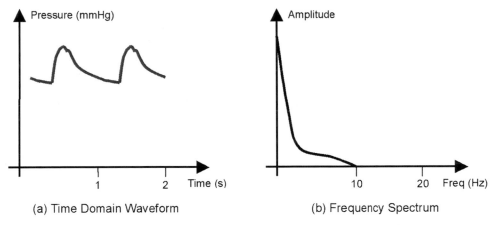

Figure 18–11. Frequency Spectrum of Blood Pressure Waveform.

Signal Processing

From the blood pressure waveform, the systolic, mean, and diastolic blood pressures are determined. In addition, the patient's heart rate can be derived as the frequency of the pressure cycle is the same as the cardiac cycle. The systolic blood pressure is obtained by using a peak detector circuit (Figure 18–12a). In order to track the fluctuating systolic pressure, a pair of peak detectors arranged in a sample and hold configuration are used. The diastolic pressure can be found by first inverting the pressure waveform and then finding the peak of this inverted waveform. Mean blood pressure is obtained using a low pass filter circuit (Figure 18–12b).

In modern monitors, the blood pressure waveform is sampled and converted to digital signal. Systolic, mean, and diastolic pressures are determined by software algorithm in the microprocessor.

Display

Liquid crystal displays (LCDs) have been replacing cathode ray tubes (CRTs) in recent years as the display of choice for medical waveform displays. In addition to waveforms, numeric information is also displayed on the medical monitor.

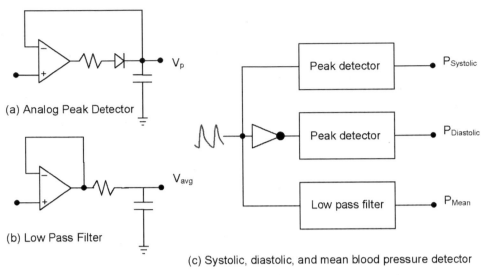

(a) Analog Peak Detector

(b) Low Pass Filter

(c) Systolic, diastolic, and mean blood pressure detector

Figure 18–12. Blood Pressure Detection from Pressure Waveform.

COMMON PROBLEMS AND CAUSES OF ERRORS

Problems in an invasive blood pressure measurement system may produce inaccurate pressure readings or distorted blood pressure waveform. These erroneous signals may cause improper diagnosis, leading to inappropriate medical intervention. Some common sources of errors are described next.

Setup Error

The most common problem in this category relates to the zeroing process. Incorrect zeroing procedure or change in vertical distance between the transducer and measurement site after initial setup produces a constant static pressure error in the measurement. It is important for the clinician to correctly perform the zeroing procedure, understand the principles, and be aware of the implications from setup variations.

Catheter Error

Although there is no active component in the catheter and it seems to be a very simple part of the blood pressure monitoring system, many artifacts and measurement errors may arise from the catheter. Some of the common problems are described next.

End pressure, whipping, and impact artifacts—The catheter in blood pressure monitoring is a small flexible tube inserted into a blood vessel with pulsating blood flow (Figure 18–13). If the blood is flowing in the same direction of the catheter, it creates a small negative pressure at the end of the catheter tip. In contrast, blood flowing toward the catheter tip will create a net positive pressure. The flow of blood may create turbulence and set the catheter tip into whipping motion. Movement of the catheter may cause it to collide with the vessel wall or valves. Whipping motion and impact of the catheter may show up as distortion in the blood pressure waveform.

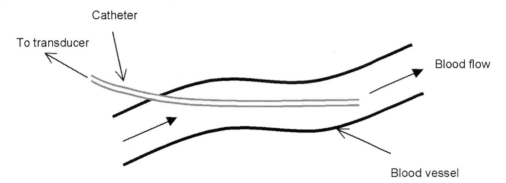

Figure 18–13. Catheter in Blood Vessel.

Air bubble, pinching, and leak—Another area of pressure waveform distortions is caused by the reduction of the frequency response of the catheter-extension tube. An air bubble in the catheter or fluid-filled extension tube reduces the cutoff frequency of the high pass filter formed by the hydraulic circuit. Pinching the line or having a leak in the line has a similar effect. Such problems in the system will attenuate the high-frequency component of the blood pressure waveform. Figure 18–14 shows the effect of such problems on the frequency response of a catheter.

Blood Clot

The purpose of the pressured infusion bag is to prevent a blood clot occurring at the tip of the catheter in the blood vessel. A total blood clot will block the transmission of the pressure signal to the transducer. A blood clot will diminish the amplitude fluctuation (difference in systolic and diastolic pressure) and lower the high-frequency response of the setup. Periodic

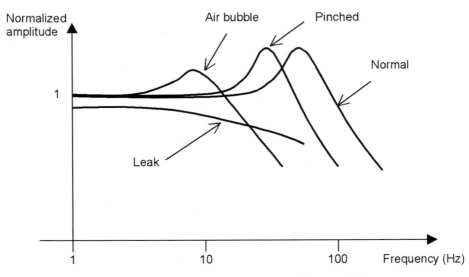

Figure 18–14. Frequency Response of Catheter Setup.

inspection of the drip chamber attached to the infusion bag to ensure a continuous flow of the heparinized saline will prevent clotting.

Transducer Calibration

Due to stringent manufacturing processes, there is no need to perform field verification of the accuracy of single-use disposable blood pressure transducers. However, blood pressure monitors must be checked periodically to ensure that they are functioning properly with amplification and frequency response according to manufacturers' specifications. In practice, a simulator is used to provide a known input to the monitor and the output is measured and compared with the specifications.

For reusable pressure transducers, a known pressure source is used to determine the sensitivity of the transducer. Most pressure monitors have a calibration factor (F) adjustment to compensate for sensitivity drift of the transducers. A simple procedure to obtain the calibration factor of a particular transducer is:

1. Apply a known pressure (P_i) to the transducer and read the pressure display (P_d) on the monitor.
2. Calculate the calibration factor by using the equation $F = \dfrac{P_i}{P_d}$.
3. Input the value of F into the calibration factor adjustment input of the monitor.
4. The monitor is now calibrated to use with this particular transducer.

Example

A 200 mmHg pressure source is used as input to determine the calibration factor of the monitor with a reusable pressure transducer. If the pressure reading of the monitor is 190 mmHg, what is the calibration factor?

Solution

Using $F = \dfrac{P_i}{P_d}$, the calibration factor is $F = \dfrac{200}{190} = 1.05$.

Hardware Problems

As with all medical devices, there is always a possibility of component failure. It is important that users be able to differentiate between normal and abnormal performance of the monitoring system. Many monitors have built-in simple test procedures to allow the users to verify the function and performance of the system. In order to ensure that the monitor is functioning according to standards or manufacturers' specifications, periodic performance verification inspections by qualified professionals are required to detect nonobvious problems such as component parameter drifts.

Chapter 19

NONINVASIVE BLOOD
PRESSURE MONITORS

OBJECTIVES

- Identify the components of a sphygmomanometer.
- Describe the principles of operation and the limitations of using a manual auscultatory method to measure systolic and diastolic blood pressure.
- Differentiate the auscultatory and oscillometric methods employed in automatic NIBP measurement.
- Describe the principles of operation and limitations of NIBP measurement using the oscillometric method.
- Identify the functional building blocks of a typical oscillometric NIBP monitor.
- Explain the principles of using Doppler ultrasound and tonometry in NIBP monitoring.

CHAPTER CONTENTS

1. Introduction
2. Auscultatory Method
3. Oscillometric Method
4. Other Methods of NIBP Measurement

INTRODUCTION

Blood pressure, an important physiological parameter, is measured routinely throughout the course of nearly all medical procedures and diagnosis. While one may measure blood pressure accurately using the invasive technique described in the previous chapter, being able to measure blood pressure noninvasively is a tremendous achievement made possible by the combination of creativity and technology.

In 1876, E. J. Marey, a French physiologist, performed the first experiment using counterpressure to measure blood pressure. Marey was investigating the interaction between the arterial pulsatile pressure with an applied external pressure. He had his assistant place his hand into a jar filled with water; the jar was sealed at the wrist. The pressure in the jar was increased incrementally and the pressure oscillation in the jar was measured at each pressure increment. Marey noticed that when the jar pressure was slightly above the systolic pressure, all the blood was driven out of the hand and no pressure oscillation was detected. He further noticed that the amplitude of oscillation began to rise as the jar pressure dropped below the systolic pressure, reached at maximum, and decreased as the pressure was further reduced. This method has since evolved into the oscillometric method of noninvasive blood pressure (NIBP) measurement–the most popular method to noninvasively measure blood pressure. The auscultatory method was introduced in 1905 by J. S. Korotkoff.

Although results from NIBP measurement may not be as accurate as invasive methods, NIBP measurement is easy, nonhazardous, and inexpensive. It provides safe and reliable trending of a patient's blood pressure in clinical settings. Today, NIBP measurement is performed in almost every medical examination. This chapter describes the principles and instrumentations of a number of common indirect methods in blood pressure measurement.

AUSCULTATORY METHOD

Indirect methods measure blood pressure without directly accessing the bloodstream. The most commonly used instrument is based on the auscultatory technique. The device used in this technique is called a sphygmomanometer, which is present in every hospital bedside, clinic, and physician's office.

A sphygmomanometer (Figure 19–1) consists of:

1. An inflatable rubber bladder enclosed in a fabric cover called the

cuff;

2. A rubber hand pump with valve assembly so that the pressure in the setup can be raised and released at a slow controlled rate; and

3. A pressure measurement device. Mercury manometers were commonly used as the pressure measurement device. However, since mercury is a hazardous material, rotary mechanical air pressure gauges have replaced mercury manometers to measure the pressure in the cuff.

In addition to the sphygmomanometer, a stethoscope is required to listen to the sounds in the artery during the measurement.

During blood pressure measurement, the pressure cuff is wrapped around the upper arm of the subject and a stethoscope is placed on the inner elbow for the operator to listen to the sound produced by the blood flow in the brachial artery. While watching the pressure gauge, the operator manually squeezes the hand pump to raise the cuff pressure until it is above the systolic blood pressure (e.g., 150 mmHg). At this pressure, the brachial artery is occluded. Since blood is not able to flow to the lower arm, no sound will be heard from the stethoscope. The cuff pressure is then slowly reduced, say, at a rate of approximately 3 mmHg per second, by opening the pressure release valve. As the cuff pressure falls below the systolic pressure, the clinician will start to hear some clashing, snapping sounds from the stethoscope. This sound is caused by the jets of blood pushing through the occlusion. As the cuff pressure continues to decrease, the sound intensity will first increase; it will then turn into a murmur-like noise and become a loud thumping sound. The intensity and pitch of the sounds will change abruptly into a muffled tone when the cuff pressure is getting close to the diastolic pressure and will disappear completely when the pressure is below the diastolic pressure.

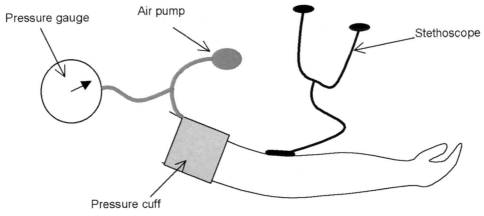

Figure 19–1. NIBP Measurement Setup Using Manual Auscultatory Method.

These sounds are called Korotkoff sounds.

The cuff pressure at which the first Korotkoff sound appears corresponds to the systolic pressure, while the disappearance of the sound corresponds to the diastolic pressure. Figure 19–2 shows the relationships between the arterial pressure and the cuff pressure during the course of measurement. This method is suitable for most patients, including hypotensive and hypertensive patients. Other than applying the cuff over the upper arm, the cuff can be placed over the thigh or the calf of the patient. In each of these applications, the Korotkoff sounds should to be detected downstream of the occlusions.

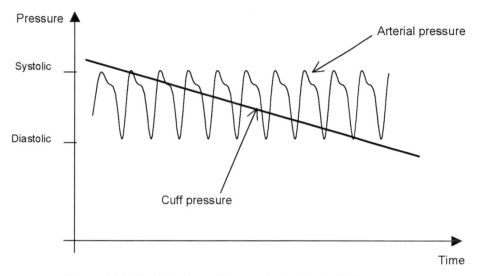

Figure 19–2. Relationships Between Arterial and Cuff Pressure.

The accuracy of this method has several limitations:

- The Korotkoff sounds are normally in the range of less than 200 Hz, where human hearing is normally less acute. Determination of the Korotkoff sounds is affected by the hearing acuity of the operator, especially when it is used on hypotensive patients or infants, where the sound levels are low.
- Inappropriate cuff size or incorrect placement can produce falsely high (undersized or loosely applied cuff) or falsely low (oversized cuff) readings. The American Heart Association (AHA) recommends that the length of the bladder under the cuff be 80% of the circumference of the patient's limb and the width of the bladder be 40% of the circumference.
- A too fast rate of cuff deflation will produce an erroneous reading.

Figure 19–3 shows an underestimation of the systolic pressure due to a too fast deflation rate.

- It is known that the Korotkoff sounds disappear early in some patients and then reappear as the cuff pressure is lowered toward the diastolic pressure. This phenomenon is referred to as the auscultatory gap.
- The auscultatory method can determine the systolic and diastolic pressures but not the mean blood pressure.

Although the sphygmomanometer is a relatively simple device, regular maintenance is still required, which includes pressure gauge calibration; cleaning; and checking for leaks on tubing, cuff bladder, valves, and the hand pump.

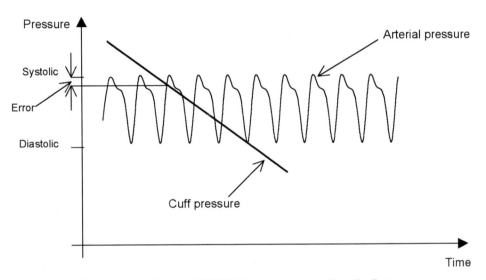

Figure 19–3. Error in NIBP Measurement on Fast Deflation.

An automatic NIBP monitor uses the same principle as the manual auscultatory method. Automation overcomes the hearing acuity limitation by employing a microphone inside the cuff to pick up the Korotkoff sounds instead of relying on human hearing. It also replaces the manual pump with an automatic pump and uses an electronic pressure transducer instead of a mechanical pressure gauge. After the cuff is applied, the NIBP monitor automatically inflates the cuff to occlude the blood vessel. The bladder pressure is slowly released while the microphone listens for the Korotkoff sounds. These processes are automatically coordinated by the monitor. The systolic and diastolic pressures are determined by tracking the bladder pressure and correlating it to the different phases of the Korotkoff sounds picked up by the microphone.

OSCILLOMETRIC METHOD

NIBP monitors using the oscillometric method are similar to the auscultatory method except the oscillometric method detects the small fluctuations of pressure inside the cuff rather than listening to the Korotkoff sounds in the auscultatory method. When the cuff pressure falls below the systolic pressure, blood breaks through the occlusion, causing the blood vessel under the cuff to vibrate. This vibration of the vessel's wall causes fluctuation (or oscillation) of the cuff pressure. The onset of the vibration correlates well with the systolic pressure, while the maximum amplitude of oscillation corresponds to the mean arterial blood pressure. When the cuff pressure is at the mean arterial pressure, the net average pressure on the arterial wall is zero (both sides of the wall are of the same pressure), which allows the arterial wall to freely move in either direction. Under this condition, the amplitude of vibration of the arterial wall caused by blood pressure fluctuation in the artery is the highest. The diastolic pressure event on the oscillometric curve is somewhat less defined. One commonly adopted approach to determine the diastolic pressure is to take the point where the amplitude of the oscillation has the highest rate of change; another approach estimates the diastolic pressure by locating the point where the cuff pressure corresponds to a fixed percentage of the maximum oscillation amplitude.

Figure 19–4a shows the relationships between the arterial blood pressure and the cuff pressure. The maximum amplitude of pressure oscillation is usually less than a few percent of the cuff pressure. To extract only the oscillatory component from the pressure signal obtained by the pressure sensor, the low-frequency component of the signal (corresponding to the slowly deflating cuff pressure) is removed by a high pass filter. The remaining oscillatory component of the signal (shown amplified in Figure 19–4b) is then used to determine the mean, systolic, and diastolic blood pressures. The cuff pressure corresponding to the maximum oscillation amplitude is taken as the mean arterial pressure. Different manufacturers of NIBP monitors may use different algorithms to determine the systolic and diastolic pressures from this oscillometric signal.

Compared to the auscultatory method, NIBP measurements using the oscillometric method are not affected by audible noise and therefore can work in a noisy environment. On the other hand, as this method relies on detecting the amplitude of pressure fluctuation, any movement or vibration can lead to incorrect readings. Furthermore, in oscillometric NIBP monitors, the diastolic pressure is only an estimated quantity. In addition, the small pressure change at the onset of oscillation (which corresponds to the systolic pressure) is difficult to detect. Of the two automatic noninvasive methods, the oscillometric method is more commonly used than the auscultatory

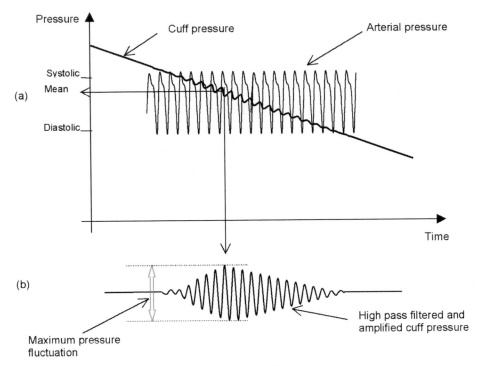

Figure 19–4. Relationships Between Arterial
and Cuff Pressure in Oscillometric Method.

method in automatic blood pressure monitors.

Figure 19–5 shows the functional building blocks of a NIBP monitor using the oscillometric method. The following descriptions explain the functions of the building blocks.

Pump and Solenoid Valve. The motorized air pump inflates the cuff pressure to a predetermined pressure so that the artery is occluded under the cuff. The solenoid valve connects the air circuits between the pump and the cuff during inflation and connects the cuff to atmosphere during deflation. The rate of deflation can be controlled by pulsing the solenoid at a certain duty cycle.

Pressure Sensor. Through the internal tubing connections, the cuff pressure is constantly monitored by the pressure sensor in the NIBP monitor.

Amplifiers and Oscillometric Filter. The signal picked up by the pressure transducer is amplified (by about 100 times). This signal consists of two sets of information: the slowly decreasing cuff pressure and the oscillatory signal. The slow varying signal is separated from the oscillatory signal by a high pass filter (with cutoff frequency of about 1 Hz). Both signals are fed to the analog to digital converter.

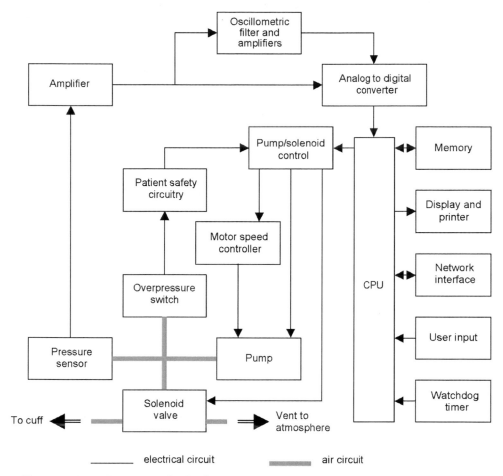

Figure 19–5. Functional Block Diagram of Oscillometric NIBP Monitor.

Central Processing Unit (CPU) and Analog to Digital Converter (ADC). The cuff pressure and oscillometric signal are digitized by the ADC and sent to the CPU to determine the mean, systolic, and diastolic pressures of the measurement. The heart rate can also be determined from the signals.

Display, Printer, Memory, and Network Interface. The measured systolic, diastolic, and mean blood pressures are shown on a display (e.g., LCD). A hard copy may be printed for charting. These data may also be time-stamped and saved in the memory of the monitor for trending or communicated via network connections to other devices.

Watchdog Timer and Overpressure Switch. An independent overpressure safety switch activates the solenoid valve to release the cuff pressure down to atmospheric pressure should excessive pressure develop in the cuff. The solenoid will also open to the atmosphere if the cuff pressure remains high for a preset duration of time. Both features are in place to prevent compression damage of the tissues under the cuff.

OTHER METHODS OF NIBP MEASUREMENT

There are many other methods to measure or estimate blood pressure noninvasively. Compared to the auscultatory or oscillometric methods, these methods are either not as accurate or more complicated or not as easy to use in clinical settings. Two of the better methods are described next.

Doppler Ultrasound Blood Pressure Monitor

This class of device makes use of the Doppler effect to detect blood flow patterns in the artery of interest. A sound transmitter and a receiver are placed inside the pressure cuff. The monitor detects the Doppler shift when the incident sound wave is reflected from the blood flow in the subject. When the artery is occluded by the cuff, the Doppler shift is zero. When the cuff pressure is slowly reduced, the arterial pressure is able to overcome the cuff pressure occlusion, causing the occlusion to snap open. This jet of blood flowing through the cuff occlusion produces a Doppler shift. There are actually two Doppler events during each cardiac cycle–the opening and closing of the blood vessel under the cuff. When the arterial pressure exceeds the cuff pressure, the blood flowing through the opening of the occlusion produces a high-frequency Doppler shift (e.g., 200 to 500 Hz). When the arterial pressure recedes toward the diastolic pressure, the blood vessel will be reoccluded. This event produces a lower frequency Doppler shift (e.g., 15 to 100 Hz).

When the cuff pressure is allowed to be bled down at constant speed from the systolic pressure, the high- and low-frequency events appear and are next to each other. As the cuff pressure continues to drop, the two events become farther and farther apart. When the cuff pressure reaches the diastolic pressure, the low-frequency event will coincide with the high-frequency event of the next cardiac cycle (Figure 19–6). The frequency shift may be coupled to a loudspeaker to allow the operator to determine the systolic and diastolic pressures. Figure 19–6 shows the Doppler events due to the interaction of the cuff pressure and blood pressure.

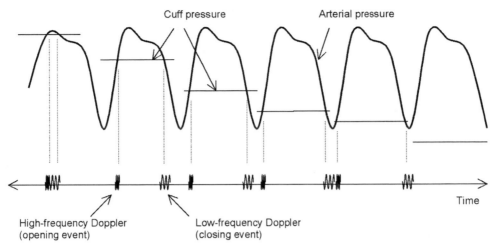

Figure 19–6. Doppler Events Due to Interaction of Cuff Pressure and Blood Pressure.

Arterial Tonometry

None of the NIBP methods discussed are able to measure the blood pressure waveform. Arterial tonometry is a continuous pressure measurement technique that can noninvasively measure pressure in superficial arteries with sufficient bony support, such as the radial artery. A tonometer is a contact pressure sensor that is applied over a blood vessel. It is based on the principle that if the sensor is depressed onto the vessel wall of an artery such that the vessel wall is parallel to the face of the sensor, the arterial pressure is the only pressure perpendicular to the surface and is measured by the sensor (Figure 19–7). Theoretically, accurate real-time blood pressure waveform

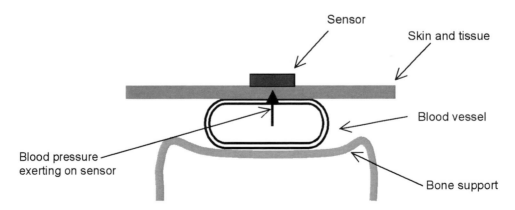

Figure 19–7. Arterial Tonometry.

can be recorded using this noninvasive technique. However, experiments showed that although this method produces good-quality pulse waveform, it tends to underestimate the systolic and diastolic pressures.

To obtain good results, tonometry requires that the contact surface be stiff and the sensor be small relative to the diameter of the blood vessel. In addition, proper sensor application is critical because if the vessel is not flattened sufficiently (e.g., due to inadequate depression), the tonometer will measure forces due to arterial wall tension and bending of the vessel. However, too much depression force may occlude the blood vessel.

Chapter 20

CARDIAC OUTPUT MONITORS

OBJECTIVES

- Define the terms *cardiac output*, *stroke volume*, and *cardiac index*.
- State the Fick principle and the indicator dilution method.
- Describe how to measure cardiac output using oxygen and heat as the "tracer."
- Explain the principle of the thermal dilution method in cardiac output measurement.
- Review the setup and the procedures to measure cardiac output using the thermal dilution method.
- Sketch the block diagram of a cardiac output monitor using the thermal dilution method.
- Identify potential sources of error in cardiac output measurement and methods to minimize errors.

CHAPTER CONTENTS

INTRODUCTION

Cardiac output is a measurement of the performance of the heart. It is also used to calculate many hemodynamic functions. The heart serves as a pump to circulate blood around the cardiovascular system. In fluid mechanics, the power produced by a pump is determined by its output pressure and volume flow rate. In the last two chapters, we have studied devices to measure blood pressure. In this chapter, we are going to study cardiac output monitor–a medical device to measure blood flow of the heart.

Although there are many direct and indirect methods to measure cardiac output, since the introduction of the Swan-Ganz catheter in the 1970s, the thermal dilution method has become a standard procedure to measure cardiac output in intensive care units, surgical suites, and cardiac care units.

The thermal dilution method in cardiac output measurement is an application of the indicator dilution method based on the Fick principle. The Fick principle was proposed by Adolf Fick and states that the rate Q of a substance delivered to an area with a moving fluid stream is equal to the product of the flow rate F of the fluid and the difference in concentration C of the substance at sites proximal and distal to the area. In equation format: $Q = F(C_d - C_p)$ or:

$$F = \frac{Q}{(C_d - C_p)}. \tag{1}$$

DEFINITIONS

For every contraction, the heart pushes a certain volume of blood into the common aorta. This volume of blood pumped by the ventricles during one ejection is defined as the stroke volume or SV. Therefore, the volume of blood pumped out from the heart per unit time is equal to the SV multiplied by the heart rate or HR. This product, which is the volume of blood pumped out by the heart per unit time, is defined as the cardiac output. Cardiac output or CO is commonly expressed in liters per minute (L/min). Therefore, CO = SV × HR where SV is in liters, and HR is in beats per minute.

For a normal adult, the resting CO is about 3 to 5 L/min. However, during intense exercise, since both the HR and SV become higher, the CO of the same individual may have increased to several times of that at rest (e.g., to 25 L/min). As with all physiological signals, the resting CO varies from person to person and is often dependent on body size. To facilitate comparison, CO is often normalized by dividing it by the weight or by the body surface area of the patient. The latter is called the cardiac index, which has a unit of L/min/m². A typical resting cardiac index is 3.0 L/min/m². One may wonder how body surface area is determined. In fact, lookup tables of body surface area based on the weights and heights of typical individuals are available. Alternatively, an empirical formula can be used to obtain the body surface area:

$$A = W^{0.425} \times H^{0.725} \times 0.007184, \qquad (2)$$

where A = total body surface area in m²,
W = body weight in kg, and
H = height in cm.

For example, the body surface area A of a 70 kg, 1.7m tall patient is

$$A = 70^{0.425} \times 170^{0.725} \times 0.007184 = 1.73 \text{ m}^2.$$

DIRECT FICK METHOD

The direct Fick method is considered to be the "gold standard" in cardiac output measurement. It uses oxygen as the indicator and assumes that the left ventricular blood flow is equal to the blood flow through the lungs. This method involves measurement of the rate of oxygen uptake of the lungs and the oxygen content of the arterial blood and venous blood. Deoxygenated blood from the right ventricle, which has the lowest oxygen concentration in the cardiovascular system, enters the lungs and picks up oxygen to become oxygenated blood. The oxygenated blood then flows via the left atrium, left ventricle, and common aorta into the arteries. According to the Fick principle, the volume blood flow F through the lung (i.e., the cardiac output) can be obtained if the rate of oxygen uptake Q and the difference in oxygen concentration C_a of the arterial blood and oxygen concentration C_v of the venous blood are known. Using these quantities, equation (1) then becomes:

$$F = \frac{Q}{(C_a - C_v)}. \qquad (3)$$

In practice, blood samples are drawn during measurement of oxygen consumption. The venous blood is drawn from the pulmonary artery and the arterial sample is taken from one of the main arteries. Oxygen content of the venous and arterial blood is determined by laboratory analysis of these blood samples. The oxygen consumption Q is calculated from the rate of gas inhalation and the difference of the oxygen concentrations in the atmospheric air and the expired air from the patient. The rate of gas inhalation is measured using a spirometer and the expired gas oxygen concentration is measured using an oxygen analyzer. The blood flow rate F, or cardiac output, is then calculated. In this method, the subject must be in a steady state throughout the period of measurement (about 3 minutes) to avoid transient changes in blood flow or in the rate of ventilation.

Example

In a cardiac output measurement using the direct Fick method, the rate of oxygen consumption was found to be 300 ml/min. Blood sample analysis shows the arterial and mixed venous oxygen contents are 200 ml/l and 140 ml/l, respectively. Calculate the cardiac output.

Solution

Using equation (3),

$$F = \frac{Q}{(C_a - C_v)} = \frac{300 \text{ ml/min}}{(200 \text{ ml/l} - 140 \text{ ml/l})} = \frac{300 \text{ ml/min}}{60 \text{ ml/l}} = 5 \text{ l/min.}$$

INDICATOR DILUTION METHOD

The indicator dilution method is a variation of the Fick principle. The indicator dilution method to measure fluid flow rate is based on the upstream injection of a tracer (or detectable indicator) into a mixing chamber and measuring the concentration-time curve (or dilution curve) of the tracer downstream of the chamber (Figure 20–1a). To obtain accurate results, the tracer is required to thoroughly mix with the fluid in the mixing chamber. Theoretically, for the same flow and same tracer injection volume, the area under the dilution curve will be the same even though the shapes of the curves are different. Figure 20–1b shows the ideal indicator dilution curve obtained by immediate mixing of the tracer with the fluid after injection and having the same fluid velocity over the entire cross section of the tube. In the ideal case (Figure 20–1b), the fluid flow rate F is proportional to the amount of tracer m injected and inversely proportional to the concentration C of the tracer and the duration T of the concentration curve, or simply:

$$F = \frac{m}{CT}.$$

Note that the product C and T is the area under the dilution curve.

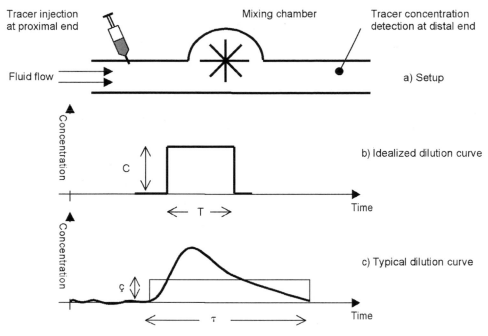

Figure 20–1. Indication Dilution Method.

Figure 20–1c shows a typical dilution curve in a realistic situation. Although it shows a rapid rise and an exponential fall in concentration, the area under the curve is still roughly the same as that of the idealistic curve (Figure 20–1b) as long as the fluid flow rate and the amount of tracer injected are the same.

$$F = \frac{m}{\zeta \tau} = \frac{m}{A},$$

where A = area under the dilution curve.

Two types of indicators may be used in indicator dilution methods—diffusible and nondiffusible indicators. A nondiffusible indicator will remain in the system for a much longer period of time than a diffusible indicator. For example, saline, which can be measured by a conductivity cell, is a diffusible indicator in cardiac output measurement. It is estimated that over 15% of the salt will be removed from the blood in its first pass through the lung. Indocyanine green is a nondiffusible indicator that can be detected using optical sensors. Experiments showed that only about 50% of it will be lost in the first 10 minutes as it circulates around the cardiovascular system. Measurements using a diffusible indicator tend to overestimate the cardiac output, while recirculation of a nondiffusible indicator may result in lower cardiac output measurements. Recirculation is the effect of increased indicator concentration when the previous bolus of indicator returns to the measurement site during subsequent measurements. Figure 20–2 shows the dilution curve affected by recirculation. The dotted line shows the normal trace of the curve if no recirculation occurs.

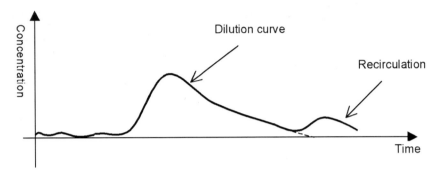

Figure 20–2. Effect of Recirculation in Indicator Dilution.

Example

In an indicator dilution method to measure cardiac output, 10 mg of indicator is injected and the average concentration of the dilution curve is found to be 2.5 mg/liter. If the indicator takes 60 seconds to pass through the detector, what is the cardiac output?

Solution

Using the equation $F = \dfrac{m}{CT}$,

the cardiac output is $\dfrac{m}{CT} = \dfrac{10 \text{ mg}}{2.5 \text{ mg/liter} \times 60 \text{ s}} = \dfrac{4 \text{ liter}}{60 \text{ sec}} = 4 \text{ l/min.}$

THERMAL DILUTION METHOD

The thermal dilution method of cardiac output measurement is based on the indication dilution method where heat is used as the indicator. In this method, a known volume of cold solution (5% dextrose or saline) is injected into the right atrium. This bolus of cold solution causes a decrease in the blood temperature when it mixes with the blood in the right ventricle. The change of blood temperature in the pulmonary artery (downstream of the mixing chamber) is measured to obtain the thermal dilution curve as shown in Figure 20–3. It shows that the temperature of blood in the pulmonary artery drops when the indicator-blood mixture passes through the temperature sensor and gradually rises back to the normal body temperature. Note that the curve is inverted for easier reading since the cold solution causes a negative change in blood temperature.

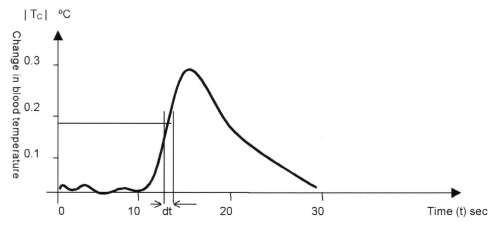

Figure 20–3. Thermal Dilution Curve.

From the thermal dilution curve, the heat loss *dH* from the blood over the time interval *dt* is:

$$dH = C_BF\rho_BT_cdt, \tag{4}$$

where C_B = specific heat capacity of blood,
F = blood flow rate (cardiac output),
ρ_B = density of blood, and
T_c = temperature change (from body temperature) of the blood at time *t*.

The total heat loss of the blood to the injectate *H* is equal to the integral of equation (4):

$$H = \int_0^\infty dH = \int_0^\infty C_BF\rho_BT_cdt = C_BF\rho_B \int_0^\infty T_cdt = C_BF\rho_BA, \tag{5}$$

where $A = \int_0^\infty T_cdt$ is the area under the thermal dilution curve.

Since the total heat loss of the blood is equal to the heat gain of the injectate (to raise the injectate temperature to body temperature), the heat gain of the injectate *Hi* can be determined from the preinjection condition of the injecte if we know the volume V_I, density ρ_I, specific heat capacity C_I and the initial temperature T_I of the injectate.

$$H_I = V_I C_I \rho_I (T_B - T_I). \tag{6}$$

Since $H = H_I$, equations (4) and (5) give

$$C_B F \rho_B A = V_I C_I \rho_I (T_B - T_I)$$

$$\Rightarrow F = \frac{V_I C_I \rho_I (T_B - T_I)}{C_B \rho_B A} \tag{7}$$

$$\Rightarrow CO = F = \frac{V_I K (T_B - T_I)}{A}, \tag{8}$$

where $K = \dfrac{C_I \rho_I}{C_B \rho_B}$ is a constant for a particular indicator.

As heat (cold saline or dextrose) is a diffusible indicator, a correction factor K_I (< 1) is multiplied to equation (7) to compensate for the warming effect of the indicator during measurement.

$$\Rightarrow CO = \frac{V_I K_I K (T_B - T_I)}{A}. \tag{9}$$

Example

In a cardiac output measurement using the thermal dilution method, 5 ml of iced 5% dextrose is injected into the right atrium to obtain the thermal dilution curve. If the area under the curve is found to be 1.80°Cs and a correction factor K_I of 0.825 is used, find the cardiac output given that $\dfrac{C_I \rho_I}{C_B \rho_B} = 1.08$ for 5% dextrose and typical blood composition.

Solution

Using 37°C as the body temperature and 0°C as the initial injectate temperature, from equation (9), the cardiac output is calculated by:

$$CO = [5 \text{ ml} \times 0.825 \times 1.08 \times (37°C - 0°C)]/1.80°Cs = 91.6 \text{ ml/s} = 5.5 \text{ l/min}$$

In practice, a special catheter called the Swan-Ganz catheter is used to inject a known volume (e.g., 5 ml) of cold dextrose into the right atrium of the heart; the temperature of the blood in the pulmonary artery is measured by a temperature sensor embedded near the distal end of the catheter to obtain the thermal dilution curve. Mixing of indicator and blood occurs in the right ventricle. A Swan-Ganz catheter is a special multilumen catheter with a distal opening, a proximal opening, a thermistor temperature sensor, and an inflatable balloon. A typical catheter is about 110 cm long and 2 to 3 mm in diameter.

Figure 20–4 shows the construction of a four-lumen Swan-Ganz catheter, and Figure 20–5 shows the position of the catheter in the cardiovascular system during cardiac output measurement. The catheter is positioned into the heart such that the injectate orifice is in the right atrium and the thermistors in the pulmonary artery. During measurement, the injectate (cold saline or dextrose) delivered into the right atrium is mixed with blood as it travels through the right ventricle into the pulmonary artery. The temperature of blood flowing through the pulmonary artery is continuously measured by a thermistor located a few centimeters from the distal end of the catheter.

The procedures to measure cardiac output using a Swan-Ganz catheter are:

1. Create an intravascular access to a vein (subclavian, internal jugular, or basilic) using, for example, the Seldinger technique.
2. Insert the distal end of the catheter into the vein and slightly inflate the balloon.

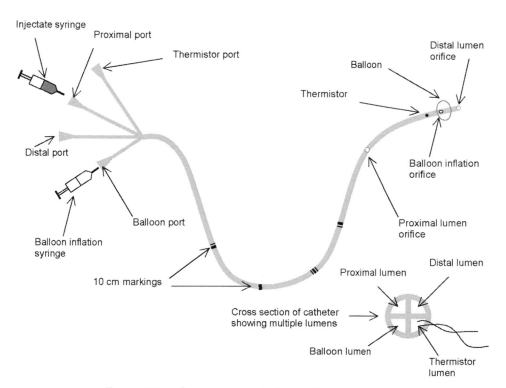

Figure 20–4. Construction of a Swan-Ganz Catheter.

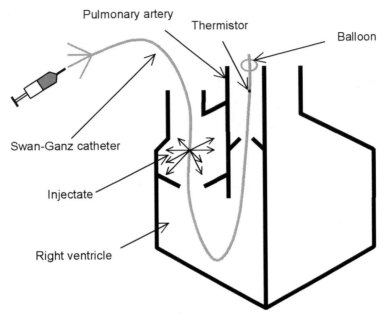

Figure 20–5. Positioning of Swan-Ganz Catheter in Heart Chambers.

3. Continue to insert the catheter into the vein. The balloon will be dragged by the blood flow to go through the right atrium, tricuspid valve, right ventricle, pulmonary valve, and into the pulmonary artery.

4. The position of the catheter can be estimated by the distant markings on the catheter and verified by:
    (a) using X-ray fluoroscopy (the tip of the catheter is radiopaque), or
    (b) monitoring the characteristic changes in blood pressure waveform at the distal lumen as it travels from the vein into the heart chambers and then into the pulmonary artery during the catheter insertion.

5. Deflate the balloon.

6. Connect the catheter to the cardiac output monitor and initialize the monitor.

7. Enter patient data.

8. Prepare injectate (saline or DW5–5% dextrose).

9. Measure injectate temperature (usually 0 to 5°C).

10. Inject a fixed volume of injectate (e.g., 5 ml) at a uniform rate (over a period of 2 to 4 sec) into the injectate port.

11. The CO monitor will display the temperature change versus time curve (thermal dilution curve) and calculate the CO using equation (6).

12. Several measurements (and averaging the results) may be required to obtain a reliable reading.

A Swan-Ganz catheter setup can also be used to monitor the pulmonary arterial wedge pressure (PAWP). The PAWP, also termed the pulmonary capillary (wedge) pressure (PCW), reflects the mean level of pressure in the left atrium. While the distal end of the catheter is in the pulmonary artery, the balloon is fully inflated to occlude the pulmonary artery. The PAWP is measured from the distal lumen by connecting a pressure transducer to the distal port of the catheter.

Note that the setup procedure to measure blood pressure using the Swan-Ganz catheter is the same as setting up an invasive pressure line as discussed in Chapter 18. A CO monitor usually consists of one or more blood pressure modules, one or more temperature modules, a computer, and interface components. The functional block diagram of a cardiac output monitor is shown in Figure 20–6. During a CO measurement, a blood pressure transducer BP Tx_1 is connected to the distal port to display the blood pressure waveform at the distal end of the catheter. This pressure waveform is a mean to allow the user to determine the position of the catheter during catheter insertion. These blood pressure modules may also be used to monitor intracardiac blood pressure. The thermistor Temp Tx 1 located near the distal end of the catheter is use to acquire the thermal dilution curve. A second thermistor Temp Tx 2 may be used to measure the injectate temperature. These pressure and temperature signals are digitized, multiplexed, and sent to the central processor to compute the cardiac output, cardiac index, blood pressures, et cetera. The thermal dilution curve and the blood pressure waveform can be viewed from the integrated display of the monitor.

Instead of using cold saline or dextrose, a nondiffusible dye (e.g., indocyanine green) may be used as the indicator. The dye dilution curve is obtained by continuously withdrawing blood from the pulmonary artery and dye concentrate measured by a calibrated optical densitometer.

PROBLEMS AND ERRORS

Any inaccuracy in equation (9) will result in an incorrect cardiac output measurement. Studies showed that CO measurement using thermodilution under ideal conditions is generally within 5% of the results obtained from other methods. To avoid single measurement error, the usual practice is to average the results of three good measurements. Potential error sources of this technique are explained next.

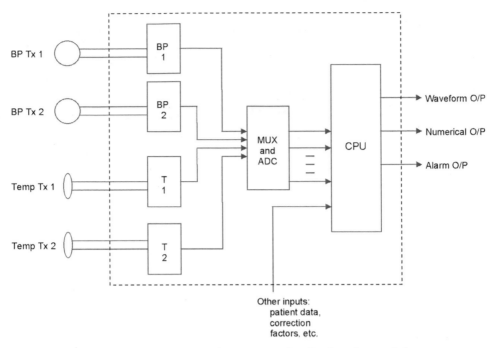

Figure 20–6. Functional Block Diagram of a Cardiac Output Monitor.

Catheter Dead Space and Injectate Warming

The CO equation assumes that all injectate enters the bloodstream and heat transfer occurs only between the injectate and blood in the right atrium. In practice, some injectate will remain in the catheter and heat is exchanged between the injectate and the wall of the catheter during injection. To minimize such errors, the first reading should be discarded because the first injection contains warm fluid in the catheter dead space. A correction factor (K_7 < 1) is multiplied to equation (8) to compensate for these errors.

Timing of Injection

Although respiratory action of the patient affects the blood pressure and flow, it is impractical to synchronize the injection with the respiratory cycle. Using an average of three or more sequential measurements can minimize the variations.

Rate of Injection

Erratic and long injection duration introduces errors in the thermal dilution curve and increases the injectate warming effect. Injection duration should be between 2 and 4 seconds and at a steady speed.

Injectate Volume

The injectate volume should be measured accurately as this will affect the calculation. A small syringe (e.g., 10 ml) is usually included in the package of the catheter. CO measurements using a small volume of injectate are more likely to be affected by injectate warming.

Injectate Temperature

Theoretically, a higher volume injectate at a lower temperature should increase the signal to noise ratio in the measurements. Studies confirmed that cardiac output measurements using injectate at room temperature produced higher variability than using injectate at 0°C (iced injectate). It is recommended that if the volume of injectate is less than 10 ml, the solution should be iced. As well, clinicians should average more measurements if room temperature injectates are used. Care should be taken to avoid warming the injectate during handling.

Thermistor Position

If the thermistor in the catheter is in contact with the wall of the pulmonary artery, the temperature reading will be higher, resulting in a lower value of A in equation (8). There will be errors in the temperature measurement if the thermistor is positioned inside the ventricle instead of inside the pulmonary artery. Inside the ventricle, the injectate may not have been thoroughly mixed with the blood.

Frequency of Injection and Recirculation

If consecutive measurements are made within a short period of time, the temperature of blood in the pulmonary artery may not have enough time to return to normal body temperature before the next bolus of injectate is introduced into the bloodstream. If too many measurements are done in a short period of time, it may lower the overall blood temperature of the patient.

This latter problem is more significant in the dye dilution method as it takes longer for the kidneys to remove the dye from the patient's bloodstream.

Intravenous Administration

Any intravenous fluid infusion will introduce below body temperature fluid into the bloodstream. This effect will create errors in the thermal dilution curve.

Chapter 21

CARDIAC PACEMAKERS

OBJECTIVES

- Define arrhythmia and list indications for artificial pacemaker implantation.
- Differentiate between endocardial and myocardial, bipolar and unipolar pacing leads.
- Define asynchronous, demand, and rate-modulated pacing.
- Describe the procedures of pacemaker implantation.
- Interpret the NBG (NASPE/BPEG) generic pacemaker codes
- State applications of external pacing.
- Differentiate between invasive and transcutaneous external pacing.
- Describe the characteristics and design of implantable pacemakers.
- Analyze the block diagram of a demand pacemaker and describe its principles of operation.
- List problems in artificial pacing.

CHAPTER CONTENTS

9. Temporary Pacing
10. Potential Problems with Pacemakers

INTRODUCTION

In 1952, Paul M. Zoll, working with engineers of the Electrodyne Company, developed a device that could stimulate the heart to contract through large electrodes placed on the chest wall. In 1957, C. Walton Lillehei and his colleagues, using an external pulse generator, successfully paced the heart by directly placing electrodes in the heart muscle. In 1958, Wilson Greatbatch developed a fully implantable pacemaker. In 1986, the U.S. Food and Drug Administration gave market approval to a rate-responsive pacemaker made by Medtronic.

A pacemaker is a therapeutic device designed to rectify some heart problems arising from irregular heart rhythms. It performs its function by applying controlled electrical stimulations to the heart. A healthy heart is stimulated to contract by electrical impulses initiated from the sinoatrial (SA) node located in the atrium near the superior vena cava. The SA node is also called the natural pacemaker of the heart. An electrical impulse generated from the SA node is conducted through the atria, causing them to contract. The impulse eventually arrives at and depolarizes the atrioventricular (AV) node located in the septal wall of the right atrium. Through the Bundle of His and the Purkinje fibers, the action potential is distributed to the myocardium, causing the ventricles to contract.

INDICATION OF USE

Normal sinus rhythm is a result of the continuous periodic and coordinated stimulation of the atria and ventricles of the heart. Failure of any part of this pathway will compromise the cardiac output. An arrhythmia is any disturbance in the rhythm of the heart with respect to rate, regularity, or propagation sequence of the depolarization wave. Depending on its nature, an arrhythmia may be mild or life-threatening. There are two kinds of arrhythmias:

1. Arrhythmias caused by disturbances of conduction, and
2. Arrhythmias caused by disturbances of the origin of the stimulation

Disturbances of conduction include:

• Slowing of the spread of conduction of the electrical stimulation in one part of the conduction system, so that part of the heart is activated significantly later than the rest, resulting in distortion of the ventricular contraction pattern

- Conduction through anomalous paths, which causes different parts of the heart muscle to contract in an uncoordinated manner
- Partial or complete blocks of the stimulation signal from the SA node to the ventricles. Heart blocks originate from some malfunctions of the heart's built-in electrical conduction system. The results of heart blocks include low heart rate, heart muscle not getting enough oxygen, and cardiac muscle becoming irritable and susceptible to irregular rhythm. A patient with heart blocks has inadequate body oxygen and low exercise tolerance, and in extreme cases, experiences loss of consciousness and convulsion due to lack of oxygen to the brain. There are three degrees of heart block:

    1st degree—long delay in signal transmission
    2nd degree—intermittent complete blockage of transmission
    3rd degree—continuous complete blockage of transmission

Disturbances of the origin of stimulation include:

- rate of SA node erratic resulting in erratic heart beat
- more than one natural pacemaker site
- high heart rate, e.g., sinus tachycardia
- low heart rate, e.g., sinus bradycardia

Pacemakers are indicated to improve cardiac output, prevent symptoms, or protect against arrhythmias related to cardiac impulse formation and conduction disorders.

TYPES OF CARDIAC PACEMAKERS

A pacemaker has two physical parts, the pulse generator and the lead system (Figure 21–1). The pulse generator produces electrical stimulation pulses. Through the lead system, these pulses are delivered to the heart muscle, causing the heart to contract. There are three types of pacemakers: implantable, external invasive, and transcutaneous. For an implantable pacemaker, both the pulse generator and the leads are placed inside the patient's body without any exposed parts. For an external invasive pacemaker, the pulse generator is located outside the patient's body, while the lead wire connecting the pulse generator and the heart muscle is inserted through a vein into the right chamber of the heart. A transcutaneous pacemaker, sometimes called an external noninvasive pacemaker, has a pair of skin electrodes placed anterior and posterior to the chest. The electrical stimulation from the

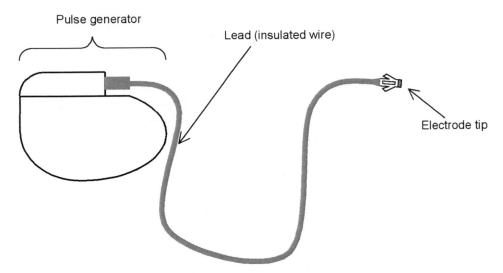

Figure 21-1. Implantable Pacemaker and Lead.

external pulse generator is conducted through the heart across the externally placed electrodes.

According to how it regulates the pacing rate, a cardiac pacemaker has three modes of operation: asynchronous, demand, and rate-modulated. A pacemaker in asynchronous mode can deliver only a fixed rate of stimulation. In demand mode, it senses the heart's activity to determine its pacing sequence. Rather than pacing at a fixed rate, a rate-modulated pacemaker can adjust its pacing rate based on the state of physical activity of the patient; therefore it is able to adjust the patient's cardiac output to meet the body's demand.

Some pacemakers can perform cardiac defibrillation. An implantable cardiac defibrillator (ICD) automatically produces a shock to the heart upon detecting ventricular fibrillation. Ventricular fibrillation is a deadly form of arrhythmia caused by completely uncoordinated contraction of heart muscle. Cardiac defibrillation is discussed in Chapter 22.

Most modern pacemakers are programmable. Parameters that can be programmed include pacing rate, mode of pacing, pacing pulse amplitude, pulse duration, sensitivity, et cetera. In addition to the simple programmable features, multiprogrammable pacemakers have built-in programmable diagnostic tests as well as the ability to log heart rhythms and pacing activities. To program or interrogate an implanted pacemaker, a pacemaker programmer or receiver is placed on the skin surface above the pacemaker. Programming commands and data are transmitted via telemetry (or electromagnetic coupling) between the programmer and the pacemaker.

PACEMAKER LEAD SYSTEM

The pacemaker lead system serves two functions. The first is to transmit pacing pulses from the pulse generator to the heart. The second is to pick up electrical activities of the heart to modify the pacing sequence. The pacemaker lead is insulated with nonconductive material (e.g., silicon) except at the tip electrode and the connector to the pacemaker. The conductor is made of corrosion-resistive wire, which is coiled to increase its flexibility. The electrode (tip of the lead wire) may be attached to the surface of the heart or inserted through a vein into the chambers of the heart. The former is called the myocardial (or epicardial) lead system and the latter is called the endocardial lead system. Figure 21–2 shows the two lead systems.

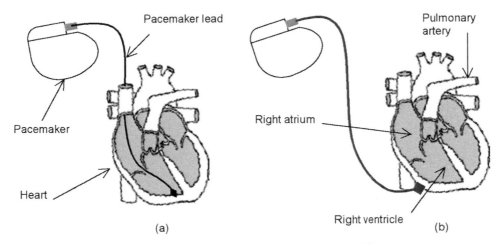

Figure 21–2. Pacemaker Lead System (a) Endocardial Lead, (b) Myocardial Lead.

To complete the conduction path, the current produced from the pulse generator, after passing through the heart tissue, must return to the pulse generator. For a unipolar lead configuration, a single conductor lead is used. The conductor in the pacemaker lead carries the pacing current from the pulse generator circuit to the heart tissue. The metal housing of the pacemaker serves as the return electrode. As there is only one conductor in the pacemaker lead, the return current must therefore return via the conductive body tissue of the patient to the metal housing and then back to the pulse generator circuit of the pacemaker. In a bipolar lead configuration, both the active and return conductors are inside the insulated lead (a dual conductor lead). The pacing current (from the electrode tip) to the heart is picked up by the return electrode located near the tip electrode and returned to the pulse gen-

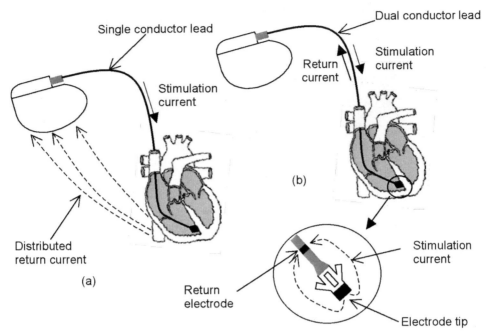

Figure 21–3. Lead Configuration: (a) Unipolar Lead, (b) Bipolar Lead.

erator via the return conductor in the pacemaker lead wire. Figure 21–3 illustrates the two configurations.

A pacemaker with two leads (one in the atrium and the other in the ventricle) to allow pacing and/or sensing of both the ventricle and the atrium is referred to as a dual chamber pacemaker (Figure 21–4). A dual chamber pacemaker can more likely restore the natural contraction sequence of the heart.

In conventional cardiac pacing, only the right atrium and the right ventricle are paced. During normal intrinsic heart contractions, both ventricles are activated at almost the same time. Under conventional (right-heart-only) cardiac pacing, contraction of the left ventricle is triggered through propagation of depolarization from the right ventricle. Such delay results in diminished cardiac output, which may cause significant problems for some patients. Biventricular pacing refers to pacing of both ventricles simultaneously to improve cardiac output. This is achieved by placing an additional lead in the lateral or posterolateral cardiac vein (located at the far side of the left ventricle). Special lead placement techniques are required as it is not easy to insert a lead into these cardiac veins.

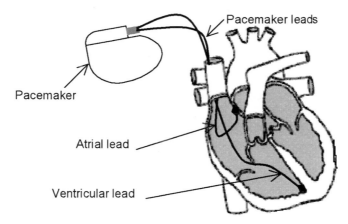

Figure 21–4. Dual Chamber Pacemaker.

IMPLANTATION OF PACEMAKER

The procedures to implant myocardial and endocardial pacemaker leads are quite different. The following descriptions summarize the two procedures.

Myocardial Pacemaker Lead

Myocardial pacemaker lead implantation is performed under general anesthesia. The procedure starts with an incision between the ribs to expose the apex of the heart. An area of the apex free from coronary arteries is chosen. The electrode tip is inserted into the heart muscle (screw-in for spiral electrode or stab-in for barb electrode) at the chosen location. The other end of the lead is tunneled under the skin down toward the abdomen. A shallow incision is made in the abdomen so that the lead can be pulled out. Correct lead placement is confirmed by verifying the pacing and sensing thresholds (often by using a pacemaker analyzer). The lead is then plugged into the pulse generator. The pulse generator is pushed into the pocket made by the incision. The two incisions are closed to complete the procedure.

Endocardial Pacemaker Lead

Endocardial pacemaker lead implantation is done under local anesthesia. The procedure starts with an incision over a vein (e.g., the right external jugular or subclavian). The pacemaker lead is passed down within the vein, into the right atrium, through the right atrioventricular valve, and into the right ventricle. Correct placement is achieved when the tip of the lead is wedged firmly between the trabeculae at the apex of the right ventricle and the lead is observed to be fixed and immobile. Fluoroscopy is often used during the procedure to ensure proper lead placement. A shallow incision is then made in an appropriate area of the upper chest (e.g., under the clavicle). A tunnel is formed under the skin of both incisions so that the connector end of the lead wire is pulled through and is accessible at the chest incision. Correct lead placement is confirmed by verifying the pacing and sensing thresholds. The lead is then plugged into the pulse generator. The pulse generator is pushed into the pocket made by the incision. The two incisions are closed to complete the procedure.

After the procedure, the pacemaker parameters are programmed according to the patient's condition. Regular patient follow-up should be scheduled to monitor the condition of the pacemaker's battery and to confirm that the programmed parameter values are appropriate. Note that the pacing threshold (minimum values to achieve pacing) will rise shortly after implantation and eventually become stabilized after about 3 to 4 months.

Figure 12–5a shows the strength duration curve of heart stimulation. In order to stimulate the heart, the stimulus must have its amplitude and duration above the curve. In the example shown, if the pulse amplitude is 1 V, the pulse width of the stimulation must be larger than 0.7 ms. A pulse duration of 1 ms or longer will be chosen. Figure 21–5b shows the variation in voltage threshold after lead implantation. In this example, the initial pacing voltage amplitude should be set to over 3 V and subsequently reduced to about 2 V after 2 months. A lower pacing amplitude and narrower pacing pulse width will prolong the battery life.

Pacemakers are presterilized in the package. If sterility is compromised, resterilization should be performed (e.g., using ethylene oxide below 60°C and 103 kPa). Most manufacturers specify not to resterilize pacemakers more than twice.

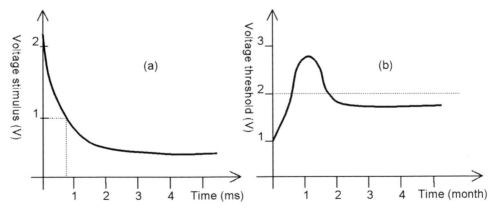

Figure 21–5. (a) Strength Duration Curve; (b) Change in Threshold After Implantation.

PACING MODE SELECTION

The pacemaker modes are defined in the NBG Code. NBG stands for the **N**orth American Society of Pacing and Electrophysiology (NASPE) and the **B**ritish Pacing and Electrophysiology Group (BPEG) **G**eneric. It is a set of codes specifying the modes of operation of implantable pacemakers. It is intended for quick identification of the functionality of the pacemaker in case a pacemaker patient requires intervention. It supersedes the older ICHD (Intersociety Commission on Heart Disease) Code. Each letter of the five-letter NBG code describes a specific type of operation. Table 21–1 describes the codes.

Although there are five letters in the NBG Code, some pacemakers may have only the first three or four letters imprinted on the pacemaker.

Table 21–1.
NBG Pacemaker Code

Position I Chamber Paced	O–None V–Ventricle A–Atrium D–Dual chamber (ventricle and atrium) S*–Single chamber (ventricle or atrium)
Position II Chamber Sensed	O–None V–Ventricle A–Atrium D–Dual chamber (ventricle and atrium) S*–Single chamber (ventricle or atrium)
Position III Mode of Response	O–None T–Triggered I–Inhibited D–Dual (triggered and inhibited)
Position IV Rate Modulation	O–None R–Rate-modulated
Position V Multi-site Pacing	O–None A–Atrium V–Ventricle D–Dual (ventricle and atrium)

*Note: Manufacturer's designation only.

The following examples illustrate how to interpret the NBG pacing code.

An *AOO* pacemaker will pace the atrium (1st letter–A) at a fixed rate (i.e., at every sensor-indicated interval) irrespective of the intrinsic rate of the heart. Figure 21–6 shows the timing sequence of such a pacemaker. AP in the diagram stands for atrial paced. The dotted line indicates the timer, which keeps track of the pacing intervals. When this timer reaches zero, a pacing pulse is generated.

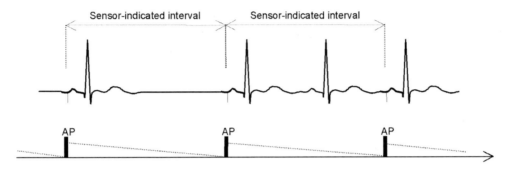

Figure 21–6. AOO Mode of Pacemaker Operation.

A *VVI* pacemaker monitors ventricular contraction (2nd letter–V). It will pace the ventricle (1st letter–V) if it cannot sense ventricular contraction (intrinsic rate slower than sensor-indicated interval). If ventricular signal is sensed, it will inhibit (3rd letter–I) the pacing action. VVI pacemakers are often used to treat patient with second degree heart block. Figure 21–7 shows the timing sequence of such a pacemaker. In the diagram, VP stands for ventricle paced and VS ventricle sensed. After the first paced ventricular contraction, the timer started to count down. It was reset by the sensed intrinsic ventricular contraction. When the timer has reached the sensor-indicated interval without sensing any intrinsic ventricular activity, a pacing pulse is generated to trigger ventricular contraction.

A *DDD* pacemaker senses both atrial and ventricular activities (2nd letter–D). When it cannot detect atrial contraction (2nd letter–D), it will trigger the atrium (1st letter–D, 3rd letter–D). After an atrial paced or intrinsic contraction, if no ventricular contraction is detected (2nd letter–D) after the AV delay interval, the ventricle will be paced (1st letter–D). If ventricular contraction is detected, the ventricular stimulation will be inhibited (3rd letter–D). A DDD pacemaker is a dual chamber pacemaker; that is, it has two leads, one in the right atrial chamber and the other in the right ventricular chamber. The timing sequence of a DDD pacemaker is shown in Figure 21–8. In the diagram, AP stands for atrial paced, AS for atrial sensed, VP for ventricular paced, and VS for ventricular sensed. If it is also a rate-modulat-

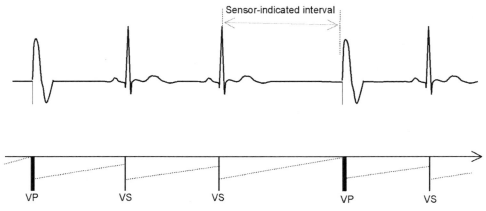

Figure 21–7. VVI Mode of Pacemaker Operation.

ed pacemaker, the pacing rate (or the sensor-indicated interval) will change with the patient's activities. Such a pacemaker will be labeled DDDR. The fourth letter indicates that it is a rate responsive pacemaker.

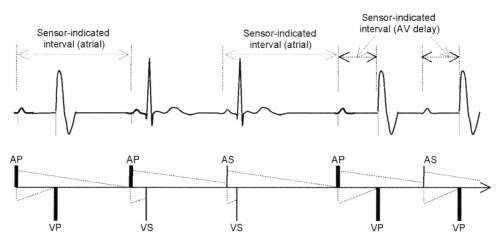

Figure 21–8. Example of DDDR Mode of Operation.

Other than the modes described by the NBG Code, most pacemakers can be switched to a magnet operation mode. Magnet mode is activated by placing a magnetized programming head or a permanent magnet over the pacemaker. During magnet operation, the pacemaker is paced asynchronously at a predetermined fixed rate. Magnet mode is usually combined with a threshold margin test and a self-diagnostic test to evaluate the integrity of the lead and pacemaker system.

PERFORMANCE CHARACTERISTICS

Table 21–2 lists some common implantable pacemaker performance parameters and their nominal values.

Table 21–2.
Performance Parameters of an Implantable Pacemaker.

Parameter	Capability	Nominal Setting
Lower rate	30 to 175 min^{-1} (±2 min^{-1})	60 min^{-1}
ADL rate	10 to 189 min^{-1} (±2 min^{-1})	95 min^{-1}
Upper sensor rate	80 to 180 min^{-1} (±2 min^{-1})	120 min^{-1}
Amplitude	0.5 to 7.6 V (±10%)	3.5 V
Pulse width	0.12 to 1.5 ms (±25 µs)	0.4 ms
Atrial sensitivity	0.25 to 4 mV (±40%)	2.8 mV
Ventricular sensitivity	5.6 to 11.2 mV (±40%)	8.5 mV
Refractory period	150 to 500 ms (±9 ms)	330 ms
Single chamber hysteresis	40 to 60 min^{-1} (±1 min^{-1})	Off
Rate limit	200 min^{-1} (±20 min^{-1})	Nonprogrammable

Lower rate is the programmed minimum pacing rate in the absence of sensor-driven pacing. The time between two consecutive pulses at the lower rate is called the escape interval.

Activities of daily living (ADL) rate is the sensor-driven target rate that the patient's heart rate is expected to reach during moderate exercise.

Upper sensor rate is the upper limit of the sensor-indicated rate during exercise.

Sensitivity is the voltage level to which the pacemaker's sense amplifiers are responsive to electrical activities in the heart.

Refractory period is the period of time following the onset of an action potential during which the heart tissue will respond to neither an intrinsic impulse nor an extrinsic impulse.

Hysteresis is a pacing operation that allows a longer escape interval after a sensed intrinsic event. By waiting a bit longer after an intrinsic impulse, it gives the heart a greater opportunity to beat on its own.

Rate limit is a nonprogrammable upper limit of the pacemaker. It is a built-in safeguard to limit the rate of the pulse generator.

In general, the *acceptable lead impedance* of the pacemaker is from about 200 to 1,000 Ω. Very often, a patient load of 500 Ω is chosen to verify pacemaker parameters.

A number of different *output waveforms* are used by different pacemaker manufacturers. See Figure 21–9 for different types of waveforms. The simplest waveform is the square pulse.

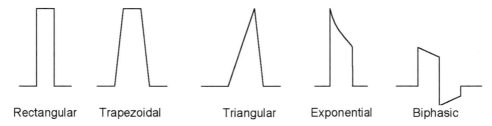

| Rectangular | Trapezoidal | Triangular | Exponential | Biphasic |

Figure 21–9. Pacemaker Output Pulses.

A lithium-iodine *battery* is commonly used in implantable pacemakers. For example, the Medtronic Sigma 213 lithium-iodine battery is rated at 2.8 V with a capacity of 0.83 Ah. Lithium silver vanadium (Li/SVO) batteries with energy density of 2.0 kJ/cm^3 are used in implantable cardiac defibrillators. In general, the lower the pacing rate, pulse amplitude, and pulse duration, the longer the battery life.

Chassis–the battery and electronic components of a pacemaker are placed inside a polypropylene container and then totally shielded by a titanium housing. The lead connectors are molded into an epoxy housing. A radiopaque ID code is placed inside the housing so that the pacemaker can be identified from a radiograph of the patient.

Example

Estimate the battery life of an implantable pacemaker given that it is pacing 100% at a rate of 70 beats per minute, with pulse width of 0.45 ms, pulse amplitude of 3.5 V, and lead impedance = 500 Ω. The useful capacity of the battery is 0.83 Ah at 2.8 V. Assume that 80% of the battery energy is used to produce the impulses.

Solution

The average output power *P* is the product of the output voltage, output current, and the duty cycle, Therefore,

$$P = \frac{V^2}{R}\frac{t_p}{T} = \frac{3.5^2 \times 0.45 \times 10^{-3}}{500 \times \dfrac{60}{70}} \, W = 13 \; \mu W.$$

The energy E of the battery is

$$E = V \times I \times t = 2.8 \times 0.83 \times 60 \times 60 = 3.4 \text{ kJ.}$$

If 80% of the energy is used to produce the impulses, the longevity t of the battery is

$$t = \frac{E}{P} = \frac{0.8 \times 3.4 \times 10^3}{13 \times 10^{-6}} \text{ s} = 0.21 \times 10^9 \text{ s} = 6.6 \text{ years.}$$

FUNCTIONAL BUILDING BLOCKS OF AN IMPLANTABLE PACEMAKER

In an implantable pacemaker, the battery occupies most of the volume of the pulse generator. The remaining space contains the electronic circuit for sensing, pacing, and communication. Pacemakers are non-field serviceable; all malfunctioned pacemakers are sent back to the factory for analysis. They will not be repaired and reused. Figure 21–10 is a functional block diagram of a dual chamber pacemaker. The descriptions of the various functional blocks follow.

- Battery Monitor–This is a voltage level detector to monitor battery level. When the battery voltage drops below a certain limit (e.g., below 2.2 V for a 2.8 V lithium-iodine battery), the pacemaker will suspend most activities (e.g., cease to collect data) and fall back to a fixed rate to conserve power. A battery replacement message will be displayed when the programmer is engaged with the pacemaker.
- Programming–The transmit/receive coil is the antenna for the programming signal. The signal from the external programmer is detected and demodulated to provide input signal to program the pacemaker parameters. Stored data from the pacemaker can be modulated and transmitted to the programmer via the transmit/receive coil.
- Atrial and Ventricular Sensing Amplifiers–The input filter and amplifier function together provide bandpass and gain characteristics to identify the intrinsic atrial and ventricular activities. The sensitivity detector circuit senses a minimum amplitude level according to the programmed sensitivity setting. A blanking circuit disables the sensing circuit for a predetermined period of time after an impulse is delivered.
- Output Circuit and Rate Limit–The output circuit is designed to deliver an electrical pulse to the heart. The pulse amplitude and duration is controlled by the digital timing circuit. The rate limit circuit operates independent of other circuits in the pacemaker. It limits the pulse rate

to a maximum value for patient safety (e.g., 185 min^{-1} for ventricular pacing).

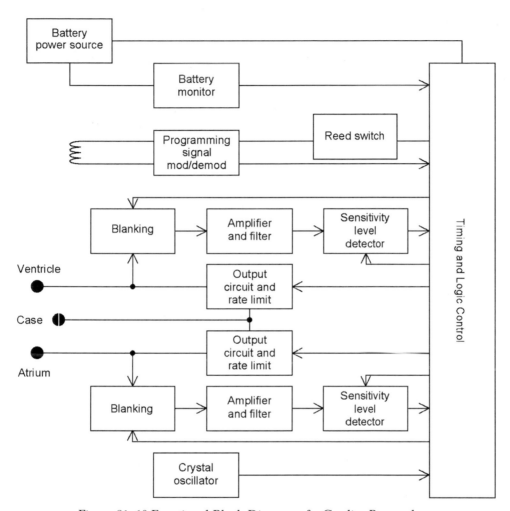

Figure 21–10.Functional Block Diagram of a Cardiac Pacemaker.

TEMPORARY PACING

Temporary cardiac pacing is achieved by employing external pacemakers. Temporary pacing is used under the following situations:

- After open-heart surgery until the heart reverts to a satisfactory condition

- For temporary pacing until a permanent pacemaker can be implanted
- When permanent pacing is not necessary such as in the case of someone recovering from myocardial infarction
- During surgery to control the heart rate

There are two types of external pacemakers: invasive and noninvasive.

External invasive pacemakers have the pulse generator located outside the patient's body. The pacing lead is inserted into the heart chamber via a venous access (endocardial lead). A return lead is attached to the ground electrode placed on the patient's skin.

External noninvasive pacemakers (also known as transcutaneous or transthoracic pacemaker) have two large-surface, pre-gelled, adhesive, disposable electrodes that conduct the stimuli through the skin and skeletal muscle to the heart. One electrode supplies a current and the other collects the current from the body. They are applied to either the anterior-posterior or anterior-anterior position of the patient's chest. External noninvasive pacing is preferred in some situations because it can be applied more quickly and easily and does not require the skills of a physician. However, each stimulating pulse causes contraction of skeletal muscle and can be painful to the patient. In demand mode, intrinsic heartbeats are generally picked up by an integrated ECG monitor using a separate set of leads and electrodes. As the electrical current must overcome the impedance of the skin and underlying tissues, and only a portion of the current flows through the heart, the pacing energy delivered by a transcutaneous pacemaker is substantially higher than that of an implantable or external invasive pacemaker (e.g., pacing current up to 20 mA and pulse width up to 20 ms in transcutaneous pacing). Table 21–3 summarizes the differences of the three types of pacemakers.

Table 21-3.
Characteristics of Different Types of Pacemakers.

	Implantable	*External Invasive*	*Transcutaneous*
Pulse Generator Placement	Inside body	Outside body	Outside body
Lead Placement	Inside body; connected to heart via a blood vessel into the heart chamber	Inserted through skin via a blood vessel into the heart chamber	Outside body; on skin posterior and anterior to the chest
Pacing Energy Level	Low	Low	High

POTENTIAL PROBLEMS WITH PACEMAKERS

Although the electronic circuits of modern pacemakers are very reliable, the pacemaker/lead system may operate inappropriately due to the following problems:

Threshold Drift–Threshold level may increase after initial implantation and may drift higher after prolonged usage. Increase in threshold may result in failure to capture.

Lead Problems–Broken lead wires, poor connections, and insulation failure may cause continuous or intermittent loss of capture, failure to sense properly, loss of sensing, cross-talk between leads, and inhibition of pacing.

Cross-talk occurs in dual chamber pacemakers when a stimulus or intrinsic event from one chamber is sensed by the other chamber (e.g., the ventricular lead senses the pacing stimulation initiated in the atrium), resulting in an inappropriate pacemaker response such as inhibition or resetting of the refractory period.

External Interference–Pacemakers may be susceptible to certain sources of electromagnetic interference (EMI). They include, but are not limited to, the following:

- Magnetic resonance imaging (MRI) scanners
- Therapeutic diathermy devices
- Therapeutic ionization radiation equipment
- Defibrillators
- Electrosurgical/cautery units
- High voltage systems and current-carrying conductors
- Radio transmitters
- Theft prevention security systems
- High power electromagnetic fields
- Ultrasound energy
- Communication equipment, such as cellular phones

If the pacemaker is inhibited or has reverted to asynchronous operation in the presence of EMI, turning off the source or moving the pacemaker away from the source may return the pacemaker to normal operation. Extremely strong EMI sources, however, may reset the pacemaker to partial or full electrical reset condition.

Muscle sensing–Electrical signals from skeletal muscle activities may be sensed and misinterpreted as heart activities. Muscle sensing may be corrected by increasing the sensitivity of the pacemaker.

Muscle stimulation–Refers to the stimulation of a muscle (other than the heart) by a pacing stimulus. Skeletal muscle stimulation only occurs with unipolar lead systems as it uses the body tissue as a return electrical path.

Diaphragmatic stimulation can occur in either bipolar or unipolar systems, usually due to electrode placement that is too close to the diaphragm or phrenic nerve.

Chapter 22

CARDIAC DEFIBRILLATORS

OBJECTIVES

• State the clinical applications of cardiac defibrillation. Sketch the damped sinusoidal, truncated exponential, and biphasic defibrillation waveforms, and analyze the basic circuits to generate such waveforms.
• Draw a block diagram of a cardiac defibrillator and explain the functions of each block.
• Describe built-in safety features, including isolated output and energy dump.
• Identify and explain the functions of critical components in a typical defibrillator.
• Explain synchronous cardioversion and its operating precautions.
• Identify common problems of cardiac defibrillators and methods to prevent the problems.

CHAPTER CONTENTS

INTRODUCTION

Fibrillation is an arrhythmia. During fibrillation, the heart muscle quivers randomly and erratically as a result of individual groups of heart muscle contracting randomly instead of synchronously. If fibrillation occurs at the ventricles, it is called ventricular fibrillation. This situation is life-threatening as it prevents effective pumping of blood to vital organs such as the brain, lungs, and the heart itself. If it occurs at the atria, it is called atrial fibrillation. Atrial fibrillation is less severe and in most cases is not fatal. However, it compromises cardiac output and will likely lead to other more severe arrhythmias. Figure 22–1 shows a normal sinus rhythm, atrial fibrillation, and ventricular fibrillation waveforms.

Prevost and Batelli in 1899 proved that an "appropriate" large, alternating current (AC) or direct current (DC) electric shock could reverse ventricular fibrillation. It was not until 1960 that open-chest defibrillation was replaced by the external defibrillation method. Today, the defibrillator is a critical life-saving medical device that is widely deployed in hospitals, clinics, ambulances, and even in public areas to treat sudden cardiac arrest.

PRINCIPLES OF DEFIBRILLATION

Fibrillation can be caused by disruption of the electroconductive pathways in the myocardial muscle such as the SA or AV nodes. It may also be triggered by an electrical shock. Passing a very large momentary electrical current through the heart causes all musculature of the heart to be depolarized for a short period of time and enter their refractory period together. This gives the SA node a chance to regain control and return to normal rhythm. Defibrillation can be external or internal. During defibrillation, an ECG monitor is necessary to detect ventricular fibrillation and thereafter monitor the heart function until the patient can be placed in a critical care environment. When defibrillation is applied externally on the patient, a larger voltage (and higher energy) is required to overcome the impedance of the body and to allow enough current to go through the heart. A typical discharge energy range is from 2 to 40 joules for internal defibrillation and 50 to 400 joules for external defibrillation.

Defibrillators/monitors can also be used for synchronized cardioversion to treat certain atrial arrhythmias such as atrial flutter or atrial fibrillation. An electrical shock applied to a nonfibrillating heart during the T wave of the heart rhythm may trigger ventricular fibrillation. During atrial flutter or atrial fibrillation, the ventricles can still contract at regular intervals, therefore

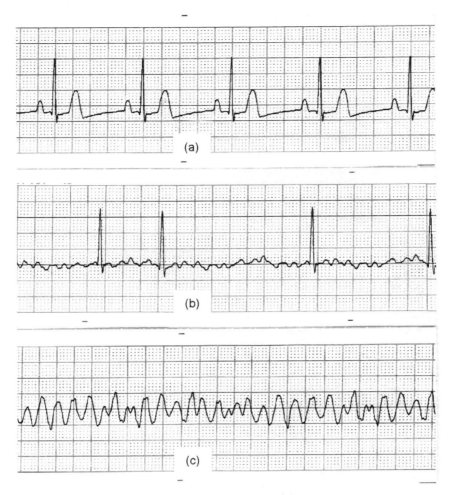

Figure 22–1. (a) Normal Sinus Rhythm, (b) Atrial Fibrillation,
(c) Ventricular Fibrillation.

producing a certain amount of cardiac output (e.g., 80% of the normal value). It would be counterproductive and could create a life-threatening situation to the patient should this countershock to correct atrial heart condition trigger ventricular fibrillation. In order to avoid discharging the energy during a T wave under cardioversion mode, the defibrillator is synchronized to discharge its energy right after the patient's R wave and before the T wave. This is achieved by detecting the R wave with the help of an ECG monitor and electronically synchronizing the energy discharge with a short delay (e.g., 30 ms) from the R wave.

An implantable cardiac defibrillator (ICD) is a pacemaker with defibrillation capability. Upon sensing ventricular fibrillation, an ICD will automatically produce a shock to the heart. An ICD can be programmed to provide defibrillation, cardioversion, antitachycardia pacing, and antibradycardia pacing.

Studies since its initial conception indicated that numerous factors can affect the effectiveness of the defibrillation procedure. These include the waveform, energy and amplitude of the electric shock, the electrode position, and interface impedance, as well as the size and weight of the patient.

DEFIBRILLATION WAVEFORMS

Early experimental defibrillators used 60 Hz alternating current (AC) and a step-up transformer to create and increase the defibrillation voltage. Bursts of several hundred volts of sine wave were applied across the chest wall for a period of 0.25 to 1 second. The desire for portability led to the development of direct current (DC) defibrillators. A DC defibrillator uses a battery as the power source so that connection to the AC outlet is not required during defibrillation. The battery may be replaced or recharged after use. It was later discovered that DC shocks were more effective than AC shocks. Until recently, defibrillators have used one of the two types of monophasic waveforms: damped sinusoidal (MDS) and monophasic truncated exponential (MTE). The MDS waveform is also called the Lown waveform. Figure 22–2 shows a typical MDS and MTE defibrillation waveform. Note that the typical MDS waveform has a small negative component; therefore, strictly speaking, it is not truly monophasic.

Monophasic waveforms require a high energy level (up to 360 J) to defibrillate effectively. A MDS waveform requires a high peak voltage (e.g., 5,000 V) to deliver such energy. The MTE waveform uses similar energy settings. However, it uses a lower voltage than the MDS waveform. In order to deliver the same amount of energy, the MTE waveform requires a longer duration. While studies had associated myocardium damages with high peak voltages, long-duration shocks have higher chances of refibrillation.

Studies in the early 1990s had shown that biphasic defibrillation waveforms are more effective than monophasic waveforms. In fact, the biphasic waveform has been the standard waveform for an implantable cardiac defibrillator (ICD) since it was introduced. With biphasic waveforms, the defibrillation current passes through the heart in one direction and then in the reverse direction. A number of biphasic waveforms are incorporated by different defibrillator manufacturers. Figure 22–3 shows one such waveform. Studies have shown that defibrillations using biphasic waveforms not only defibrillate as well as traditional monophasic waveforms but also are associated with better postshock cardiac function, fewer postshock arrhythmias,

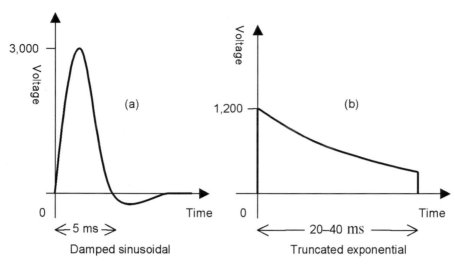

Figure 22–2. Monophasic Defibrillation Waveforms.

and better neurological outcomes for survivors. In addition, biphasic defibrillators at lower energy settings have been shown to produce the same results as traditional high energy monophasic defibrillators. One manufacturer recommends that escalating energy shock protocols traditionally used in monophasic defibrillation are not required in monophasic defibrillation. Instead, a setting of 150 J is recommended to be used for the first and all subsequent shocks.

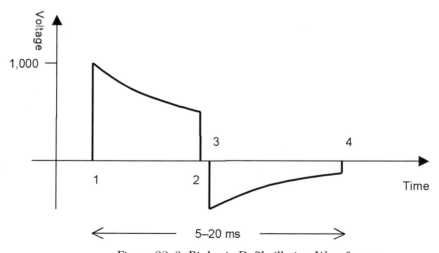

Figure 22–3. Biphasic Defibrillation Waveforms.

WAVEFORM SHAPING CIRCUITS

Figure 22–4 shows a simple functional block diagram of a DC cardiac defibrillator. The main component of a defibrillator is the energy storage capacitor. The capacitor is charged by the charging circuit, which is powered from the power supply. The charge control circuit monitors the amount of energy stored in the capacitor. It terminates the charging process when adequate energy has accumulated. The discharge control releases the stored energy from the energy storage capacitor when the user activates the discharge buttons. The waveform shaping circuit produces the particular type of waveform to effect defibrillation. Three of the more common waveform shaping circuits are discussed in this section.

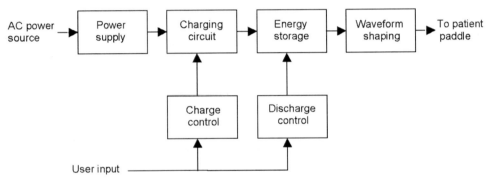

Figure 22–4. Block Diagram of a DC Defibrillator.

Monophasic Damped Sinusoidal Waveform

Figure 22–5 shows a simplified circuit to produce a damped sinusoidal defibrillation waveform. It consists of the energy storage capacity C, a step-up transformer, a rectifier, a charge relay, a discharge relay, and a wave shaping inductor L. During charging, the charge relay is energized, and AC voltage from the power source is stepped up to the desired level by the step-up transformer. The charging circuit (a full wave rectifier in this example) converts AC to a DC charging voltage. The capacity C is being charged up by this high-level DC voltage until enough energy is stored in the capacitor. The energy Ec stored in the capacitor is related to the voltage across the capacitor according to the equation:

$$Ec = \frac{1}{2}CV^2. \tag{1}$$

The voltage across the capacitor is monitored to determine the amount of energy stored. The charge relay is deenergized when sufficient energy is stored in the capacitor. When the operator pushes the discharge buttons, the discharge relay is energized. The energy stored in the capacitor flows through the inductor L into the patient. For ease of analysis, the patient load R is considered to be a resistive load of 50 Ω. The current discharging through this LRC circuit produces the damped sinusoidal waveform (Figure 22–2a).

Example

A cardiac defibrillator is designed to deliver up to 400 joules of energy during discharge. If a capacitor of 16 µF is used as the energy storage capacitor, what is the minimum voltage across the capacitor at full charge?

Solution

Using equation (1),

$$V = \sqrt{\frac{2E}{C}} = \frac{2 \times 400}{16 \times 10^{-6}} = 7,000 \text{ V}.$$

The minimum voltage across the capacitor is 7,000 V.

In practice, not all energy stored in the capacitor is delivered to the patient during discharge. Some energy, for example, is lost as heat in the discharge circuit. The energy delivered to the patient E_D is always less than the energy stored in the capacitor E_C. Assuming that the patient load is a constant resistive load, the energy delivered to the patient E_D for an MDS waveform defibrillator is given by:

$$E_D = \int_{t=0}^{t=\infty} \frac{V^2}{R} \, dt = \frac{1}{R} \int_{t=0}^{t=\infty} V^2 \, dt.$$

A typical value of the waveform shaping inductor to produce an MDS waveform is 50 mH. The function of the resistor R_L is to limit the initial inrush current into the capacitor when the charge relay is first energized. Without R_L, the large inrush current may damage components in the charging circuit. A typical value of R_L is 3 kΩ, which will limit the initial inrush current to a worst case of 2.3 A (7,000 V divided by 3 KΩ).

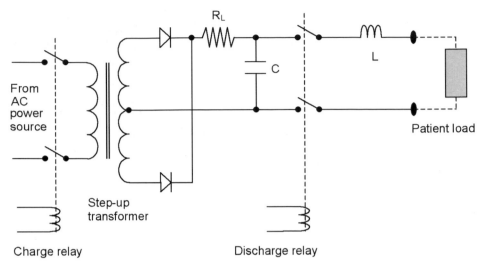

Figure 22–5. Simple MDS Defibrillator Circuit.

Monophasic Truncated Exponential Waveform

Figure 22–6 shows a simplified circuit of a monophasic truncated exponential waveform defibrillator. This circuit is identical to the circuit described above except that there is no waveform shaping inductor in the discharge circuit. A typical value of the energy storage capacitor is 200 µF. Without the inductor, the discharge circuit is an RC instead of a LRC circuit where R is the patient load. An RC discharge will produce an exponential decay curve (Figure 22–2b). Instead of allowing sufficient time to discharge all energy stored in the energy storage capacitor, a MTE defibrillator will terminate the discharge when enough energy is delivered to the patient. During defibrillation, the voltage across the paddles is monitored and the amount of energy discharged into the patient E_D is determined by:

$$E_D = \int_{t=0}^{t=T} \frac{V^2}{R} \, dt = \frac{1}{R} \int_{t=0}^{t=T} V^2 \, dt.$$

Biphasic Truncated Exponential Waveform

Figure 22–7 shows a simplified circuit of a biphasic truncated exponential waveform generator. A bank of switches is added to the previously described MTE circuit. By closing and opening the biphasic switches S1 to S4, a biphasic waveform (Figure 22–3) is produced. Table 22–1 shows the switching sequence of the switches and relays for the charging, discharging, and energy dumping functions. In the table, an "X" denotes switch closure.

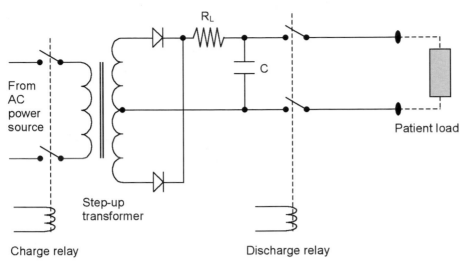

Figure 22–6. Simple MTE Defibrillator Circuit.

There are four phases in the discharge sequence: positive (P1), zero (P2), negative (P3), and discharge (P4).

During the charging period, the charge relay is energized, and switch SC is closed so that the capacitor (e.g., a 200 μF metalized polypropylene capacitor) is charged by the charging circuit. SC will open when enough charge is stored in the capacitor. In the positive phase of the discharge sequence, S1, S4, and SD are closed. The flow path of the current from the capacitor is:

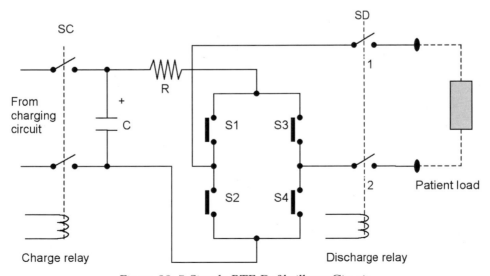

Figure 22–7. Simple BTE Defibrillator Circuit.

R→S1→SD-1→patient→SD-2→S4 and back to the capacitor. During the zero phase, only SD is closed. This zero phase provides a time separation to ensure that S1 and S4 are opened before S2 and S3 are closed. If all fours switches are closed at the same time, a short circuit on the output circuit will result. In the negative phase, S2 and S3 are closed. The current flow path from the capacitor is: R→S3→SD-2→patient→SD-1→S2 and back to the capacitor. After enough energy is discharged, all biphasic switches and SD are closed to remove the remaining charge stored in the energy storage capacitor. The previously described phases complete the discharge sequence. If the capacitor is charged but defibrillation is not necessary, the energy stored in the capacitor must be removed for safety reasons. All modern defibrillators have a programmed dumping sequence to remove the stored charge if defibrillation is not performed within a set time (e.g., after 60 seconds) and also when another energy level is selected (to avoid high residue energy stored in the capacitor). To dump the stored energy, all biphasic switches are closed to allow the energy to discharge through the resistor R.

Table 22–1.
Biphasic Waveform Generator Switching Sequence.

	SC	S1	S2	S3	S4	SD	
Charging	X						
P1 (1–2)		X			X	X	Positive
P2 (2–3)						X	Zero
P3 (3–4)			X	X		X	Negative
P4 (4–5)		X	X	X	X	X	Discharge
Energy dump		X	X	X	X		

SC and SD are mechanical switches. In fact, these are the contacts of high current relays (or contactors). The biphasic switches S1, S2, S3, and S4 are solid-state switches. S4 is usually a high-voltage, high-current switch (such as an insulated gate bipolar transistor) that is designed to interrupt the circuit at any current level. S1, S2, and S3 are usually silicon controlled rectifiers. The function of the resistor R is to limit current during capacitor discharge or energy dump. Some manufacturers may introduce an additional inductor to modify the shape of the waveform. For example, one manufacturer used a 5 Ω, 700 μH inductive resistor to serve both functions.

FUNCTIONAL BUILDING BLOCKS OF DEFIBRILLATORS

Figure 22–8 shows the functional block diagram of a DC defibrillator. After the user selects the energy setting and pushes the charge button, the charge control circuit energizes the charge relay. The voltage across the energy storage capacitor is monitored during charging. Using equation (1), the charge relay is deenergized when the voltage across the capacitor is equal to the voltage corresponding to the selected defibrillation energy level. The charging sequence is then completed. The discharge relay is energized once the user pushes the discharge buttons on the defibrillator paddles (both buttons, one on each paddle, must be activated to prevent inadvertent discharge). The energy stored in the capacitor is then released through the waveform shaping circuit to the patient's chest to perform defibrillation. The energy being delivered to the patient is determined by the voltage and current monitors ($E_D = V \times I \times t$). When the total delivered energy has reached the user selected value, the discharge relay is deenergized.

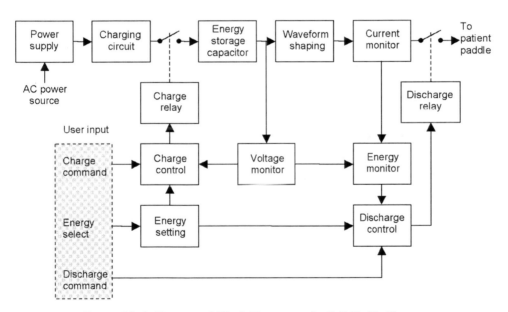

Figure 22–8. Functional Block Diagram of a DC Defibrillator.

Due to portability requirements, an internal rechargeable battery is used as the primary energy source of DC defibrillators. The capacity of a fully charged battery is usually sufficient to perform 20 to 80 defibrillation discharges. Defibrillators are always plugged into the AC mains on standby. AC voltage is rectified to charge the battery. When fully charged, the battery charge is maintained using a trickle charge system. During the charging phase, the low-voltage DC from the battery is first converted to a high-frequency (e.g., 25 kHz) AC voltage by an inverter. This AC voltage is then stepped up to a higher voltage, say, 7,000 V, and rectified to charge the energy storage capacitor. The functional block diagram of the power supply and charging circuit is shown in Figure 22–9.

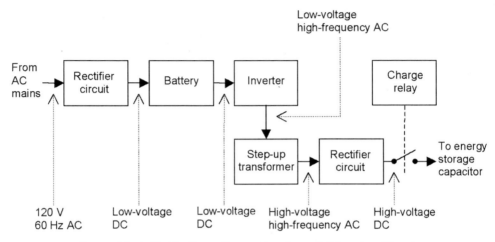

Figure 22–9. Defibrillator Power Supply and Charging Circuit.

OUTPUT ISOLATION AND ENERGY DUMPING

A defibrillator produces an electrical shock on the patient to correct heart arrhythmia. If during the delivery of an electrical shock, the operator inadvertently touches the discharge paddles or the patient, the shock may cause burns or trigger ventricular fibrillation to the operator. Such injuries to the operator can be prevented by isolating the output of the defibrillator from ground. Figure 22–10a shows a nonisolated defibrillator output circuit. When an operator who has a ground connection is in contact with the output while the energy is discharged, a current will flow through the operator to ground and return to the energy storage capacitor. Figure 22–10b shows an isolated defibrillator output circuit. During shock delivery, the energy storage capacitor is not connected to ground. Theoretically, even when the operator is touching a defibrillator paddle, no current will flow through the operator as there is no return path for such current. In practice, however, a small current still flows through the operator.

Isolated output can also prevent secondary burn to the patient. For a grounded output circuit, a secondary burn occurs when the patient is in contact with ground; such ground connection will provide a alternative return path for the discharge current. It will cause a burn at the ground contact site if sufficient current flows through this patient ground path.

After the energy storage capacitor is charged, if no defibrillation is necessary after a period of time, the charge in the capacitor will be dumped through a high power resistor. This is a safety feature to ensure that no hazardous high voltage is present in the unit for the safety of the users. In addition, if another energy level is selected, the charge stored in the capacitor will be released before it receives its new charge. This is to prevent accumulation of charge in the capacitor, especially if the new selection is of lower energy.

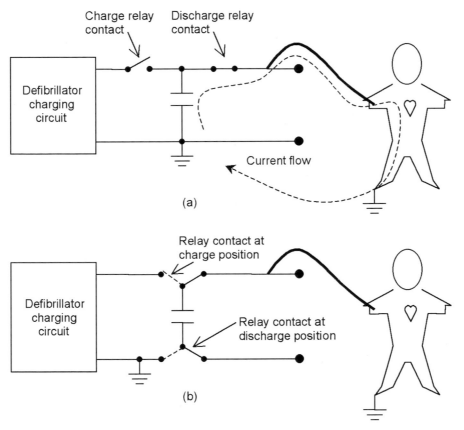

Figure 22–10. (a) Nonisolated Output, (b) Isolated Output.

CARDIOVERSION

Cardiac defibrillators are useful in correcting ventricular fibrillation. However, the defibrillation shock may trigger ventricular fibrillation in a healthy heart. During atrial fibrillation or atrial flutter, only the atrial muscle is contracting erratically. Studies have shown that a defibrillation pulse applied during the refractory period (T wave) of the ventricles may induce other more severe arrhythmias such as ventricular fibrillation. Therefore, a synchronization circuit is required in cardioversion to avoid such complications.

The window of discharge for safe cardioversion is immediately after the QRS complex and before the T wave. A cardioversion synchronizing circuit consists of an R wave detector and a time delay circuit to synchronize the discharge within this safety window (Figure 22–11). An enabling signal is sent to the discharge control about 30 ms after detection of the R wave. When the synchronous cardioversion feature is selected, care should be taken to check whether the machine is able to lock onto the R wave (usually, successful detection of the R wave is highlighted on the ECG display). The user may have to increase the ECG sensitivity level to provide sufficient R wave amplitudes for the R wave detector to lock onto the signal.

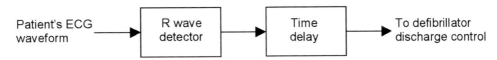

Figure 22–11. Cardioversion Synchronous Module.

DEFIBRILLATOR OPERATION AND QUALITY ASSURANCE

The procedures for safe operation of a cardiac defibrillator are:

1. Apply electrolyte gel to the defibrillator paddles (for better patient electrical contact and to reduce risk of burn by lowering the skin resistance).
2. Set energy level and press the charge button.
3. Allow capacitor to charge until a ready signal is given.
4. Press the paddles against the patient's chest.
5. Clear the patient area.
6. Press the defibrillator discharge buttons.
7. Check the patient's ECG waveform.

8. Repeat the above procedures if no sinus rhythm is detected (usually with a higher energy setting).

Because a defibrillator delivers a high-voltage therapeutic pulse to critically ill patients, reliability of the device is crucial. A defibrillator should be tested regularly to ensure its performance. Most hospitals require daily user testing. Depending on the hospital's protocol, testing includes functional checks and may include checking for correct energy delivery. Often, extensive performance verifications, including battery capacity and defibrillation energy accuracy, are done periodically (e.g., every 3 months) by biomedical engineering personnel. When not in use, a defibrillator should always be plugged into the AC wall outlet to ensure that the internal battery is charged and ready for use.

COMMON PROBLEMS

Problems with defibrillators can be divided into two groups: hardware problems and operational problems.

Hardware Problems

- Batteries are considered as high-maintenance components in a defibrillator. Failure of batteries prevents successful defibrillation, causing death. Common battery problems include battery not fully charged, battery failure, and cell memory failure in some batteries. Common batteries used in defibrillator are nickel-cadmium (NiCad), sealed lead acid, and nickel metal hydride (NiMH).
- Electronic components in general are quite reliable.
- Due to the need to deliver high-energy discharge pulses, relay failure is not uncommon in defibrillators. Relay contacts (especially the discharge relay) may be pitted from arcing which creates high resistance at the contact; or fused due to excessive heat from high discharge current.
- Common problems with the energy storage capacitor are excessive leakage (which prevents the capacitor from maintaining the energy level), and short circuit due to insulation breakdown.

Hardware problems can be prevented by periodic performance assurance inspections and battery analysis.

Operational Problems

- Users not familiar with the operation of the defibrillator
- Incorrect application of conductive gel, causing high paddle-skin resistance; high current density; or current shunt path, which may lead to unsuccessful defibrillation or patient injuries
- Incorrect paddle placement resulting in current not passing through the heart
- Electrical shock to staff from gel spill, staff touching patient, or staff touching paddles

Most user errors can be prevented by proper in-service training, periodic practice, and equipment standardization.

Problem Unique to Synchronous Cardioversion

- Unit not picking up R wave properly (missing or too low R wave level due to poor skin contact or too low sensitivity setting)

To prevent problems or hazards, the following must be done by the users regularly:

- Receive proper user in-service training.
- Perform operational check by charging and discharging into dummy load (e.g., weekly).
- Plug unit into wall outlet to maintain battery charge when not in use.
- Clean unit, especially paddles, after every use to prevent dried gel and dirt from building up.
- Check quantities and expiration dates of all supplies (e.g., conductive gel, ECG electrodes) that are with the unit.
- Send unit periodically to biomedical engineering for complete functional and calibration check.

Chapter 23

INFUSION DEVICES

OBJECTIVES

- State the applications of IV infusion.
- Describe the setup and identify the components of a typical gravity flow manual infusion system.
- List the common problems encountered in manual gravity flow infusion.
- Differentiate between infusion pumps and infusion controllers.
- Analyze the pumping mechanisms of common infusion pumps.
- Evaluate the safety and convenient features of modern infusion pumps.
- Draw a functional block diagram of an infusion pump and describe its operation.
- Review performance verification procedures of infusion pumps.
- Identify factors affecting the accuracy of infusion pumps.

CHAPTER CONTENTS

1. Introduction
2. Purpose of IV Infusion
3. Types of Infusion Devices
4. Manual Gravity Flow Infusion
5. Infusion Controllers
6. Infusion Pumps and Pumping Mechanisms
7. Common Features
8. Functional Block Diagram
9. Performance Evaluation
10. Factors Affecting Flow Accuracy

INTRODUCTION

Infusion devices are used to administer fluid into the body either through intravenous (IV) or epidural routes. Infusion devices for IV administration are commonly referred to as IV devices. As the venous pressure is below 50 mmHg (about 0.6 mH_2O), a 1-meter water column is sufficient to allow gravity to overcome the venous blood pressure and drive the solution into the blood vessel. Manual gravity flow IV infusion is used extensively in health care facilities for general-purpose infusion. To allow more controlled and accurate fluid delivery, more sophisticated devices have been developed. A number of infusion devices are available for different applications. This chapter studies the principles and applications of a few of these devices.

PURPOSE OF IV INFUSION

In general, four types of solutions are administered intravenously.

1. Water–Usually in the form of saline or dextrose, to prevent patient dehydration.
2. Medications and electrolytes–IV administration of drugs and electrolytes produces precise and fast-acting effects as it sends the drug directly into the bloodstream without going through the process of digestion and absorption. Examples include IV cardiovascular drugs, chemotherapy drugs, et cetera.
3. Nutrition–Although parenteral nutrition can be delivered through enteral feeding, total or partial parenteral nutrition is administered by IV infusion to patients when their normal diet cannot be ingested, absorbed, or tolerated for a significant period of time.
4. Blood–Blood infusion may be performed by an IV infusion device. However, some may require special infusion sets to avoid problems associated with the relatively high viscosity of blood and potential hemolysis of blood cells.

IV infusion is a procedure commonly performed in health care facilities. Infusion devices can be found in most parts of a hospital, including the emergency department, medical imaging areas, operating rooms, and so forth.

TYPES OF INFUSION DEVICES

Many different types of infusion devices are available in the market. Each has its own characteristics and serves some special applications. In general, infusion devices can be divided into two main groups: gravity flow infusion devices and infusion pumps. A gravity flow infusion device relies on the gravitational force exerted by a liquid column to push the fluid via a venous access into the patient's bloodstream, whereas an infusion pump has a motorized pumping mechanism to generate the positive pressure. Within the gravitation group are the manual gravity flow sets and the infusion controllers. There are two types of pumps in the infusion pump group: volumetric and syringe. Within the volumetric pump group are three different pumping mechanisms: piston cylinder, diaphragm, and peristaltic pumping mechanisms. Figure 23–1 shows the different types of infusion devices.

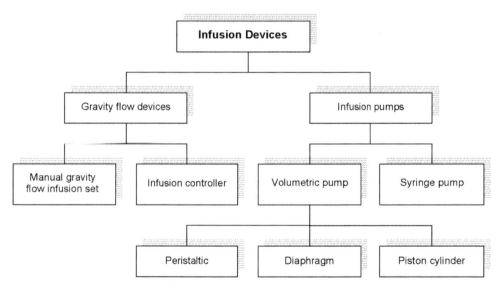

Figure 23–1. Types of Infusion Devices.

MANUAL GRAVITY FLOW INFUSION

The simplest infusion device is the manual gravity flow infusion set. Figure 23–2 shows a typical gravity flow infusion set. It consists of a long flexible PVC tubing with a solution bag spike at one end and a luer lock connector at the other end. The following sections describe the functional components of a gravity flow infusion setup.

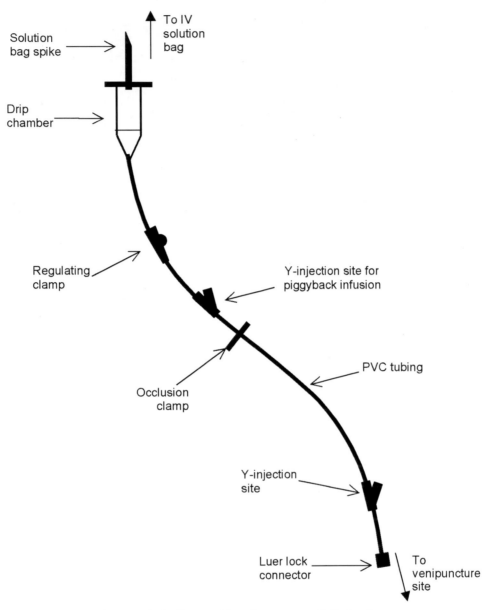

Figure 23–2. Gravity Flow Intravenous Infusion Set.

IV Solution Bag

The solution bag contains the IV solution and comes in different sizes (e.g., 500 cc, 1 liter, etc.). The bag is usually hung on an IV pole about 1.5 m above the infusion site to create enough pressure to overcome the venous pressure to cause infusion. Solution-filled glass bottles instead of disposable bags are used in some developing countries.

Solution Bag Spike

The solution bag spike is a sharp-ended tubing connecting the set to the IV solution bag. This sharp spike is pushed through the seal of the solution bag to allow solution to flow from the bag into the line.

Drip Chamber

The drip chamber is a clear compartment that permits the clinician to see the solution drops coming down from the solution bag. The size of the drop nozzle is designed so that each drop of solution is 1/20 ml (or 1/60 ml for slow flow rate sets). By counting the number of drops within a known time interval, a nurse can calculate the volume flow rate of the infusion.

Regulating Clamp

The regulating clamp is used to control the volume flow rate of infusion. It is also known as a roller clamp. By squeezing the roller over the flexible PVC tubing, it changes the cross-sectional area of the lumen, thereby controlling the infusion flow rate.

Y-injection Site

The Y-injection site provides a point of access into the infusion line. Drugs or other solutions can be injected into the infusion fluid by puncturing the injection port with a needle. To infuse a second solution when an infusion line has already been established (e.g., medication, blood plasma, etc.), a setup called piggyback infusion is used (Figure 23–3a). In this setup, since the secondary solution bag is located at a higher level than the primary solution bag, only the solution from the second bag will flow downstream through the Y-injection site. Flow of the primary solution will resume automatically when the secondary solution bag becomes emptied.

Occlusion Clamp

An occlusion clamp is used to totally occlude or shut down the infusion flow. Unlike the roller clamp, an occlusion clamp either fully opens the infu-

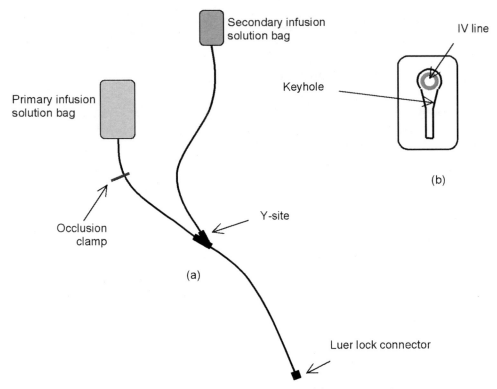

Figure 23–3. (a) Piggyback Infusion Setup, (b) Occlusion Clamp.

sion line or totally occludes the line. It is constructed from a piece of thick plastic with the infusion line threaded through a keyhole-shaped opening in the middle (Figure 23–3b). The line is fully open when the PVC tubing is at the larger opening of the keyhole. If the line is pushed to the narrow end, the clamp will occlude the tubing and shut off the flow.

Luer Lock Connector

A luer lock connector is a special twist lock mechanism to ensure a secure connection. To set up an IV infusion, a catheter is inserted into a vein; the other end of the catheter is a male luer lock connector. After the IV line is primed, it is connected to the catheter using the luer lock connector.

The procedure to prime the IV line is:

• Suspend the IV solution bag on the IV pole.
• Open the bag containing the IV line following sterile supplies handling procedure.
• Insert the solution bag spike of the line into the IV bag.

- Open the roller clamp and the occlusion clamp to allow the solution to flush all the air from the line.
- Remove air bubbles trapped in the Y-injection site by inverting and gently tapping it with a finger.
- Close the roller clamp and connect the luer lock at the end of the line to the luer lock at the catheter.
- Squeeze and release the drip chamber compartment to fill about one-third of the chamber with the IV solution.
- Slowly open the roller clamp to set up the desired solution flow rate (by counting the drops using a stopwatch).

Example

A nurse is observing the drop rate in the drip chamber to set the infusion flow rate on a manual gravity flow infusion set. How many drops per minute should be counted in the drip chamber if an infusion flow rate of 60 ml/hr is required? Assume that a 20 drops/ml nozzle is used in the drip chamber.

Solution

At a flow of 60 ml/hr, 60×20 drops will come down from the nozzle in 1 hour. Therefore, there will be $60 \times 20/60 = 20$ drops from the nozzle in 1 minute.

As the fluid to be infused flows directly into the bloodstream, infusion sets are sterilized inside their packages and are single-use disposable devices. With proper handling, infusion fluid from the solution bag flows only inside the infusion line, thereby maintaining the sterility of the system. A major drawback of manual gravity flow infusion is the low flow rate accuracy. As the mechanism to regulate the infusion flow rate (roller clamp) relies on compressing the PVC tubing of the infusion set, the rate of infusion cannot be precisely controlled. Figure 23–4 shows the change in flow rate after initial setup when there is no user intervention. This decrease in flow is due primarily to the nonperfect elastic nature of the material of the infusion line. The flow rate also changes with the level of fluid in the solution bag (the height of the liquid column). Experiments have shown that the flow rate can drop by about 40% within a couple of hours after initial setup. To overcome such a problem, as a normal practice, a nurse must recheck the flow rate after initial setup and adjust the regulating clamp to reestablish the desired flow rate.

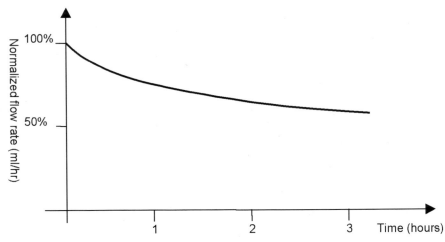

Figure 23–4. Flow Rate Change in Gravity Infusion.

INFUSION CONTROLLERS

An infusion controller overcomes the problem of flow rate variation by automatically adjusting the regulating clamp. Figure 23–5 shows the setup of an infusion controller. An infusion controller monitors the flow rate by counting the drops in the drip chamber. A typical drop sensor consists of an infrared light-emitting diode (LED) and an infrared light-sensitive transistor, each located on the opposite side of the drip chamber. A fluid drop from the solution bag interrupts the optical path and produces an electrical pulse. The flow rate is computed from the drop rate and the drop size. The calculated flow rate is then compared to the setting. If it is lower than the setting, the pinching force of the pinch mechanism will be released to allow more fluid to flow through. If it is higher, it will increase the pinching force to reduce the flow. Such a feedback mechanism maintains a constant flow rate equal to the setting. Although it automatically regulates the fluid flow rate, an infusion controller still relies on gravitational force to generate the infusion. If there is some restriction in the infusion line, the gravity pressure created by the liquid column may not be sufficient to produce the desired flow rate.

INFUSION PUMPS AND PUMPING MECHANISMS

An infusion pump contains a motor-driven pumping mechanism to produce a net positive pressure on the fluid inside the infusion line. With the

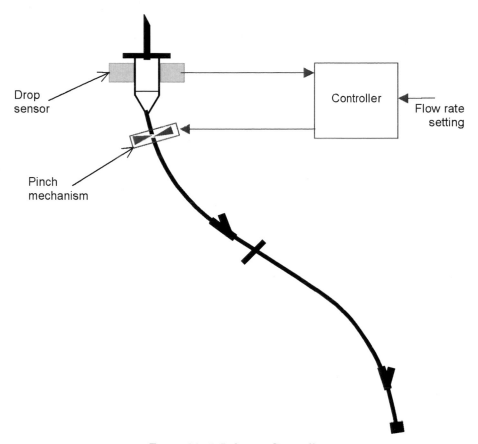

Figure 23–5. Infusion Controller.

pumping mechanism, infusion pumps produce a more controlled and consistent flow than infusion controllers. Infusion pumps can be divided into two types: volumetric pumps and syringe pumps.

Three common pumping mechanisms are used in volumetric infusion pumps. They are piston cylinder, diaphragm, and peristaltic. A syringe pump uses a screw and nut mechanism to drive the plunger of a syringe; it is also called a screw pump. The following sections describe these pumping mechanisms.

Piston Cylinder Pumps

The pumping mechanism of a piston cylinder pump consists of a cylinder, a piston, and valves that are mechanically linked to the piston motion. A stepper motor drives a cam to move the piston in and out of the cylinder in a reciprocal motion. Figure 23–6a shows that when the piston is moving downward, it creates a negative pressure inside the cylinder. The valve, which is linked to the cam, will be in such a position that the input port to the cylinder is opened and the output port is closed. Fluid from the IV bag will therefore be drawn into the cylinder. When the piston is moving upward (Figure 23–6b), the valve will close the input port and open the output port, allowing IV solution in the cylinder to exit through the output port. The stroke distance and the diameter of the piston determine the stroke volume, and the infusion flow rate is equal to the stroke volume times the cam's rotational speed.

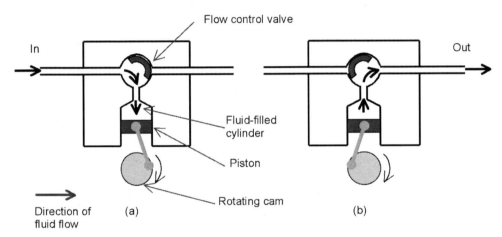

Figure 23–6. Piston Cylinder Infusion Mechanism.

Diaphragm Pumps

The pumping mechanism of a diaphragm pump is similar to that of a piston cylinder pump except that the stroke motion is replaced by a moveable diaphragm. In the illustration shown (Figure 23–7), when the diaphragm moves to the left, the intake valve is open to allow fluid to enter the fluid chamber. When it moves to the right, fluid is forced out of the chamber. Repeating the action provides a continuous flow of fluid.

Peristaltic Pumps

A peristaltic pump employs a protruding finger mechanism to occlude the flexible IV tubing. Its pumping action is similar to one using the thumb and index finger to squeeze on a plastic tubing filled with fluid and then running the fingers along the tube. This action will force the fluid to move along

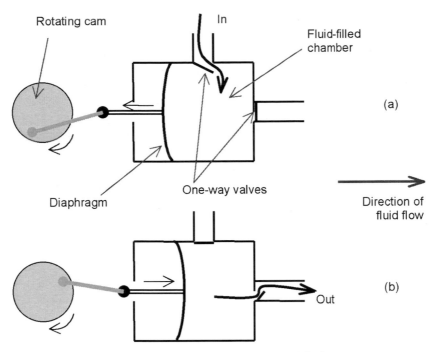

Figure 23–7. Piston Diaphragm Infusion Mechanism.

the direction of the finger motion. Repeating this action will produce a continuous fluid flow.

Figure 23–8a shows the pumping mechanism of a rotary peristaltic infusion pump. In a rotary peristaltic pump (or roller pump), the rotor has several protruding rollers. The flexible IV tubing is placed inside a groove on the pumping mechanism housing with one side open to the rotor. The rollers on the rotating rotor push the tubing against the wall of the groove. The protruding rollers, while occluding the tubing, move in one direction along the IV tubing, creating a continuous fluid flow in the direction of motion of the rollers.

Instead of rotating the protruding rollers over the IV tubing, the protruding fingers in the linear peristaltic infusion pump sequentially occlude the IV tubing. Figure 23–8b shows the positions of the protruding fingers of a linear peristaltic pump at three sequential time instances. These coordinated motions of the protruding fingers produce a continuous flow of fluid in the direction shown. The driving mechanism of a linear peristaltic pump is shown in Figure 23–9. To create a linear peristaltic motion, cams with eccentric axes are attached to a rotating cam shaft (Figure 23–10a) such that when a shaft rotates, it moves the protruding finger up or down according to its eccentric angle of rotation (Figure 23–10b).

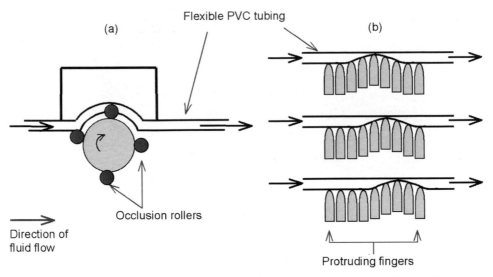

Figure 23–8. Peristaltic Infusion Mechanism. (a) Rotary Peristaltic; (b) Linear Peristaltic.

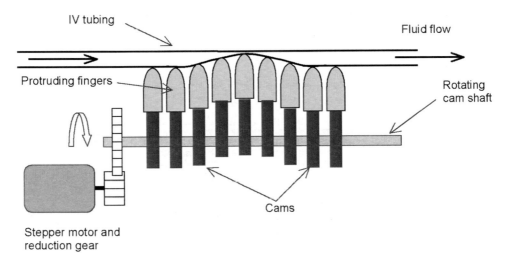

Figure 23–9. Linear Peristaltic Pump Driving Mechanism.

Syringe Pumps

A syringe pump has a long screw mounted on the pump support. The screw is rotated by a stepper motor and gear combination. The screw is supported by two bearings to allow smooth operation. As the screw rotates, it moves a nut threaded onto the screw in the horizontal direction (Figure 23–11). The nut is attached to a pusher connecting to the plunger of a

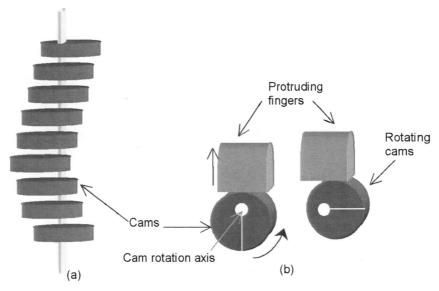

(a)

(b)

Protruding fingers

Rotating cams

Cams

Cam rotation axis

Figure 23–10. Linear Peristaltic Plunger Driving Mechanism.

syringe, which is loaded with the solution to be infused. The flow rate of the fluid coming out of the syringe depends on the rotational speed of the screw and the cross sectional area of the syringe body. In mathematical terms, the volume flow rate of a syringe pump is:

$$F = R \times t \times A,$$

where:
F = volume flow rate in cubic centimeters per minute,
R = rotational speed of the screw in revolutions per minute,
t = screw pitch in cm, and
A = cross-sectional area of the syringe plunger in cm^2.

Syringe pumps are often used in high-accuracy, low-flow rate applications (e.g., 0.5 to 10 ml/hr) and when more uniform flow pattern is required. It is also used to infuse thicker feeding solutions. A patient-controlled analgesic (PCA) pump is a special syringe pump designed to allow patients to self-administer boluses of narcotic analgesic for pain relief.

In general, piston cylinder infusion pumps and syringe pumps produce a more accurate and consistent flow output. However, during low flow rate settings, piston pumps (both piston cylinder and diaphragm) produce boluses of infusion rather than a smooth flow pattern. Figure 23–12a shows the flow pattern of a piston cylinder pump at a low flow rate setting (e.g., 10 ml/hr); a bolus in the diagram corresponds to the flow of one stroke of the piston. A bolus type of infusion may not be suitable for some applications such as

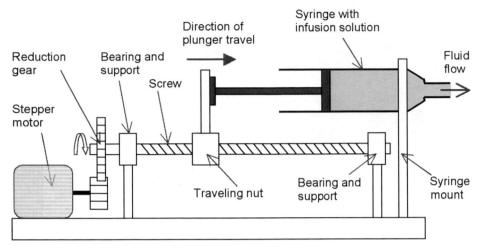

Figure 23–11. Syringe Pump.

administering medications to small infants. Under ideal conditions, a syringe pump will produce a uniform flow with little fluctuation. A peristaltic pump, with its multiple protruding finger pumping action, produces a flow pattern with less fluctuation than piston pumps as shown in Figure 23–12b.

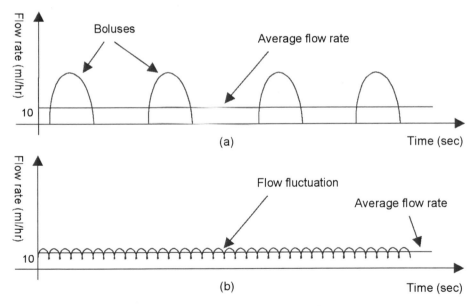

Figure 23–12. Low Flow Rate Infusion Flow Pattern.

COMMON FEATURES

Some common features found in general-purpose infusion pumps are described in the following sections. Depending on the design application, an infusion pump may have other additional features.

Flow Rates

The flow rate of a general-purpose infusion pump can be set within a range from 1 to 999 ml/hr with an accuracy of ±5 to 10%. For neonatal pumps, the range is 0.1 to 99 m/hr with an accuracy of ± 2%.

Volume To Be Infused (VTBI)

A VTBI of 1 to 9,999 ml can be programmed such that the pump will stop after this volume has been delivered. Usually, when VTBI is reached, an audible tone will sound to alert the clinician. The pump will switch to its KVO rate.

Keep Vein Open (KVO)

When infusion has stopped, in order to prevent blood clot at the venipuncture site, a slow infusion rate of about 1 to 5 ml/hr is maintained to flush the catheter to prevent blood clotting.

Occlusion Pressure Alarm

A pressure sensor inside the pump monitors the pressure of infusion. A high pressure indicates occlusion downstream of the pump. An alarm is set to notify the clinician to check the IV line. Downstream occlusion may be due to clot IV catheter or pinching of the IV line (e.g., by the patient rolling over the line). In some infusion pumps, the occlusion pressure alarm may be adjusted to activate between 1 and 20 psi.

Fluid Depletion (or Upstream Occlusion) Alarm

When the IV bag is empty, a negative pressure will develop upstream of the pump. An alarm to indicate such a condition can prevent air from entering the IV line and being infused into the patient.

Infusion Runaway (or Free Flow) Prevention

Most modern pumps have a built-in mechanism to prevent free flow of solution into the patient. Free flow can occur when the IV line is removed from the pump while the occlusion clamp and roller clamp are both open. When the pump is used to administer a potent drug to a patient, free flow can impose serious risk to the patient if a large dose of such medication is infused into the patient. A mechanical interlock on the IV line to shut off the line when it is pulled out from the pump will prevent this.

Air-in-Line Detection

To prevent air embolism in patients, air-in-line detectors are built into infusion pumps to detect air bubbles in the IV lines. Infusion will stop and an alarm will sound when a large air bubble is detected during infusion.

Dose Error Reduction System

This is a software algorithm that checks programmed doses against preset limits specific to certain drugs and clinical location profiles. It alerts clinicians if the programmed dose exceeded the preset limits. For example, drug X used in area A has a dose limit of 20 mcg/kg/hr. If the dose, based on the programmed flow rate and drug concentration, exceeds 20 mcg/kg/hr, infusion will not start and an alarm will sound.

Battery Operation

Most pumps are powered by internal rechargeable batteries so that the pump may be moved around with the patient during use. A battery low detector circuit will alert the user if the battery is running low and must be recharged.

FUNCTIONAL BLOCK DIAGRAM

Figure 23–13 shows a functional block diagram of a volumetric infusion pump. The user input/output interfaces are shown on the left-hand side of the diagram. User selectable inputs include:
- Infusion flow rate
- Volume to be infused (VTBI)

- Keep vein open (KVO) enable selection
- Pump start/stop control

The CPU, based on the input settings, controls the speed of the stepper motor driving the pumping mechanism to deliver the set infusion rate. The rotational speed of the pump driver is monitored by a LED/optical transistor slit detector. Based on this rotational speed, the volume of infusion is computed and compared to the VTBI setting. If KVO is enabled, the motor speed will be reduced to the KVO rate when VTBI has been reached.

The pressure in the IV line is monitored by a pressure sensor pressing on the IV tube inside the pump. When the pressure exceeds the occlusion pressure, the CPU will shut down the pump and sound an alarm.

Air bubbles in the IV line are detected by an ultrasound transmitter and receiver pair. The attenuation of ultrasound in air is higher than that in water.

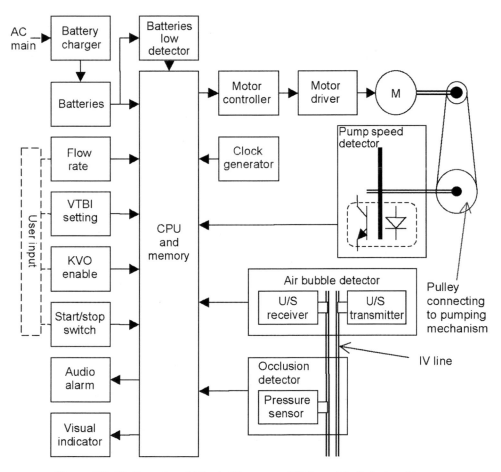

Figure 23–13. Functional Block Diagram of Volumetric Infusion Pump.

When an air bubble passes through the detector, the intensity of ultrasound detected by the receiver will decrease. The duration of this decreased signal corresponds to the size of the air bubble in the line. The CPU will stop infusion and sound an alarm if a large air bubble is detected.

PERFORMANCE EVALUATION

An important performance parameter of an infusion device is its flow rate accuracy. The flow rate of an infusion pump can be calculated by measuring the volume of solution delivered over a period of time. For example, a measuring cylinder can be used to collect the fluid infused over a period of, say, 5 minutes at a certain flow rate setting. Such a method is generally acceptable for most general-purpose infusion devices. However, this method will not be appropriate to measure the accuracy of very low flow rate settings due to the fact that it will take a very long time to collect enough solution to obtain an accurate volume measurement (e.g., it takes 2 hours to collect 10 ml of solution at 5 ml/hr setting). Evaporation of fluid in the collection container will also affect the accuracy of such low volume long duration measurement. In addition, this measure gives only the average flow rate over a period of time. No information regarding the flow pattern is obtained (flow fluctuation, bolus effect, etc.).

Another parameter to be measured is the occlusion alarm pressure. This pressure is measured by connecting the IV line to a pressure meter and then starting the infusion. The pressure inside the line will quickly build up until it reaches the occlusion pressure alarm limit. It is important to leave an air buffer between the liquid line and the pressure meter should the meter not be able to measure wet pressure.

Example

A measuring cylinder is used to collect fluid from an infusion pump during a flow rate performance evaluation test. During the test, 9.6 mL of fluid is collected over a period of 5 minutes. If the flow rate setting of the infusion pump is 120 ml/hr, what is the accuracy of the pump?

Solution

From the test, 9.6 ml of fluid is infused in 5 minutes. Therefore, the calculated pump flow rate is 9.6 ml/5 min = 1.9 ml/min = 115 ml/hr. Therefore, the percentage error of the infusion pump is $\dfrac{120 - 115}{120} \times 100\% = +4.2\%$

FACTORS AFFECTING FLOW ACCURACY

Other than electronic component failures and mechanical wear and tear, the following common factors affect the flow accuracy of infusion pumps.

Too high backpressure in the IV line can reduce the flow rate. Normal backpressure depends on the flow rate, the diameter and length of the IV tubing, and the viscosity of the IV fluid. The smaller the inside lumen and the longer the tubing, the higher the backpressure. Backpressure increases with increase flow and fluid viscosity. Backpressure may also be created when the IV tube is kinked. When the backpressure is too high, the pumping mechanism may not be able to overcome such pressure. For example, during high backpressure, if the occlusion pressure created by the protruding fingers on the IV tubing is not high enough, fluid may leak backwards at the location of occlusion.

Another potential problem associated with high backpressure is bolus infusion. As the flexible IV tubing is slightly elastic, its diameter will increase under high backpressure. Upon clearing the occlusion, the IV tubing will recoil to its original diameter thereby releasing the stored fluid along the length of the tubing. Therefore, a large bolus of fluid may be infused into the patient.

For IV pumps using the peristaltic pumping mechanism, as the flow rate depends on the inner diameter of the IV tubing, variation of the inner diameter will change the rate of infusion. It is therefore important to ensure that the inner diameter dimension of IV lines used with peristaltic infusion pumps are manufactured within acceptable tolerance. In addition, as the section of IV tubing under the protruding fingers is being compressed for a period of time with prolonged use, the shape and therefore the inner diameter of the tubing will change. In order to avoid inaccuracy, manufacturers often recommend that users move a different section of tubing under the pumping mechanism every several hours.

Theoretically, a syringe pump should produce an accurate and uniform flow pattern. In practice, however, under very low flow rate applications, the plunger may stick to the side of the cylinder until the pusher delivers enough force to overcome the static friction. Once the plunger is free, it will advance rapidly and stop, thereby pushing a bolus of solution into the patient. This sudden start and stop movement can repeat itself during low flow rate infusion.

In general, among different pumping mechanisms of volumetric infusion pumps, the piston cylinder pump is the most accurate but most expensive due to the special infusion set with the piston cassette. The linear peristaltic pump is very commonly used in general IV infusion since it has a fairly accurate infusion rate. In addition, most peristaltic pumps can use ordinary gravity infusion sets and are therefore less expensive to operate than those that require dedicated infusion sets.

Chapter 24

ELECTROSURGICAL UNITS

OBJECTIVES

- Describe the tissue response to electrosurgical current in terms of desiccation, fulguration, and cutting.
- Identify the characteristics of the cut, coagulation, and blended electrosurgical waveforms.
- Explain the constructions and functions of active bipolar and monopolar electrodes, and the dispersive return electrode.
- Sketch the block diagram of an electrosurgical generator and explain the functions of each block.
- Analyze ESU waveform generation circuits.
- Perform quality assurance testing on an ESU generator.
- Identify the potential hazards of electrosurgery and safety precautions during electrosurgical procedures.

CHAPTER CONTENTS

1. Introduction
2. Principle of Operation
3. Modes of Electrosurgery
4. Active Electrodes
5. Return Electrodes
6. Functional Building Blocks and ESU Generators
7. Output Characteristics
8. Quality Assurance
9. Common Problems

INTRODUCTION

An electrosurgical unit (ESU) delivers high-frequency electrical current through an active electrode to produce cutting and coagulation effects on tissues. The frequency of electrosurgery for cutting is between 100 kHz and 5 MHz, which is within the radio frequency (RF) band. When appropriately modulated, this RF frequency can cut through tissues and cauterize bleeding blood vessels. The simultaneous cutting and hemostatic effect make ESU useful for procedures on tissues with capillaries and on patients receiving a high dose of anticoagulant drugs.

Electrosurgical units using spark-gap generators have been used since the 1920s. Most ESUs today use solid-state technology with microprocessor-controlled output for better results and improved safety. Argon-enhanced ESU systems, using a jet of argon gas to cover the surgical site during electrosurgery, can provide rapid and uniform coagulation over a large bleeding surface and are therefore useful in surgeries on organs such as the liver, spleen, and lung. ESUs are also used in endoscopic procedures to perform ablation, desiccation, cauterization, and removal of tissues. Special handpieces are designed for different ESU procedures.

PRINCIPLE OF OPERATION

An ESU is a RF generator. Two electrodes, one called active and the other called passive, are used to apply the RF current from the ESU to the patient. At the beginning of the procedure, the passive electrode (or return electrode) is attached to the patient's body. The surgeon then applies the active electrode to the surgical site to achieve the surgical effect. The active electrode is usually a very small tip electrode, while the return electrode has a large contact surface area with the patient. The high-frequency current passing through the tissue creates the surgical effect. The surgical effect is due to heat created by the RF current at the tissue–active electrode interface. The degree of heating in the tissue depends on the resistivity of the tissue as well as on the RF current density (the resistivity of soft tissue is about 200 Ωm). Figure 24–1 shows a typical setup of an electrosurgical procedure.

Different current densities create different effects on living tissues. Table 24–1 shows typical tissue effects at different levels of RF current density.

In practice, a current density much higher than 400 mA/cm^2 at the surgical site is necessary to produce electrosurgical effect. However, to prevent tissue injury beyond the surgical site, the current density must be limited to below 50 mA/cm^2 in tissues outside the surgical site. This is achieved by

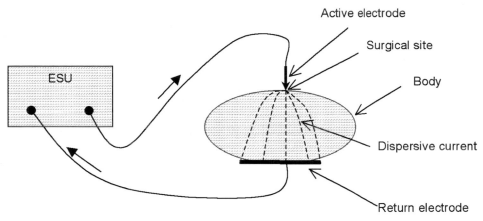

Figure 24–1. Electrosurgery Setup.

Table 24–1.
Tissue Effect of RF Current Density.

Current Density	Tissue Effect
> 50 mA/cm^2	Reddening of tissue
> 80 mA/cm^2	Pain and blistering
> 100 mA/cm^2	Intense pain
> 400 mA/cm^2	Second-degree burn

attaching a large surface area electrode on the opposite side of the active electrode so that the return current is dispersed over a larger area within the patient's body. Figure 24–1 shows the active electrode applied to the surface of the tissue and the flow of current inside the tissue when the return electrode is placed far from the active electrode. The density of the RF current flowing in the tissue closest to the active electrode is the highest, and it decreases rapidly (inversely proportional to the square of the distance from the surgical site) at locations farther from the active electrode site.

Three different tissue effects can be created by an electrosurgical current at the active electrode site: desiccation, cut, and fulguration.

Desiccation

When a relatively small RF current flows through the tissue, it produces heat and raises the tissue temperature at the surgical site. Heat will destroy and dry out the cells. This process may produce steam and bubbles and eventually turns the tissue a brownish color. This mechanism of tissue damage is called desiccation. It is achieved by placing the active electrode in contact with the tissue and setting the ESU output to low power. As desiccation is created by the heating (I^2R) effect, any current waveform may be used for desiccation.

Cut

By separating the active electrode by a small distance (about 1 mm) from the tissue and maintaining a few hundred volts or higher between the active and return electrodes, RF current may jump across the separation, producing sparks. Sparking creates intense heat, causing cells to explode. Such destruction of cells leaves behind a cavity. When the active electrode moves across the tissue, this continuous sparking creates an incision on the tissue to achieve the cutting effect. In general, a high-frequency (e.g., 500 kHz) continuous sine wave is used to create the cutting effect. Cutting usually requires a high power output setting.

Fulguration

To produce fulguration, the energized active electrode first touches the tissue and then withdraws a few millimeters to create an air gap separation. As the active electrode moves away from the tissue, the high voltage creates an electric arc jumping across the active electrode and the tissue. This long arc burns and drives the current deep into the tissue. Intermittent sparking does not produce enough heat to explode cells, but it causes cell necrosis and tissue charring at the surgical site. Fulguration coagulates blood and seals lymphatic vessels. To achieve fulguration, most manufacturers use bursts of a short-duration damped sinusoidal waveform. The sinusoidal waveform is usually the same frequency used for cutting (e.g., 500 kHz), and the repetition frequency for the bursts is much lower (e.g., 30 kHz). A higher voltage waveform is required to maintain the long sparks. Although the peak voltage is higher, fulguration produces less power than cutting due to its low duty cycle.

Table 24–2 summarizes the three mechanisms of electrosurgery.

MODES OF ELECTROSURGERY

The cut mode in electrosurgery applies a continuous RF waveform (sinusoidal or near sinusoidal) between the active and return electrodes. The coagulation mode uses bursts of a higher voltage damped RF sinusoidal waveform (to create fulguration tissue effect). Instead of switching back and

Table 24–2.
Mechanism of Electrosurgery.

Tissue Effect	*Active Electrode*	*Power*	
Desiccation	Heat dries up tissue, produces steam and bubbles. Turns tissue brown.	Monopolar or bipolar. In contact with tissue.	Low
Cut	Sparking produces intense heat, explodes cells leaving cavity. Incision on tissue caused by continuous sparking.	Monopolar. Electrode separated from tissue by a thin layer of steam.	High
Fulguration	Intermittent sparking does not produce enough heat to explode cells. Heat causes necrosis to tissue. High voltage drives current deep into tissue, chars tissue to carbon	Monopolar. Electrode separated by an air gap.	Medium

forth between cut and coagulation during a procedure, most ESUs have one or more blended modes, which allow simultaneous cutting and coagulation. A blended waveform has a lower voltage level but a larger duty cycle than the coagulation waveform. Figure 24–2 shows an example of the cut, blended, and coagulation output waveforms of an ESU. A blended mode with a larger duty cycle will have more cutting effect than one with a lower duty cycle.

The setup shown in Figure 24–1 with the active electrode and the large surface return electrode is called a monopolar operation. Instead of placing a separate return electrode away from the surgical site, a bipolar handpiece has both the active and return electrodes grouped together (e.g., an ESU forceps). Biopolar electrodes are often used to perform localized desiccation on tissue. In Figure 24–3, the ESU is switched to bipolar coagulation mode to cauterize a section of a blood vessel before it is cut apart to avoid profuse bleeding.

Table 24–3 lists the characteristics of different modes of ESU operations. The crest factor (last column) is defined as the peak voltage amplitude of the ESU waveform divided by its root mean square voltage. For a continuous sine wave, the crest factor is 1.41. Since a pure sine wave has little or no hemostatic effect on tissues, most manufacturers use a lightly modulated sine wave to achieve a small degree of hemostatic effect in the cut mode. The crest factor of the coagulation waveform is the highest (about 9) since it has the largest peak voltage but the smallest duty cycle. In general, the higher the crest factor, the more hemostatic effect the ESU waveform will have on tissues.

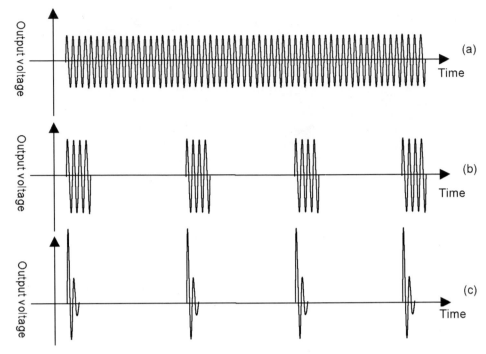

Figure 24-2. ESU Output Waveforms. (a) Cut, (b) Blended, (c) Coagulation.

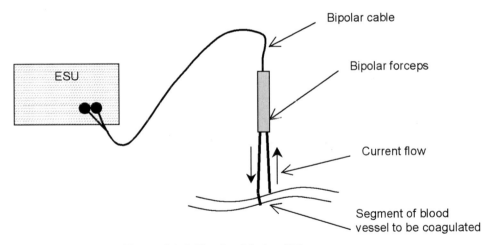

Figure 24–3. Bipolar Mode of Electrosurgery.

Table 24–3.
Characteristics of ESU Operation Modes.

	Effect	*Waveform*	*Voltage*	*Power*	*Crest Factor*
Monopolar					
Cut	Pure incision plus slight hemostatic effect	Continuous unmodulated sine wave to lightly modulated sine wave	Low	High	~1.41 to 2
Coagulation	Desiccation or fulguration	Burst of damped sine wave	High	Low	~9
Blended	Cut and coagulation	Burst of medium duty factor sine wave	Medium	Medium	Between cut and coagulation
Bipolar					
Coagulation	Desiccation	Continuous unmodulated sine wave	Lowest	Lowest	1.41

ACTIVE ELECTRODES

ESU active electrodes for monopolar operations come in different forms and shapes. The most common active electrode is the flat blade electrode, which can be used to perform cutting and coagulation. Some of the other commonly used active electrodes are needle, ball, and loop electrodes. Ball electrodes are usually used for desiccation (by pressing the electrode against the tissue and passing the RF current through the tissue). Loop electrode, with its conductive wire loop, is used to remove protruded tissues such as a nodule. The metal tips of the electrodes (Figure 24–4b) are usually single-use disposable units. The electrode handles may be multiple use or single use. The handle part of the electrode may have a switch to activate the ESU. A foot switch operated by the surgeon may be used instead of the hand switch. The combination of an ESU handle and a tip (Figure 24–4a) is often referred to as an ESU pencil (or a hand-switched ESU pencil if a switch is located on the handle).

RETURN ELECTRODES

While the function of the active electrode is to create the surgical effects, the return electrode (or passive electrode) in monpolar ESU operation pro-

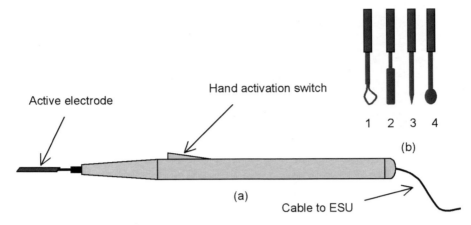

Figure 24–4. (a) Hand-Switched ESU Pencil with a Flat Blade Electrode;
(b) Monopolar Tips: 1) Loop, 2) Flat Blade, 3) Needle, 4) Ball.

vides the return path for the ESU current. As mentioned earlier, the maximum RF current density level to avoid causing any tissue damage is 50 mA/cm². A large surface area electrode (e.g., 100 cm²) is therefore required to limit the current density below this safe level in tissues away from the surgical site, including those in contact with the return electrode.

There are many types of return electrodes for ESU procedures. Bare metal plates placed under and in contact with the patient were used in early days. However, it was noted that burns (primarily heat burns) and tissue damage sometimes occurred at the return electrode sites. Investigations revealed that the primary cause of such patient injuries was due to poor electrode–skin contact or insufficient contact surface area between the electrode and the patient (part of the electrode not in contact with the patient). It was also noted that burns often appeared in the form of rings at the skin surface. Laboratory experiments showed that the current density at the skin–return electrode interface is highest around the rim of the electrode. Figure 24–5 shows the current density distribution of such an experiment. This occurrence is due to the fact that electrons are negatively charged particles; when they are allowed to freely move in a conductive medium, they will repel each other and therefore more will end up at the perimeter of the medium, in this case at the perimeter of the return electrode. This phenomenon is known as the "skin effect" in electrical engineering, where the current density of high-frequency current in a conductor is very much higher at the surface of the conductor than in its core.

Today, conductive gel pads are used for ESU return electrodes. A conductive gel pad electrode has a self-adhesive surface to avoid shift and falloff and is flexible to fit the contour of the patient's body. Return electrodes are designed so that, under normal use, no skin burn will occur at the return electrode site. To ensure patient safety, technical standards are in place specifying the performance of return electrodes. For example, the ANSI/AAMI HF18 Standards stipulate that the overall tissue-return electrode contact resistance shall be below 75 Ω. In addition, no part of the tissue in contact with the return electrode shall have more than a 6°C temperature increase when the ESU is activated continuously for up to 60 seconds with output current up to 700 mA.

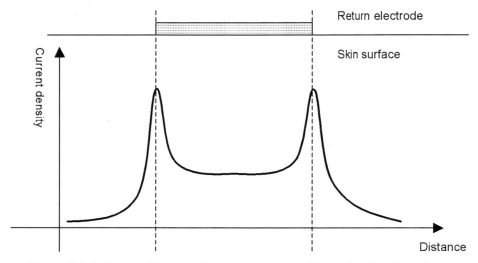

Figure 24–5. Current Density Crossing the Return Electrode–Skin Interface.

Due to problems associated with burns, special monitoring devices are often built into ESUs to monitor the integrity of the return electrode path. If the integrity is breached, an alarm will sound and the ESU output will be disabled to prevent patient injury. Two levels of monitoring are often available for high output power ESU (e.g., output greater than 50 W). The first is return electrode monitoring and the second is return electrode quality monitoring.

Return Electrode Monitor (REM)

A REM system monitors the return path of the electrode to the ESU. It detects the continuity of the return electrode cable from the electrode to the ESU. In a typical REM system, a double conductor cable and a low-frequency (relative to the ESU output frequency; e.g., 140 KHz) low-current (e.g., 3 mA) isolated source from the ESU are used to measure the resistance of the return cables (Figure 24–6a). A high resistance (e.g., > 20 Ω) will trigger the REM alarm.

Return Electrode Quality Monitor (REQM)

REM measures only the continuity of the return electrode cable, not the quality of contact between the electrode and the patient, whereas REQM monitors both. Figure 24–6b illustrates the principle of the REQM. In REQM, a dual conductive pad electrode is used. The right-hand side diagram in Figure 24–6b shows the cross-sectional view of the electrode–skin interface. The small monitoring current flows from the ESU REQM circuit to one of the conductive pads, passes through the two electrode–skin interfaces, and returns to the ESU via the second pad. Too high a REQM resistance (e.g., greater than 135 Ω) suggests poor electrode–skin contact or open circuit return cable; too low a resistance (e.g., less than 5 Ω) suggests a short circuit between the two conductive pads. In addition, some machines may sound an alarm if the REQM detects a large change in the resistance (e.g.,

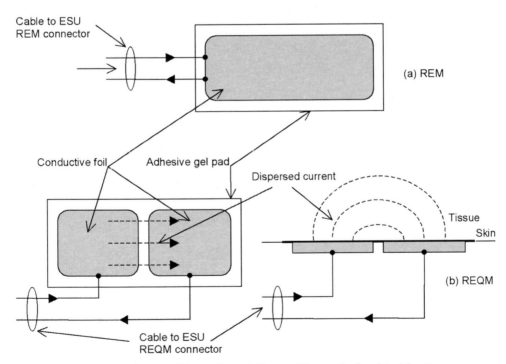

Figure 24–6. Return Electrode and Return Electrode Quality Monitors.

resistance increase by more than 40% from the initial reference value).

FUNCTIONAL BUILDING BLOCKS OF ESU GENERATORS

The spark gap ESU generator developed in the 1920s consists of a step-up transformer T1, which increases the 60 Hz 120 V line voltage to about 2,000 to 3,000 V (Figure 24–7). As the sinusoidal voltage at the secondary of T1 increases from zero, electrical charge accumulates in the capacitor C1 and the gas inside the spark gap (a gas discharge tube) starts to ionize until an arc is formed between its electrodes. Arcing (or sparking) of the spark gap resembles closing of a switch in the series resonance circuit formed by C1, L1, and the impedance of the spark gap. The fundamental frequency of the arcing current is approximately equal to the resonance frequency of L1/C1. The voltage amplitude of this high-frequency oscillation will decay until the arc is extinguished. Proper choice of L1 and C1 produces an RF damped sinusoidal waveform that occurs twice within one period of the 60 Hz input signal. This RF damped sinusoidal waveform is coupled to the output circuit by induction between L1 and L2. The output level is selected by the taps selection on L2. The RF chokes L3 and L4 (or RF shunt capacitor C4) are used to block the RF signal from entering the power supply. Spark gap gen-

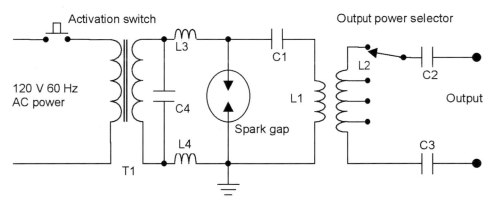

Figure 24–7. Spark Gap ESU Generator.

erators are primarily used for coagulation or cauterization.

Spark gap ESUs were commonly used until the early 1980s, when they began to be replaced by solid-state generators. In a solid-state ESU, the RF frequency (e.g., 500 kHz) and the burst repetition frequency (e.g., 30 kHz) are generated by solid-state oscillators. The shape of the ESU waveform (cut, blended, or coagulation) is created by combining the frequencies of these two oscillators. The waveform is then amplified by a power amplifier and a step-up transformer. The output of an ESU can go up to 1,000 watts, 9,000 volts (peak to peak open circuit voltage), and 10 amperes. Figure 24–8 shows

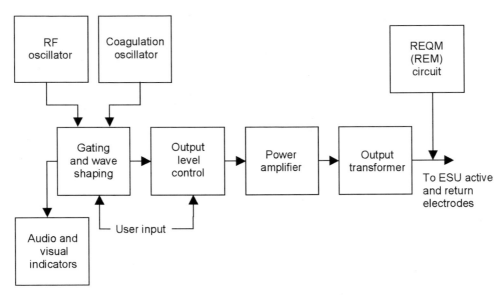

Figure 24–8. Functional Block Diagram of an ESU.

the simplified functional block diagram of a solid-state ESU.

The output stage of an ESU is shown in Figure 24–9. In the circuit, the waveform created by the gating and wave shaping circuit is fed into the base of a power amplifier Q1, and the output of the amplifier connects to the primary winding of the output transformer T1. The transformer and the power amplifier circuit are connected to a 200 V DC power source. For high-power output ESUs, a number of power transistors connected in parallel form the output circuit. Each of these transistors shares a portion of the output power. The ESU waveform, after steps up by the output transformer to several thousands volts, is fed across the active and return electrodes via a pair of capacitors C1 and C2. These capacitors behave like a short circuit to RF but block low-frequency (60 Hz) leakage current to the patient.

The ESU output circuit shown in Figure 24–9 is considered an isolated output ESU as there is no connection from the patient circuit (the secondary of the output transformer) to the power ground. Theoretically, for an isolated output ESU, a person touching the active electrode but not the return electrode will not get a shock or burn when the ESU is energized. However, due to the high frequency and nonzero leakage capacitance, if the person also touches a grounded object, some RF current will flow from the active

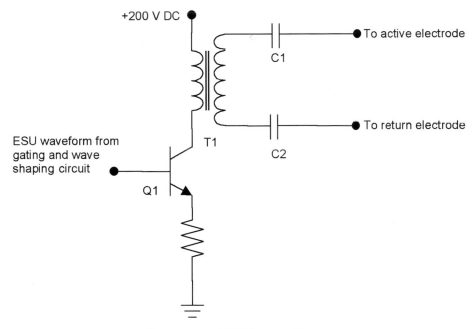

Figure 24–9. ESU Output Circuit.

electrode to the person and return to the ESU via this ground leakage path. High-frequency leakage current may be on the order of magnitude of a few tens of mA.

OUTPUT CHARACTERISTICS

Table 24–4 lists the output characteristics of a typical ESU. Figure 24–10 illustrates the output characteristics of the ESU cut waveform at different values of patient load. Note that according to the output characteristics, the ESU is rated to produce 300 W of output only when the patient load is at 300 Ω. The output power is reduced to 180 W when the patient load becomes 800 Ω. According to the ESU output characteristics, the output power decreases as the patient load increases. As the tissue impedance depends on the type of tissue as well as the condition of the tissue, this may create problems during the operation as the output power at a particular setting will fluctuate with the tissue impedance. To overcome this problem, some manufacturers have produced ESUs that can measure the tissue impedance and automatically restore the output power to the set value.

In most electrosurgical procedures, the active electrode is energized only

Table 24–4.
ESU Output Characteristics.

Mode	Waveform	Max. P-P Open Circuit Voltage (V)	Rated Patient Load (Ω)	Output Power (at rated load) (W)
Cut	500 kHz sinusoidal	3,000	300	300
Blend 1	500 kHz burst of sinusoidal at 50% duty cycle repeating at 30 kHz	3,500	300	250
Blend 2	500 kHz burst of sinusoidal at 37.5% duty cycle repeating at 31 kHz	3,700	300	200
Blend 3	500 kHz burst of sinusoidal at 25% duty cycle repeating at 30 kHz	4,000	300	150
Coagulation	500 kHz burst of damped sinusoidal repeating at 30 kHz	7,000	300	120
Bipolar	500 kHz sinusoidal	800	100	70

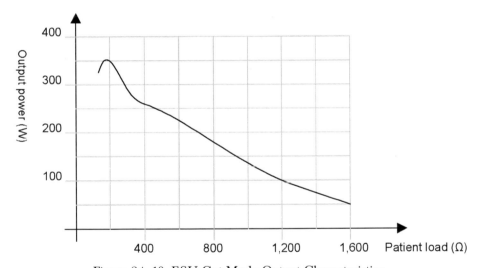

Figure 24–10. ESU Cut Mode Output Characteristics.

intermittently and each activation lasts for a short period of time (e.g., 15 seconds for cutting in general surgery). Table 24–4 shows the peak to peak open circuit voltage of different modes of operation. However, when the current starts to flow (i.e., an arc has been established), the voltage across the active and return electrodes will drop substantially.

QUALITY ASSURANCE

Since an ESU delivers high-energy therapeutic current, it is essential to ensure that the machine is safe and is operating according to its designed specifications. Other than general electrical safety inspection, the following performance tests should be carried out periodically.

Output Power Verification Test

The output power of an ESU should be measured against the manufacturer's specifications. Figure 24–11 shows the setup to measure the ESU output power. The output waveform can be sampled across the sample resistor R_s and displayed on the oscilloscope. The output voltage V_0 of the ESU is calculated from the resistance values by the equation:

$$V_0 = \frac{R + R_s}{R_s} V_s.$$

If the output voltage is a sine wave, the power output may be calculated from the equation:

$$P = \frac{V_0^2}{R + R_s}.$$

Note that the load resistance R_L is equal to $(R + R_s)$ and both should be special noninductive resistors and of sufficient power rating to withstand the

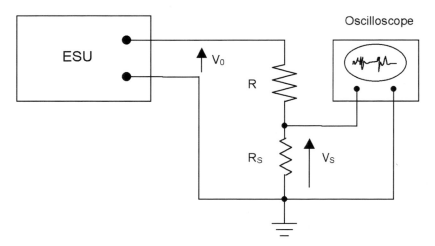

Figure 24–11. ESU Output Power Measurement.

ESU output.

High-Frequency Leakage Test

High-frequency leakage refers to the current flowing from either the active electrode to ground or the return electrode to ground when the ESU output is activated. Ideally, the amount of leakage current should be zero. However, due to the nature of the high frequency, a significant amount of capacitive leakage current will flow between the active electrode and ground as well as between the return electrode and ground. Figure 24–12b shows the setup to measure the high-frequency leakage from the active electrode to ground. To measure the leakage from the return electrode to ground, the load resistor is connected to the return electrode connection of the ESU and the active electrode connection is left open. The allowable leakage found by measuring the power dissipated by the load resistance R_L (e.g., less than 4.5 W for $R_L = 200\ \Omega$). Percentage isolation is a common value to represent the degree of isolation. It is defined as:

$$\% \text{ Isolation} = \left(1 - \frac{P_{\text{isolation}}}{P_{\text{normal}}}\right) \times 100\%.$$

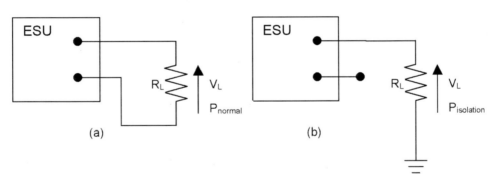

Figure 24–12. ESU Isolation Test.

Some manufacturers (and standards) call for the %Isolation to be greater that 80% for a load resistance R_L within the range of 100 to 1,000 Ω. Special testers with built-in potential dividers, variable patient load, and switchable configurations are available to facilitate these measurements.

COMMON PROBLEMS

Problems associated with electrosurgery may be grouped into four different categories:
- Burns
- Fire
- Muscle/nerve stimulation
- Electromagnetic interference

Burns

Skin burns at the return electrode site are one of the more common safety problems for patients under electrosurgical procedures. The main causes of skin burn are poor electrode–skin contact, inadequate site preparation, and pressure points on the electrode contact surface (which creates a low resistance pathway for the current).

- Internal tissue burns are caused by the concentration of ESU current along a low resistance path such as a metal implant or a pacemaker lead wire near the active or return electrodes sites.
- For grounded ESUs or ESUs with isolation failure, RF current may flow through a secondary ground path on the patient (e.g., a patient's arm may receive a burn at the location where it is touching a grounded object).
- In endoscopic or laparoscopic procedures, an insulation failure on the shaft of the ESU handpiece will cause tissue burn when such failure creates a secondary conduction path between the active electrode and the tissue.
- Too high a power setting and too long an activation period (e.g., during a liver tumor ablation procedure) when an undersized return electrode was used or the return electrode was not properly applied.
- Patient or staff burns by an activated ESU pencil when it was inadvertently energized (e.g., someone accidentally stepped on the ESU foot activation switch) while touching the patient or a staff member.

Fire and Explosion

An electrosurgical procedure produces sparks and arcing. The sparks may ignite flammable materials such as body hair, cotton drapes, or a pool of alcohol used for disinfection. This situation is worsened under an enriched oxygen environment, which is commonly found in operating room areas.

There have been incident reports on cases of explosion inside the abdominal cavity when the ESU ignited flammable bowel gas inside the patient.

Muscle and Nerve Stimulation

The reason ESU frequency is above 100 kHz is to avoid muscle and nerve stimulation. Under normal circumstances, muscle and nerve fibers are not triggered by current lower than 100 kHz. However, studies have shown that arcing may produce lower frequency current, which can stimulate nerve or muscle fibers. As a precaution, it is contraindicated to perform electro-surgery near major nerve fibers.

Electromagnetic Interference (EMI)

An ESU is a RF source. Although the machine may be shielded to prevent radiation and conduction of EMI, the electrodes and cables act as antennae to broadcast the RF frequencies. Older medical devices, with lower electromagnetic immunity, can be adversely affected by the EMI from electrosurgery. Devices may reset, produce errors, or switch to another mode of operation under EMI influence. Improperly grounded devices are especially vulnerable to EMI.

Chapter 25

RESPIRATION MONITORS

OBJECTIVES

- Explain the mechanics of breathing.
- Describe common respiration parameters.
- Explain the principle of operation and construction of medical spirometers.
- Define standardized gas volume in BTPS.
- Explain the principles of respiration monitoring using the impedance pneumographic and thermistor methods.
- Sketch a block diagram of a respiration monitor using the method of impedance pneumography and explain the functions of each block.
- List factors affecting signal quality, accuracy, and patient safety in respiratory monitoring.

CHAPTER CONTENTS

INTRODUCTION

The primary function of the lungs is to exchange gas between the inspired air and the venous blood. Air is inhaled by voluntary or involuntary action and is presented to one side of the membrane of the alveoli; venous blood is on the other side of the membrane. Gas exchange between air and blood occurs across this membrane. In the process, carbon dioxide is removed and oxygen is introduced into the bloodstream. For a normal adult, this gas-blood barrier is less than 1 μm and has a total surface area of about 100 m^2.

Disturbances of the respiratory system can be caused by a number of factors within the system or by other disorders. Diagnosis of respiratory disorders therefore can provide information about the well-being of the respiratory system as well as other organs or body functions. The rhythmic action of breathing is initiated in the respiration centers of the pons and medulla. The level and rate of respiration are controlled by the partial pressure of carbon dioxide and oxygen as well as the pH of the arterial blood. For example, a decrease in blood pH (e.g., due to increases in metabolism), increased accumulation of carbon dioxide in the arterial blood, and arterial hypoxemia will increase ventilation.

This chapter introduces some methods of monitoring respiration pattern and parameters in the clinical environment.

MECHANICS OF BREATHING

The lung is elastic and will collapse if it is not held expanded. At the end of expiration or inspiration, the pressure inside the lung (or alveolar pressure) is the same as the atmospheric pressure, whereas the pressure outside the lung (or intrapleural pressure) is below atmospheric pressure. This negative pressure keeps the lung inflated. If air is introduced into the intrapleural space, the lung will collapse and the chest wall will move outward. This disorder is called pneumothorax.

The most important muscle for inspiration is the diaphragm. When it contracts, the abdominal contents are forced downward and forward. This action increases the vertical dimension of the chest cavity. In addition, the external intercostal muscles contract and pull the ribs upward and forward, causing a widening of the transverse diameter of the thorax. In normal tidal breath (or passive breathing), the diaphragm descends by about 1 cm, but in forced breathing, a total descent of up to 10 cm may occur. Under active breathing (e.g., during heavy exercise), the abdominal muscles play an important role in expiration by pushing the diaphragm upward. The internal intercostal muscles assist active expiration by pulling the ribs downward and inward, thus further decreasing the volume of the thoracic cavity. Diseases that cause problems in these muscles or the nerves that innervate these muscles create disorders in breathing.

PARAMETERS OF RESPIRATION

Parameters of respiration include lung capacities, respiration rate, intrathoracic pressure, airway resistance, and lung compliance (or lung elasticity). In addition to these parameters, respiration waveform as well as end-tidal carbon dioxide concentration and its variations can all provide useful information in the assessment and disease diagnosis of the respiratory and related systems.

Figure 25–1 shows the volumes and capacities of respiration. The tidal volume (TV) measures the volume of inspired or expired gas during normal breathing. It is about 500 ml for a normal adult at rest. Inspiratory reserve volume (IRV) is the maximum amount of gas that can be inspired from the end-inspiratory level (or peak of the tidal volume). The sum of TV and IRV forms the inspiratory capacity (IC). The expiratory reserve volume (ERV) is the maximum amount of gas that can be exhaled from the end-expiratory level (or trough of the tidal volume). The sum of IC and ERV, which is the maximum volume of gas that the lung can expel or inhale, is the vital capacity (VC). The residual volume (RV) is the amount of gas remaining in the lung at the end of maximum expiration. This is the amount of gas that cannot be squeezed out, or anatomic dead space, of the lung. The total lung capacity (TLC) is the sum of RV and VC. These parameters, as well as the ratios of some of them (e.g., RV/TLC), are used to assess the healthiness of the respiratory system.

Airway resistance measures the ease of airflow during inspiration and expiration through the bronchi and bronchioles. This is expressed as the pressure difference between the mouth and the alveoli per unit of air flow. The normal value is about 1 to 2 cmH₂O per liter per second of flow at normal flow rate. This resistance becomes higher at higher flow rates. Lung compliance measures the ability of the alveoli to expand and recoil to its original state during inspiration and expiration. The normal lung at rest expands by about 200 ml when the intrapleural pressure falls by 1 cmH₂O. Therefore, the compliance of the lung is 200 ml/cmH₂O. At high lung volumes, the lung is less easy to expand and thus its compliance falls. When the airway is restricted, the air resistance increases. When the lung becomes more fibrous, it loses its compliance.

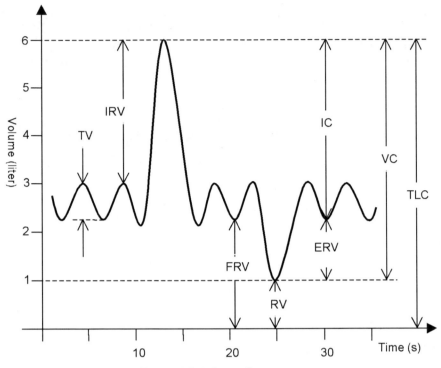

Figure 25–1. Lung Capacities.

To produce work to move the chest wall and force air along the airways, the respiratory muscle must consume oxygen. In normal subjects, the work of breathing is very small except in large ventilation during heavy exercise. However, in patients with obstructive lung disease, the resistance to airflow is very high even at rest and therefore the work of breathing can be 5 or 10 times its normal value. Under these conditions, the oxygen cost of breathing may become a significant fraction of the total oxygen consumption. Patients with a reduced compliance of the lung also have a higher work of breathing due to the stiffer structures. These patients tend to use shallower but more frequent breaths to reduce their oxygen cost of ventilation. However, the air exchange is not efficient in shallow breathing due to the fixed volume of air in the anatomic dead space in the lung, bronchi, and bronchioles.

One of the most useful tests in a pulmonary function laboratory is the analysis of a single forced expiration. The patient makes a full inspiration and then exhales as hard and as fast as possible into a spirometer (a flow and volume measurement device). The volume measured is called the forced vital capacity (FVC). FVC is usually less than the vital capacity (VC), which is obtained at slow expiration. The volume exhaled within the first 1 second is called the forced expiratory volume, or FEV_1. In obstructive lung disease (such as emphysema), due to high airway resistance, both FEV_1 and the ratio FEV_1/FVC are reduced. In restrictive lung disease (such as sarcoidosis), due to the limited lung expansion, FVC is low, but because the airway resistance is normal, the ratio FEV_1/FVC is high. Another index that can be derived from a forced expiration is the maximal midexpiratory flow ($FEF_{25-75\%}$), which is obtained by dividing the volume between 75% and 25% of the FVC by the corresponding elapsed time. This is a sensitive parameter to detect airway obstruction in early chronic obstructive lung disease. Figure 25–2 shows typical records of forced expiratory volume measurements. FEV_1 is a useful screening procedure to assess lung function and the efficacy of bronchodilator therapy, and in following the progress of patients with asthma or chronic obstructive lung disease.

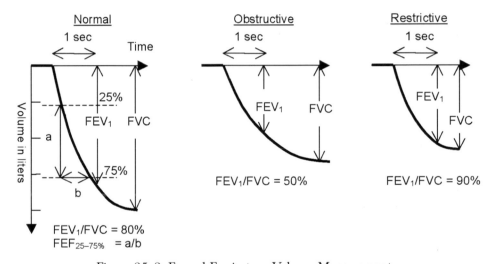

Figure 25–2. Forced Expiratory Volume Measurement.

The functional residual volume (FRV) is the volume of air in the lungs at the end of expiration which is also the volume of air remaining in the lungs between breaths. It is an important lung function as it changes markedly in some pulmonary diseases. FRV is measured using an indirect method called the helium dilution method. In this method, a container of known volume (V) is filled with a mixture of air and helium of concentration C_{iHe}. The patient first breathes normally for a few cycles. At the end of the last expiration (the volume of gas inside the lungs is the FRV), the patient starts and continues to breathe from the container. After several breaths, the gas in the container is diluted and mixed thoroughly with the gas in the lung. If the helium concentration of the mixed gas is C_{fHe}, FRV can be calculated from the equation:

$$FRV = \left(\frac{C_{iHe}}{C_{fHe}} - 1 \right) V.$$

During inspiration, some of the air that a person breathes never reaches the alveoli for gas exchange to take place. This air is called the dead space air. During expiration, this volume of air expires to the atmosphere before the air from the alveoli. The nitrogen method is used to measure the dead space volume. In this method, the patient first breathes normal air and suddenly takes a breath of pure oxygen. This intake of pure oxygen fills the entire dead space volume and some mixes with the alveolar air. The patient then expires through a nitrogen meter to produce a nitrogen concentration curve as shown in Figure 25–3. The initial expired air that comes from the dead space consists of pure oxygen. After a while, when the alveolar air reaches the nitrogen meter, the nitrogen concentration rises and then levels off. The concentration of nitrogen is plotted against the volume of expired air. The measurement terminates at the end of the expiration. The nitrogen concentration curve divides the graph into two regions with areas A_1 and A_2 as shown. One can derive that the volume of dead space air V_D can be calculated from the equation:

$$V_D = \left(\frac{A_1}{A_1 + A_2} \right) V_E,$$

where $V_E =$ the total volume of the expired air.

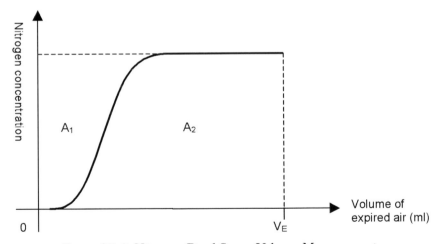

Figure 25–3. Nitrogen Dead Space Volume Measurement.

SPIROMETERS

A spirometer is a device to measure the flow and volume of gas moving in and out of the lungs during inspiration and expiration. There are two categories of spirometers: one senses volume and the other senses flow. A volume-sensing spirometer has a container to measure the gas volumes; gas flow rate can be calculated from the volume-time information. A flow-sensing spirometer has a flow transducer placed in the gas flow pathway to measure the flow rate of gas. Gas volume can be derived from the flow-time information. Figure 25–4 shows the functional block diagram of a spirometer. The patient circuit allows the patient to breathe in and out of the spirometer; the transducer converts the volume or flow to an electrical signal. The processor computes the respiratory parameters from the collected information and displays them on the output device such as a visual display or paper chart recorder.

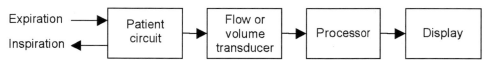

Figure 25–4. Block Diagram of a Spirometer.

Volume Transducers

Three commonly used volume transducers for respiration measurement are shown in Figures 25–5 and 25–6. The water-sealed inverted bell spirometer (Figure 25–5) moves up and down according to the respiration of the patient. The low friction water seal and the counterweight attached to the inverted bell reduce the resistance and backpressure, thereby allowing accurate volume and flow measurements. A pen, which writes on a rotating drum, is mechanically linked to the inverted bell. A rolling seal with a horizontally mounted bell (Figure 25–6a) can also be used as the volume transducer in a spirometer. The horizontal mounting of the bell eliminates the need for a counterweight and therefore simplifies the construction of the spirometer. A third type of volume-measuring transducer is a bellow (Figure 25–6b). As gas moves in and out of the bellow, it inflates or deflates the bellow. The moving bellow can move a pen to record the changing volume on a paper chart.

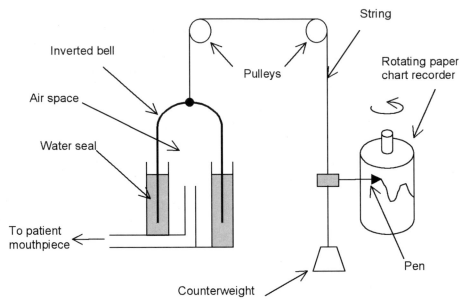

Figure 25–5. Water-Sealed Inverted Bell Spirometer.

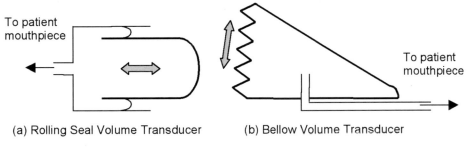

(a) Rolling Seal Volume Transducer   (b) Bellow Volume Transducer

Figure 25–6. Volume Transducers.

Flow Transducers

Spirometers using flow transducers with no moving parts are commonly used to minimize errors due to mechanical wear and tear. Figure 25–7 shows the block diagram of such a spirometer. Many different flow transducers can be used; examples are hot air anemometer, differential pressure flow transducer, et cetera. (see Chapter 7 for principles of flow transducers). Modern spirometers are microprocessor-based and have built-in compensations for temperature and pressure fluctuations. As patients breathe into the spirometer, care must be taken to avoid contamination of the internal part of the spirometer. Some of these protective measures are disposable mouthpiece and disposable patient breathing circuit, bacterial filter, and heated transducer chamber to prevent condensation.

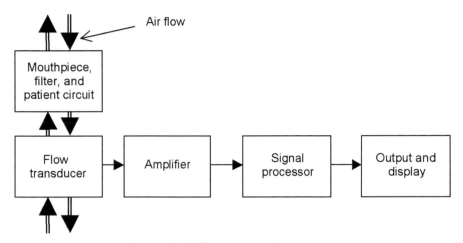

Figure 25–7. Flow-Sensing Spirometer.

The volume of gas in the lungs is at body temperature and atmospheric pressure, and is saturated with water vapor (BTPS). In respiratory volume measurements, in order to compare the volumes to those in blood, correction must be made to the volume obtained by a spirometer at ambient temperature and atmospheric pressure. The following equation derived from the gas laws can be used for the correction of the volume to body temperature of 37°C and a saturated vapor pressure of 47 mmHg.

$$V (BTPS) = V_t \times \left[\frac{273 + 37}{273 + t} \right] \times \left[\frac{P_B - P_{H_2O}}{P_B - 47} \right],$$

where t = temperature of the gas in spirometer in °C,
V_t = volume collected at t °C,
P_B = barometric pressure in mmHg, and
P_{H_2O} = water vapor pressure (mmHg) of the gas in the spirometer at t °C.

In practice, the temperature and pressure corrections can be obtained from published tables.

RESPIRATION MONITORS

Clinical bedside monitoring of respiratory function is useful to assess the need for further respiratory intervention such as the introduction of mechanical ventilation. It is also a useful tool in evaluating the maturity of the regulatory functions of the respiratory system in neonatal development. The breathing rates as well as the waveform of breathing are the two parameters to be measured in respiratory monitoring. In addition, the time elapsed of no breathing, or apnea, is also monitored. Respiration rate for a normal adult ranges from about 12 to 16 breaths per minute. Breathing rates for neonates are much higher (about 40 bpm). An apnea alarm is usually set at 20 seconds.

There are a number of methods to obtain the respiratory waveform and calculate the respiration rate. The common methods are the impedance method, which measures the electrical impedance across the patient's chest, and the thermistor method, which detects the airflow in the patient's airway.

Heated Thermistor Method

This method measures the change in temperature of a heated thermistor placed in the patient's breathing airway. A thermistor is placed in the air path of the nostril as shown in Figure 25–8 or in a breathing circuit. A current source produces a constant current to heat the thermistor so that its temperature is above the ambient temperature but less than the body temperature. When there is no air flowing across the thermistor, the voltage across the thermistor remains unchanged. During expiration, the warm air from the lung heats the thermistor. The voltage across the thermistor will then decrease with its resistance. During inspiration, the colder outside air cools the thermistor, which causes the voltage across the thermistor to increase. The variation of voltage across the thermistor will vary with the airflow of respiration. This voltage is recorded and plotted against time.

Impedance Pneumographic Method

During inspiration, the volume of the thoracic cavity increases and air is pulled into the lung. The impedance across the chest therefore becomes higher. During expiration, the chest volume decreases and pushes air out of the lung. The impedance across the chest therefore becomes lower. In the impedance pneumographic method, the monitor derives the respiration waveform and the breathing rate by measuring the change in impedance between a pair of electrodes applied on the chest of the patient.

To measure the impedance across the chest, a constant current I is applied across the chest through a pair of electrodes. The voltage V measured across the electrodes is therefore proportional to the chest impedance Z ($V = I \times Z$). Figure 25–9 shows the setup to monitor respiration using the impedance pneumographic method.

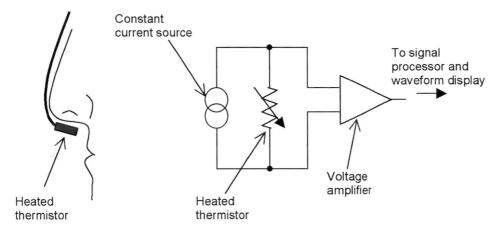

Figure 25-8. Heated Thermistor Respiration Monitor.

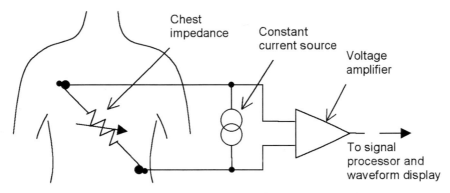

Figure 25-9. Impedance Pneumographic Respiration Monitor.

In order to prevent muscle and nerve stimulation, the injected current must be small and of high frequency. In general, monitors use frequencies higher than 25 kHz and current amplitudes below 50 µA. In fact, the output of the amplifier in Figure 25-9 is an amplitude modulated signal with the carrier frequency equal to the frequency of the applied current. The amplitude variation of the modulated signal is proportional to the impedance change due to respiration. Figure 25-10 shows the respiration impedance waveform, the current source waveform, and the waveform of the detected voltage across the chest.

In most applications, respiration monitors using the impedance methods employ the same sets of electrodes for ECG monitoring. Note that the impedance across the electrodes depends on the tissue impedance and the electrode–skin interface and is on the order of hundreds of ohms or kilo-ohms. However, the variation of the impedance due to respiration lies in the

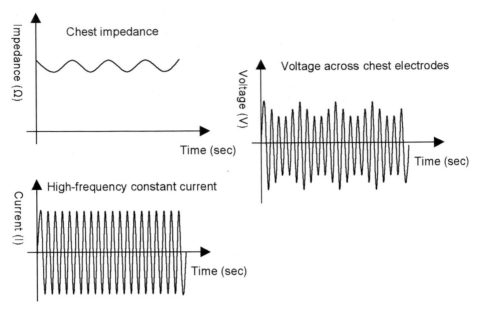

Figure 25–10. Impedance Pneumographic Respiration Monitor Waveforms.

range of 0.1 to 4 ohms. As a result, the signal is very sensitive to electrode and body movement. In addition, since tissue impedance is frequency-dependent, any fluctuation in frequency will create a change in the measured chest impedance. In order to minimize these errors, the applied current must have constant amplitude and be derived from a very stable frequency source.

Figure 25–11 shows the functional block diagram of a respiration monitor using the impedance method.

The respiration monitor is part of the ECG/respiration monitor using the

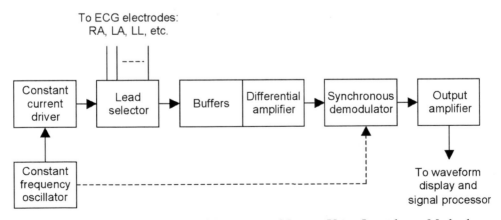

Figure 25–11. Block Diagram of Respiration Monitor Using Impedance Method.

same set of ECG skin electrodes applied to the patient. The lead selector of the respiration monitor selects a pair of electrodes from the set of ECG electrodes. The high-frequency current (e.g., 50 kHz) flowing through the patient's chest from one electrode to another creates a voltage of the same frequency with amplitude equal to the product of the current and impedance across the chest. This voltage is captured to derive the respiration waveform and breathing rate. The voltage signal is first buffered so that it will not affect the ECG part of the monitor. The synchronous demodulator then removes the high frequency from the measured voltage and recovers the respiration waveform.

Chapter 26

MECHANICAL VENTILATORS

OBJECTIVES

- Explain the applications of mechanical ventilation.
- Differentiate between positive and negative pressure ventilators.
- Classify ventilators based on the methods used to terminate inspiration.
- Explain the types of breaths delivered by a ventilator, its modes and submodes, and the ventilation parameters.
- List some of the common operator controls, alarm settings, and emergency modes in positive pressure ventilation.
- Sketch a block diagram of a positive pressure ventilator and explain the functions of each block.
- Analyze the pneumatic diagram, trace gas flow, and identify basic components of a positive pressure ventilator.

CHAPTER CONTENTS

INTRODUCTION

Ventilators provide assistance to patients who cannot breathe on their own or who require assistance to maintain a sufficient level of ventilation. Patients may require ventilation support due to illness (e.g., asthma, CNS disorder), injuries, congenital defects, postoperative conditions, or the influence of drugs (e.g., under general anesthesia).

The first mechanical ventilator was developed in 1927 by Philip Drinker of the United States. It was known as the "iron lung" for treating victims of poliomyelitis in the early 1950s. The iron lung is basically an airtight metal chamber enclosing the entire body of the patient except that the head is outside the chamber. The chamber is separated from the outside atmosphere by an air seal around the neck of the patient. To create inspiration, the pressure inside the metal chamber is reduced to below atmospheric pressure. As the outside pressure is higher than the chamber pressure, air is drawn into the patient's lungs through the patient's airway. Expiration is achieved by returning the chamber to atmospheric pressure.

The iron lung is classified as a negative pressure ventilator as the inspiratory phase of the respiratory cycle is created by a negative pressure. Today, positive pressure ventilators are used to avoid having to enclose the entire patient's body in a pressure chamber. A positive pressure ventilator uses a mask, an endotracheal tube, or a tracheostomy tube to connect the machine to the patient's airway. The lungs are inflated by positive pressure during inspiration; expiration occurs upon release of the pressure. This chapter describes the principles of operation, design, and construction of positive pressure mechanical ventilators.

TYPES OF VENTILATORS

Intermittent positive pressure breathing (IPPB) therapy is a method to assist spontaneous breathing by applying a positive pressure during inspiration and allowing passive expiration by removal of the inflated pressure. It is believed by some that IPPB can reduce the work of breathing, promote bronchopulmonary drainage, and provide more efficient delivery of bronchodilator drugs.

Mechanical ventilators overcome respiration deficiencies by assisting spontaneous breathing or completely taking over the breathing of the patient. A positive pressure ventilator inflates the lungs by elevating the pressure in the airway to achieve adequate alveolar gas exchange. Expiration is achieved by opening the airway to the atmosphere so that the gas in the lungs is passively released to the atmosphere. Portable ventilators are used in step-down units, extended care facilities, and homes. Home use portable ventilators are often used 24 hours a day and are set up and operated by the patient or home caregivers. Portable ventilators should be user-friendly and are much simpler in operation than critical care ventilators. For some patients who cannot tolerate the high inspiratory pressure and rapid airflow, high-frequency ventilators are used. These ventilators cycle at rates much higher than normal spontaneous respiration but deliver lower inspiratory volume for each breath.

Mechanical ventilators are classified according to how they terminate the inspiration phase of the ventilation cycle. Four parameters can be monitored and used to terminate inspiration: pressure, volume, time, and flow.

1. A pressure cycled ventilator monitors the pressure in the airway and ends the inspiration when a certain preset pressure is reached.
2. A volume cycled ventilator measures the volume of gas delivered to the patient and ends the inspiration when a preset volume has been delivered.
3. A time cycled ventilator tracks the time of inspiration and ends the inspiration when a preset time is reached.
4. A flow cycled ventilator senses the pressure in the airway and ends the inspiration when the inspiration flow falls to a preset level.

Figure 26–1 shows typical pressure and flow waveforms of positive pressure mechanical ventilation measured in the airway of a patient. At the start of the inspiratory phase, the airway/lung pressure increases rapidly until sufficient gas has entered the lungs. The gas flow rate also decreases as the pressure builds up. During the expiratory phase, the airway is opened to the atmosphere. The alveolar pressure drops and gas is pushed out of the lungs.

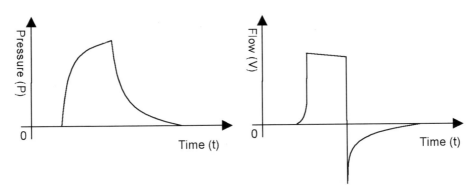

Figure 26–1. Ventilation Pressure and Flow Waveforms.

MODES OF VENTILATION

When a patient is undergoing positive pressure mechanical ventilation, there are two types of allowed breath: spontaneous breath and mandatory breath. In a spontaneous breath, the breathing parameters are determined by the patient's condition. However, in a mandatory breath, all breathing parameters are determined by the machine. A ventilator-initiated mandatory (VIM) breath is initiated by the ventilator timing circuit, whereas a patient-initiated mandatory breath (PIM) is initiated by the patient. In a PIM, the patient attempts to breathe, and the breathing action creates a small negative pressure in the lungs and airway. Upon detecting this small negative pressure change, the machine will deliver a positive pressure breath to help the patient to breathe. A PIM breath is distinguished from a VIM breath by the slight negative pressure before the onset of the positive inspiratory pressure (Figures 26–2a and b). The pressure waveform for a spontaneous breath is characterized by the small negative inspiratory pressure and small positive expiratory pressure (Figure 26–2c).

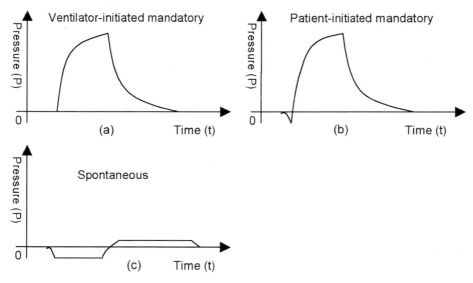

Figure 26–2. Mandatory and Spontaneous Breaths.

The modes of ventilation specify the characteristics of breaths delivered by a positive pressure ventilator in response to the patient's breathing attempts. Some of the common modes of ventilation are briefly explained below. Their typical pressure waveforms are shown in Figure 26–3.

- Controlled mandatory ventilation (CV)–Consists of ventilator-initiated mandatory (VIM) breaths at prescribed time intervals. The CV mode is for patients who cannot breathe by themselves.
- Intermittent mandatory ventilation (IMV)–Consists of VIM breaths at prescribed time intervals but allows the patient to breathe spontaneously between the controlled breaths.
- Continuous mandatory ventilation (CMV)–Consists of a mix of VIM breaths at prescribed time intervals or mandatory breaths initiated by the patient (PIM).
- Synchronized intermittent mandatory ventilation (SIMV)–produces VIM breaths at prescribed time intervals if there is no patient breathing initiation. The VIM breaths will be synchronized with the patient's inspiration effort to generate a PIM breath. The patient is allowed, within the s-phase window, to breathe spontaneously after a PIM breath. If the patient initiates a breath after the s-phase, the ventilator will generate a PIM breath. By decreasing the ventilation rate, carbon dioxide will build up in the patient's blood, stimulating the respiratory control centers, and trigger the patient to initiate mandatory (PIM) and spontaneous breaths. This is used to gradually return the work of breathing to the patient; the process is called "weaning."
- Continuous positive-airway pressure (CPAP) ventilation–in the CPAP mode, all breathing is spontaneous. A continuous positive pressure is maintained throughout the breathing cycle. It is used to give supplemental oxygen and raises baseline pressure to prevent the collapse of the small airway and alveoli.

In addition to the ventilation modes described above, the following submodes are commonly found in critical care ventilators.

- Positive end-expiratory pressure (PEEP)–PEEP is used with mandatory breaths; it maintains the lung at a positive pressure at the end of expiration (Figure 26–3). It is often used to increase the patient's arterial oxygen saturation without increasing the inspired $O_2\%$.
- Apnea–Apnea is the cessation of breathing. When the apnea alarm is activated, the ventilator will measure the duration of no breathing. On detection of an apnea, the ventilator will automatically go into a preset ventilation pattern stored under the apnea submode.
- Pressure support–pressure support creates an elevated baseline pressure during a spontaneous inspiration. By elevating the pressure during inspiration, the patient does not have to create the entire pressure gradient to obtain a meaningful tidal volume. Thus, this mode will reduce the patient's inspiratory work while still allowing the patient to control many other breathing parameters.

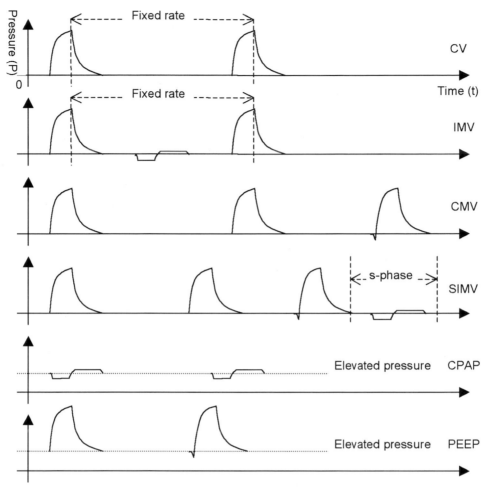

Figure 26–3. Modes of Ventilation.

- Sigh–a sigh is a breath delivered by the ventilator that differs in duration and pressure from a normal breath. The profile of a sigh is often user-programmable.

VENTILATION PARAMETERS AND CONTROLS

The basic parameters of ventilation are pressure, flow, volume, and time. These parameters are interrelated during mechanical ventilation.

- Pressure–Pressure is the driving force against the resistance of the patient circuit and airway that causes flow. Unit of measurement is in centimeters of water (cmH_2O).

- Flow–Flow is the rate of gas at which the tidal volume is delivered. A higher flow selection will require a higher pressure to create given the same air resistance in the breathing circuit and patient's airway. A higher flow will take less time to deliver the required tidal volume. The unit of flow measurement is liters per minute (LPM).
- Volume–Volume measures the quantity of gas. It is usually displayed as minute volume (total inspired gas volume in 1 minute), which is the tidal volume times the respiration rate in breaths per minute. The unit of volume measurement is liters (L) and minute volume is liter-minute.
- Time–Time is associated with how frequently a breath is delivered and also with the time of inspiration and expiration. The unit of measurement for breathing rate is breaths per minute (bpm). A decimal value is used to indicate the I:E ratio, the ratio of inspiratory to expiratory time in a breathing cycle.

As these parameters are measured outside the patient's body under different conditions than inside the lungs, it is important to correct these parameters to body temperature, sea level pressure, and gas saturated with water vapor (BTPS) before they are used to compare with preset parameters or to control ventilation.

Operator control parameters (with typical setting ranges) that can modify the ventilation pattern of a mechanical ventilator include:

- Ventilation mode (CV, IMV, SIMV, etc.)
- Inspiratory flow waveform (square, descending ramp, etc.)
- I:E ratio (0.2–1)
- Tidal volume (0.1–2.5 L)
- Peak flow (120–180 LPM)
- Respiratory rate (0.5–70 bpm)
- Sensitivity (0.5–20 cmH_2O above PEEP)–for sensing patient-initiated breathing effort
- Inspired air O_2 concentration (21–100%)
- Manual breath (or sigh) (0.1–2.5 L not exceeding twice tidal volume, 1–3 sighs per hour)
- PEEP/CPAP pressure (0–45 cmH_2O)

Some common safety alarm features and settings are:

- High pressure limit (10–120 cmH_2O)
- Low inspiratory pressure (3–99 cmH_2O)
- Low PEEP/CPAP pressure (0–45 cmH_2O)
- Low exhaled tidal volume (0–2.5 L)
- Low exhaled minute volume (0–60 L)
- High respiratory rate (0–70 bpm)

- Low oxygen/air inlet pressure (35 psig)
- Apnea interval (10–60 sec)
- I:E ratio (>1)

Some emergency modes of ventilator operation are:

- Apnea ventilation–Delivers preset ventilation when apnea is detected.
- Backup ventilation–Should the ventilator fail to provide the ventilation to the patient, backup ventilation function will be activated. For example, activation of backup air compressor to take over failed medical gas supplies.
- Safety valve open–If ventilator fails, the patient breathing circuit is open to the atmosphere to allow spontaneous breathing and manual bagging.

BASIC FUNCTIONAL BUILDING BLOCKS

Figure 26–4 shows a block diagram of a positive pressure mechanical ventilator. The following paragraphs describe the functional building blocks.

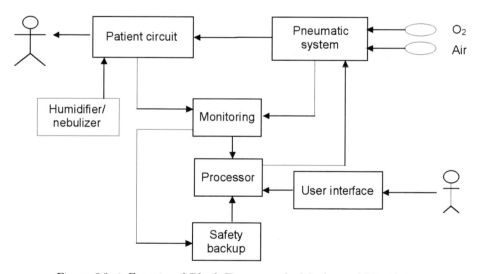

Figure 26–4. Functional Block Diagram of a Mechanical Ventilator.

- Medical air/oxygen supplies–Medical gas from wall outlets provides the sources of air and oxygen necessary to produce the breathing gas mixture delivered to the patient. For some ventilators, compressed gas cylinders are used as backup gas supplies in case of wall supplies failure.

- Pneumatic system–The pneumatic system regulates the gas pressure, blends the air and oxygen to desired proportion, and controls the ventilation flow profile according to the control settings.
- Patient circuit–It physically connects the pneumatic system to the patient. It supplies the inspired gas to the patient and removes the expired gas from the patient. It has one or more check valves to separate the inspired and expired gas flow and contains bacteria filters to prevent contamination.
- Processor–According to the user input and the information from the sensors, the processor produces control signals to the pneumatic circuit to produce breaths with desired characteristics.
- Monitoring–It measures the performance of the pneumatic system and feeds information back to the processor. Pressure and flow sensors at different locations of the pneumatic circuit are used to monitor and control ventilation parameters. Oxygen sensors are used to monitor the correct air/oxygen mixture being delivered to the patient.
- User interface–It allows users to set up ventilation parameters and displays system and patient information.
- Safety/backup–This system protects the patient under ventilation. It alerts the operator when preset conditions are violated and may initiate backup responses preset by the operator. In case of extreme circumstances, such as a loss of a gas source, the safety/backup system may take control of the pneumatic system and override settings previously selected by the operator.
- Humidifier (optional but often required)–Humidifiers are used to increase the water moisture content in the breathing gas before it is delivered to the patient. During normal breathing, the inspired gas is warmed and moisturized as it is passing through the airway. During mechanical ventilation, prolonged inhalation of dry gas will cause patient discomfort and may damage the airway tissues. When a humidifier is used, the inspired gas in the patient circuit is bubbled through a reservoir of warm water to pick up moisture before entering the patient's airway. To prevent heat damage to the airway tissues, the temperature of the inspired gas must be monitored (by a temperature sensor) to ensure that it is below 42°C.
- Nebulizers–Nebulizers are used to deliver medication into the patient's airway during ventilation. The size of the vapor droplets determines the site of deposition. Larger droplets deposit in the upper airway, while tiny droplets (<1 µm) are deposited in the alveoli. Jet venturi or ultrasound transducers are commonly used to produce tiny

droplets of water in the inspired gas. However, a nebulizer has the potential to deliver too much water and overhydrate the patient.
- Air compressor (optional)–It produces a 50 psig, 21% O_2 air source. It is used as a backup to the medical air supply to allow the patient to breathe in case of medical air supply failure. The compressor will cut in automatically when it detects a low pressure in the medical air supply line.

PNEUMATIC SYSTEM DIAGRAM

Figure 26–5 shows a typical pneumatic system diagram of a positive pressure mechanical ventilator together with the patient breathing circuit and the medical gas supplies.

Medical air from the piped gas wall outlet is connected to the ventilator via a water trap and coarse filter to remove water condensation and particulates from the hospital's gas supply system. The inlet to the ventilator consists of another filter and a pressure sensor. The pressure sensor will switch off the air supply line and sound an alarm if the pressure becomes too low (e.g., <35 psig). A check valve allows the gas to flow in only one direction, thereby preventing any contamination of the gas supply due to reverse flow. Medical air, which is usually about 50 psig from the wall outlet, is reduced to a lower pressure (e.g., 10 psig) by the air regulator before being mixed with oxygen in the oxygen/air blender. In addition to creating the desired breathing gas mixture, the flow control within the blender generates the flow pattern and controls the ventilation rate. A flow sensor (e.g., hot air anemometer) monitors the volume flow rate of the air supply. (The oxygen supply line before the blender is identical to that of the air supply line.)

The patient circuit consists of an inspiratory limb and an expiratory limb connected at a Y-connection. The breathing gas, which contains the desired proportion of air and oxygen, exits the ventilator via a bacteria filter and check valve into the inspiratory limb of the breathing circuit. The gas mixture picks up moisture from the humidifier and medication (if needed) from the nebulizer before entering the patient's lungs. During the inspiration phase, the exhalation valve is closed to allow the inspired gas to inflate the lungs. During the expiratory phase, the flow control valve stops the supply gas flow, the exhalation valve opens to the atmosphere, and the thoracic cavity collapses and forces the gas to exhale from the lungs through the expiratory limb of the patient breathing circuit.

As the exhaled gas from the lungs is at body temperature and saturated with water vapor, water will condense from the gas as its temperature becomes lowered in the expiratory limb of the breathing circuit. The bacte-

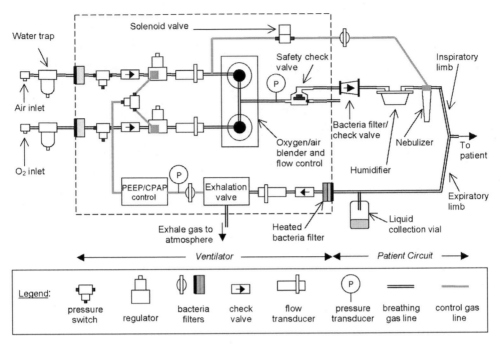

Figure 26–5. Pneumatic System Diagram of Mechanical Ventilator.

ria filter prevents contamination of the ventilator circuit components by the exhaled gas from the patient. However, a wet filter has a much lower efficiency to remove bacteria from the expired air. To prevent water condensation at the bacteria filter, a heater is required to warm the expired gas. A collection vial is also connected to the inlet of the expiration compartment of the ventilator to remove water condensation and sputum from the patient's exhaled gas before reaching the filter. A check valve is installed in the expiratory limb to prevent reverse gas flow. A flow sensor measures the exhaled gas flow before it is vented to the atmosphere.

An elevated baseline pressure can be created by imposing a pressure on the main expiratory gas flow in the expiratory limb of the patient breathing circuit. Under CPAP or PEEP mode, the CPAP/PEEP controller exerts a pressure on the valve seat of the exhalation valve. Only exhaled gas with pressure higher than the CPAP/PEEP pressure can be vented to the atmosphere.

SAFETY FEATURES

A mechanical ventilator is a critical life-supporting device for a patient who cannot breathe by himself or herself. Malfunctioning of any part in the system can threaten the life of the patient. Many safety features are built into the system. Some of the common safety features are:

- Disconnection alarm–A disconnection alarm is an alarm to detect disconnection of the breathing circuit from the ventilator or the patient. Pressure sensors detect a sudden drop in pressure in the patient circuit. Care must be taken not to lower the pressure limit too much to avoid false alarm (e.g., due to pressure fluctuation). Too low a setting may not be sensitive enough to trigger an alarm if the disconnection is at the distal end of the circuit.
- Air leak alarm–Excessive air leak in the system (especially in the patient breathing circuit) will compromise ventilation. Most ventilators utilize flow sensors to compare the inspired and expired gas flow volume. For a leak-free system, the volume of inspired gas over a period of time is equal to that of the expired gas. In the system shown in Figure 26–5, the inspired gas flow is measured by the flow sensors in the air and oxygen supply lines. The sum of these two flow sensors should be the same as the flow measured by the flow sensor in the expiration circuit. Note that all volumes must be adjusted to BTPS before making the comparison.
- High pressure alarm–A high pressure alarm can alert the user to a kink or obstruction in the patient breathing circuit. It can also prevent lung damage from inadvertent high pressure being developed in the breathing lines.
- Loss of power–Although breathing gas is derived from the medical gas wall outlets, most critical care ventilators employ electronic or microprocessor circuits for control and alarm. In case of a power loss, the ventilator should sound an alarm to alert the clinicians. The ventilator and the patient circuit should be designed such that manual ventilation can be performed on the patient in a power failure situation. The unit should have a battery backup memory to store all the machine settings and data so that it can be powered up immediately without having to undergo lengthy initialization and programming after power has been restored.
- Loss of gas supplies–Ventilators should be designed to allow automatic switch-over of oxygen to medial air if there is no supply of oxygen (and vice versa). Similar to a loss of power, the ventilator should allow manual ventilation when all gases are lost. Some ventilators have a built-in electrical air compressor to supply compressed air to the gas

lines in case the hospital gas supply has failed or is not available.

- Power-up self-test–Many critical care ventilators have a power-up self-test to check most operational conditions, including electronic diagnostic and leakage test of the pneumatic circuit. The compliance of the system, including the patient breathing circuit, is measured during the test to ensure accurate calculation of all breathing parameters.

Chapter 27

ULTRASOUND BLOOD FLOW DETECTORS

OBJECTIVES

- Describe the properties of ultrasound.
- Define the equations of sound propagation and Doppler effect in ultrasound.
- State the principles of Doppler and transit time blood flow measurement techniques.
- Sketch a block diagram of a Doppler blood flowmeter and describe the functions of each block.

CHAPTER CONTENTS

1. Introduction
2. Ultrasound Physics
3. Transit Time Flowmeter
4. Doppler Flowmeter
5. Functional Block Diagram of a Doppler Flowmeter

INTRODUCTION

Blood flowmeters and detectors are used to measure and evaluate the flow of blood in blood vessels. An ultrasound blood flow detector can be used noninvasively to locate and assess the degree of vascular restriction. For example, an ultrasound blood flow detector is used to perform postoperative assessment after vascular surgery or in detecting carotid artery occlusion by examining the pattern of dominant periorbital collaterals. In addition to detecting flow, some ultrasound blood flowmeters can noninvasively quantify the velocity and the volume of blood flow in blood vessels.

ULTRASOUND PHYSICS

Sound is a mechanical longitudinal (or compression) wave in which particles move back and forth parallel to the direction of wave travel. Ultrasound is sound beyond the upper audible frequency limit of human beings (i.e., of frequency 20 kHz or higher). Low-intensity (e.g., < 0.1 W/cm^2) ultrasound is absorbed by human tissue without known damage. However, high-intensity ultrasound (e.g., 500 W/cm^2) can cause tissue injury due to heating effects. In addition, with appropriate frequency and setup, ultrasound can create shock wave and cavitation in tissues.

The wavelength λ of ultrasound is equal to the velocity c of sound in the medium divided by its frequency f, or

$$\lambda = \frac{c}{f}. \tag{1}$$

Listed below are the propagation speeds of ultrasound in different media. In diagnostic ultrasound, the average velocity of sound in soft tissue is 1,540 m/s or 1.54 mm/µs. This average velocity is used in distance calculation and in assessing the propagation of sound in body tissue.

Table 27–1.
Propagation Speed of Ultrasound.

Medium	Propagation Speed (m/s)
Air	300
Water	1,480
Soft tissue	1,440 to 1,640
Fat	1,450
Bone	2,700 to 4,100

The distance of sound travel is equal to the velocity times the time of travel or $d = vt$.

When an ultrasound source and a receiver are moving at velocities of V_s and V_r, respectively, as shown in Figure 27–1, the apparent frequency f_r of the ultrasound signal detected by the receiver is different from the source frequency f. The difference, called the Doppler shift, depends on the source fre-

Figure 27–1. Doppler Effect.

quency as well as the velocities of the source and the receiver. This is known as the Doppler effect.

In the case of the arrangement in Figure 27–1, the frequency of the received ultrasound is:

$$f_r = \left(\frac{C - V_r}{C - V_s}\right) f, \tag{2}$$

where V_r = velocity of the receiver away from the source,
V_s = velocity of the source in the same direction as V_r,
f = frequency of the source, and
C = speed of sound (in air = 330 m/s).

The Doppler shift is defined as the change in frequency when the source and receiver are moving relative to each other. The Doppler shift is:

$$f_D = f_r - f = \left[\left(\frac{C - V_r}{C - V_s}\right) - 1\right] f. \tag{3}$$

Example

What is the Doppler shift when the source is stationary and the receiver is moving toward the source at 100 m/s in air? (C = 330 m/s).

Solution

Using equation (3), substituting C = 330 m/s, V_r = –100 m/s, and V_s = 0.0,

$$f_D = \left(\frac{330 + 100}{330 - 0.0}\right) f - f = (1.3 - 1) \, f = 0.3 \, f.$$

TRANSIT TIME FLOWMETER

A transit time flowmeter computes the flow velocity by measuring the time difference between the sound traveling upstream and downstream of the flow. Figure 27–2 illustrates the principles of an ultrasound transit time flowmeter to measure blood flow in a blood vessel. An ultrasound transmitter and a receiver are positioned at an angle θ external to the blood vessel. To start the measurement, the ultrasound transmitter A emits a short pulse. The time for the sound to reach receiver B is measured. In the next phase, ultrasound transmitter B emits a sound pulse. The time it takes to reach receiver A is again recorded. The velocity of blood flow in the vessel depends on the difference between the two recorded times. Below is the derivation:

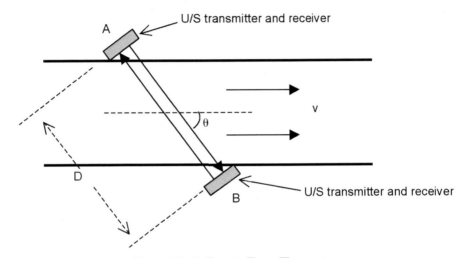

Figure 27–2. Transit Time Flowmeter.

In the downstream transmission, the time for the sound to travel from point Λ to B is:

$$T_{AB} = \frac{D}{C + v\cos\theta} \text{ (downstream)},$$

where D = the distance between the ultrasound transducers,
C = the velocity of sound in the medium,
θ = the angle between the direction of sound travel with the direction of blood flow, and
v = the velocity of blood.

In the upstream transmission, the time for the sound to transmit from point B to A

$$T_{BA} = \frac{D}{C - v\cos\theta} \text{ (upstream)},$$

The time difference ΔT between the upstream and downstream transmission is:

$$\Delta T = T_{BA} - T_{AB} = \frac{D}{C - vCos\theta} - \frac{D}{C + vCos\theta} = \frac{2DvCos\theta}{C^2 - v^2Cos^2\theta}$$

$$\text{if } C \gg v, \Delta T = \frac{2Dv\,Cos\theta}{C^2}$$

$$\Rightarrow v = \frac{C^2\,\Delta T}{2DCos\theta}. \tag{4}$$

DOPPLER FLOWMETER

Doppler flowmeters make use of the Doppler effect to determine the velocity of flow. For the setup shown in Figure 27–3, instead of a moving source and a moving receiver as shown in Figure 27–1, both transmitter and receiver are stationary. The sound wave is reflected from a moving reflector traveling at the same speed as the fluid flow. In blood flow measurement, the

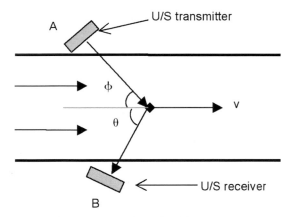

Figure 27–3. Doppler Flowmeter.

fluid is blood and the reflector is a red blood cell.

From the doppler shift equation (equation 3)

$$f_D = \left(\frac{C - VCos\theta}{C + VCos\phi} - 1\right) f_s$$

$$= -\frac{V\,(Cos\theta + Cos\phi)}{}\,f_s.$$

Note that the negative sign indicates a decrease in frequency.

$$\text{If } C >> V\cos\phi, \quad f_D = -\frac{V\,(\cos\theta + \cos\phi)}{C}\, f_s. \qquad (5)$$

$$\text{If } \theta \text{ and } \phi \text{ are both zero, } f_D = -2\,\frac{V}{C}\, f_s.$$

Example

For the ultrasound Doppler blood flowmeter as shown in Figure 27–3, if $\theta = \phi = 60°$, $V = 100$ cm/s, $f_s = 5$ MHz, and $C = 1.5 \times 10^5$ cm/s, what is the magnitude of the Doppler shift?

Solution

$$f_D = 5 \times 10^6 \times \frac{100}{1.5 \times 10^5} \times (\cos 60° + \cos 60°)\ \text{Hz} = 3.3\ \text{kHz}.$$

Note: The above results showed a single frequency shift. In a real situation, as blood cells travel at different velocities, the backscattered ultrasound received will be of a broad frequency range.

In practice, an ultrasound Doppler blood flowmeter has the transmitter and receiver together so that the probe (containing both the transmitter and receiver) can be placed on the surface of the skin or on top of a blood vessel during blood flow velocity measurements. The Doppler shift in this case becomes:

$$f_D = -2\,\frac{V\,\cos\phi}{C}\, f_s.$$

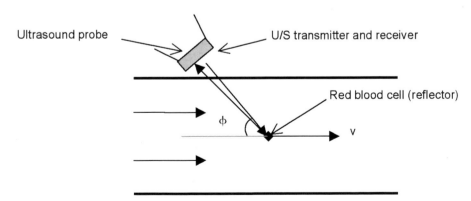

Figure 27–4. Doppler Blood Flowmeter.

FUNCTIONAL BLOCK DIAGRAM OF
A DOPPLER BLOOD FLOWMETER

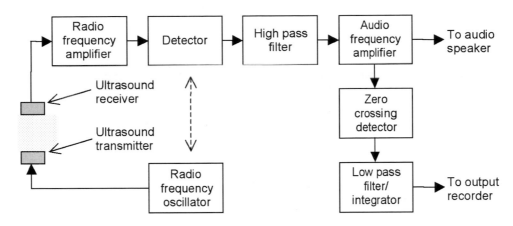

Figure 27–5. Doppler Blood Flowmeter Block Diagram.

Figure 27–5 shows a functional block diagram of an ultrasound Doppler blood flowmeter.

The radio frequency oscillator generates the RF (e.g., 5 MHz) excitation signal to the ultrasound transmitter. The receiver detects the ultrasound reflected from the moving red blood cells in the blood vessel. The RF frequency and the Doppler angle can be chosen such that the Doppler shifts due to the traveling blood cells are in the audio frequency range (see preceding example). If all the blood cells are moving at one constant velocity, the frequency of the received signal will have only one frequency, which is equal to the transmitter frequency plus the Doppler shift $(f_s + f_D)$. However, as blood flow is pulsatile and blood flow velocity is not the same across the blood vessel, f_D is not a single value and will occupy a range of frequency. The signal received is a frequency-modulated signal with the Doppler shift proportional to the blood flow velocity. The detector is an FM demodulator that removes the transmitter frequency f_s from the signal. In most cases, the output also contains a large amplitude low-frequency wave caused by the blood vessel-wall-motion. This vessel-wall-motion artifact can easily be removed by a high pass filter. An audio frequency amplifier intensifies this signal and sends it to an audio speaker. Figure 27–6a shows the output from the detector and filter. As the Doppler shift is in the audio frequency range, the clinician can hear the flow pattern of the blood in the blood vessel. A high pitch (large Doppler shift) corresponds to fast-moving blood and a low pitch corresponds to low blood flow. The Doppler shift (which is proportional to the blood flow velocity) can be converted to an analog flow velocity signal by passing it through a zero crossing detector and a low pass filter or integrator. The outputs from the zero crossing detectors and the low pass filter (representing the flow velocity) are shown in Figures 27–6b and 27–6c.

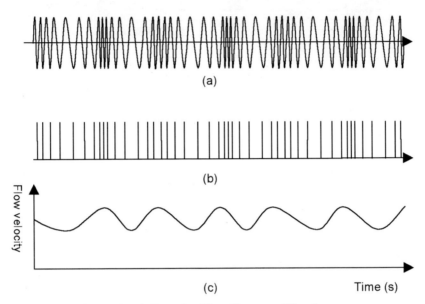

Figure 27–6. Doppler Flow Detector Waveforms.

Chapter 28

FETAL MONITORS

OBJECTIVES

- Describe the clinical significance of fetal heart rate and maternal uterine activities during labor.
- Describe and contrast different methods of monitoring fetal heart rates, including direct, ultrasonic, maternal abdominal, and phono methods.
- Describe and compare external and intrauterine methods of monitoring uterine activities.
- Explain the construction and principle of transducers and sensors used in fetal monitoring.
- Sketch a simple block diagram of a fetal monitor.

CHAPTER CONTENTS

1. Introduction
2. Monitoring Parameters
3. Methods of Monitoring Fetal Heart Rate
4. Methods of Monitoring Uterine Activities

INTRODUCTION

Electronic fetal monitoring provides graphical and numerical information to assist the clinician to assess the well-being of the fetus. During labor, the fetal heart rate often accelerates and decelerates in response to the uterine contractions and fetal movements. Characteristics of these patterns may reveal labor problems such as fetal hypoxia or decreased placental blood flow. Examining these patterns may indicate alternative courses of labor (e.g, cesarean section or forceps delivery) or drug therapy (e.g., administering labor-inducing or labor-prohibiting drugs).

Antepartum (before birth) monitoring is used to monitor the development of the fetus in the uterus. Intrapartum monitoring includes monitoring the status of the mother and fetus as well as the progress of labor. Maternal monitoring includes measurements of the mother's vital signs such as heart rate, respiratory rate, blood pressure, temperature, oxygen saturation level, and uterine activity. Fetal monitoring refers to the monitoring of the fetal heart rate (FHR) and the maternal uterine activity (UA) during labor and delivery. Fetal monitors were first available in the late 1960s. Today, fetal monitoring is used in more than 60% of deliveries in North America.

MONITORING PARAMETERS

The two primary parameters in fetal monitoring are fetal heart rate (FHR) and uterine activities (UA). Other parameters that may be monitored are the maternal ECG and %S_aO_2. Normal fetal heart rates fall within the range of 120 to 160 beats per minute (bpm) during the third trimester of pregnancy and fluctuate from the baseline rate during contractions. Fetal heart rate may reveal the conditions of the fetus during labor and delivery. Figure 28–1 shows a typical recording of FHR. Some abnormal FHR conditions and their indications are:

- Tachycardia (high heart rates)—may be caused by maternal fever, fetal hypoxia, immaturity of fetus, anemia, or hypotension
- Bradycardia (low heart rates)—may be caused by congenital heart lesions or hypoxia
- Variation—too much fluctuation indicates stress or hypoxia

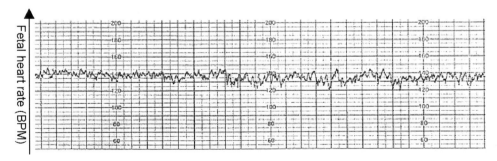

Figure 28–1. Fetal Heart Rate.

Uterine activity refers to the frequency and intensity of the contractions of the uterus. During labor, the smooth muscles of the uterus contract rhythmically, thereby increasing the pressure of the amniotic fluid and forcing the fetus against the cervix. UA indicates the progress of labor. Figure 28–2 shows a typical recording of UA.

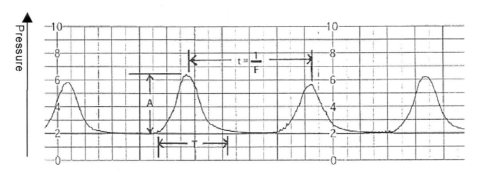

Figure 28–2. Uterine Activities.

The usual characteristics of uterine activities are:

- Frequency (F)–less than once in 3 minutes is slow progress of labor
- Duration (T)–under 45 seconds of contraction is slow progress of labor
- Amplitude (A)–above 75 mmHg usually indicates active labor
- Shape–the shape of the contraction pressure is normally bell-shaped. An irregular shape may indicate labor pushing, fetal movement, maternal respiration, or blocked catheter
- Rhythm–couplets and triplets indicate abnormal activities
- Resting tone (pressure between contraction)–about 5 mmHg for non-labor and rise to 20 mmHg for induced labor

METHODS OF MONITORING FETAL HEART RATE (FHR)

Fetal heart rate may be obtained by listening to the heart sound of the fetus, directly connecting electrodes to the fetus, applying electrodes on the abdomen of the mother, or using Doppler ultrasound. The three methods are described in the following sections.

Direct ECG (DECG)

Direct ECG is an invasive method that connects a spiral electrode to the scalp of the fetus. During application, the electrode is inserted through the vulva. While pushing against the scalp of the fetus, the clinician applies a 360 degree turn to the spiral electrode so that the electrode is screwed and secured into the skin of the scalp (Figure 28–3a). The electrode can be applied only when the head of the fetus is accessible; that is, only after the amniotic sac has ruptured. The other electrode is usually a skin electrode applied to the thigh of the mother. As the procedure is invasive, it may cause complications (e.g., infection) to the fetus.

Phono Method

The FHR may be derived by listening to the fetal heart sound. Although a microphone can be used, this is usually done manually by the obstetric nurse or physician using a stethoscope placed on the abdomen of the mother. The weak fetal heart sound is usually buried among the louder maternal heart sound and other sounds (such as sound from bowel movement) within the mother's body. The advantage of this method is that it is noninvasive and does not require expensive equipment.

Abdominal ECG

Abdominal ECG is obtained by applying skin electrodes on the abdomen of the mother (on fundus, pubic symphysis, and maternal thigh). The electrodes are attached to a normal ECG machine so that the waveform and heart rate are displayed. As the electrodes will inevitably pick up the maternal ECG, careful electrode positioning to capture the fetal ECG and differentiate them from the maternal signal is required.

Ultrasound Method

Another noninvasive method to monitor FHR employs a Doppler ultrasound detector. A beam of continuous wave ultrasound (e.g., 2 MHz) from an ultrasound transmitter/receiver pair is applied to the abdomen of the mother (Figure 28–3b). If the ultrasound beam crosses the fetal heart, the Doppler shift detected from the reflected sound will record the motion of the fetal heart wall and thus can be processed to obtain the FHR (see principle of Doppler blood flow detector in Chapter 27). This method provides an accurate beat-to-beat measurement of the heart rate provided that the ultrasound beam covers the fetal heart. To avoid picking up movement artifacts from other organs, a narrow sound beam is preferred. However, with a narrower sound beam, the transducer position must be checked from time to time to ensure that the sound beam is focused on the fetal heart. In addition, it requires good skin–transducer contact (achieved by application of ultrasound gel) to obtain good signal. Although more complicated and expensive, a pulsed Doppler with time gating can provide better quality signal than a continuous wave Doppler unit.

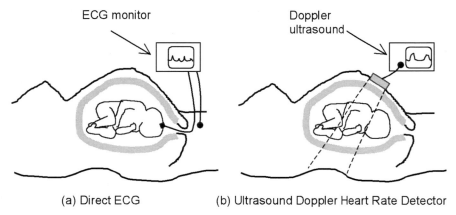

(a) Direct ECG   (b) Ultrasound Doppler Heart Rate Detector

Figure 28–3. Fetal Heart Rate Monitors.

METHODS OF MONITORING UTERINE ACTIVITIES (UA)

Intrapartum uterine activities may be obtained by using an external pressure transducer applied on the abdomen of the mother, or by inserting a fluid-filled catheter into the uterus. The former is an indirect and noninvasive method, while the latter is direct and invasive.

External Pressure Transducer Method

By placing a pressure transducer on the abdomen close to the fundus and secured by a belt wrapped around the abdomen (Figure 28–4a), the pressure in the uterus during contractions can be monitored. The pressure exerted on the transducer varies roughly in proportion to the strength of the contraction. The transducer is often referred to as the TOCO transducer. The advantage of this method is its noninvasiveness. However, it has low accuracy (about 20% error) and it requires frequent repositioning and retightening of the belt.

Intrauterine Pressure (IUP) Method

The pressure obtained in this method is more accurate than using the TOCO transducer. It is a direct pressure measurement method using a setup similar to direct blood pressure monitoring. A fluid-filled catheter is inserted into the uterus after the amniotic sac is ruptured. The catheter is connected to a disposable (or reusable) pressure transducer (Figure 28–4b). The pressure inside the uterus is displayed on a blood pressure monitor. Although this method is more accurate, it is invasive. Care should be taken to ensure that there is no obstruction or occlusion of the catheter during labor and that the transducer and setup are properly zeroed before use (see Chapter 18 on blood pressure monitors for reasons and methods of pressure transducer zeroing).

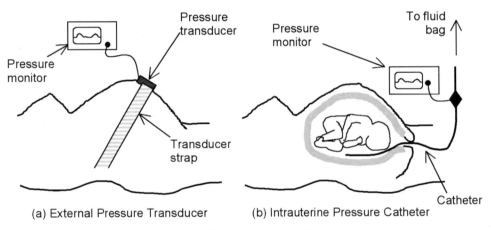

(a) External Pressure Transducer   (b) Intrauterine Pressure Catheter

Figure 28–4. Uterine Activity Monitoring.

Chapter 29

INFANT INCUBATORS, WARMERS, AND PHOTOTHERAPY LIGHTS

OBJECTIVES

- Describe the clinical functions of infant incubators and warmers.
- List typical features of an infant incubator.
- Sketch a functional block diagram of a typical infant incubator.
- Explain the construction and major components of an infant incubator.
- Identify potential hazards associated with infant incubators.
- Describe the mechanism of phototherapy and its clinical functions.
- Identify the light spectrum and intensity for effective phototherapy.
- State functional features and parameters of phototherapy light source.
- Analyze factors affecting effective output of phototherapy light.

CHAPTER CONTENTS

1. Introduction
2. Purpose
3. Principles of Operation
4. Potential Safety Hazards
5. Functional Components and Common Features
6. Phototherapy Lights

INTRODUCTION

An infant incubator provides a controlled environment to warm the infant by regulating the air temperature within the incubator chamber. In additional to air temperature, the humidity and oxygen content within the chamber can be regulated. A phototherapy light is used to break down excessive concentration of bilirubin in the newborn. These devices are found in neonatal care units to treat preterm or sick infants.

PURPOSE

At birth, an infant's body temperature tends to drop significantly due to heat loss from the body. Heat loss can be through conduction (contact with other objects), convection (heat carry away by air circulation), radiation (heat loss to cooler environment due to infrared radiation from the warm body), and evaporation (latent heat loss from the lungs and skin surface). Most term neonates regulate their body temperature naturally to some extent. However, preterm neonates, with thinner skin and higher surface to volume ratio, tend to lose more heat and can easily become hypothermic. Infant incubators and radiant warmers are used to reduce heat loss. An infant warmer radiates heat to the infant by using an external heat lamp (e.g., a quartz bulb) directed to the infant. Incubators usually have better temperature regulation than infant warmers and provide a controlled environment where infants can receive the therapies they need. However, the enclosed chamber of an incubator is less convenient for accessing the infant than the open design of an infant warmer.

PRINCIPLES OF OPERATION

An infant incubator consists of an infant compartment enclosed by a clear plastic hood. The infant lies on the mattress inside the infant compartment. Access doors and ports through the hood allow relatively easy access to the infant for feeding, examination, and treatment. A blower and heater underneath the mattress provide forced circulation of warm air inside the compartment to warm the infant. An infant incubator usually has two modes of temperature control: skin temperature and air temperature. In the skin temperature mode, a temperature senor is attached to the skin of the infant. The skin temperature signal is compared to the preset value to turn the heater on and off. In the air temperature mode, a temperature sensor is located inside the hood of the incubator to measure the air temperature. This measured value is compared to the preset value to turn the heater on or off. To provide better temperature regulation, proportional heating control instead of a simple on-off control is used.

In a proportional heating control circuit, the heater can be turned on at lower than the maximum power rating. During initial startup, when there is a large difference (ΔT) between the measured and set temperatures, the heater is switched on at full power. When the difference becomes smaller, the heater will run at a lower power setting. This control approach reduces the fluctuations of temperature within the incubator compartment. Figure 29–1 shows an example of the power and temperature relationships of a four-level proportional heater controller of an infant incubator. When the temperature difference ΔT is larger than 6°C, the heater is running at 100% power, as the air inside the incubator becomes warmer, the power of the heater is reduced. When the temperature inside the incubator is less than the preset temperature by less then 2°C, the heater is running at only 25%.

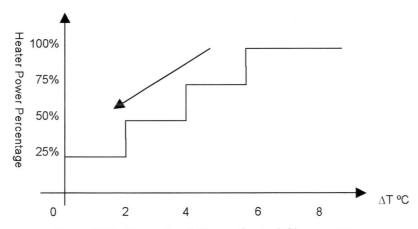

Figure 29–1. Proportional Heater Control Characteristics.

Proportional heating control can be implemented by using several banks of heaters (e.g., using four 250 W heaters instead of one 1,000 W heater) or, if a single heater is used, by varying the duty cycle of the heater supply power. The latter can be designed to produce a continuous variation of heater power according to the measured temperature difference.

Most incubators allow users to vary the relative humidity inside the units. Humidity can be controlled by adjusting the amount of airflow through a reservoir of water underneath the mattress or by using an external humidifier. Most incubators have an oxygen inlet to create an elevated oxygen level within the incubator. Some have a built-in oxygen controller to maintain an elevated level of oxygen inside the chamber.

POTENTIAL SAFETY HAZARDS

In most cases, infants inside incubators are premature with poor regulation. Deaths and injuries to infants have been linked to temperature regulation failures causing incubator overheating and infant hyperthermia. A detached skin sensor under the skin temperature control mode detects air instead of skin temperature, which will lead to overheating. Periodic checking of heat sensor mode, temperature setting, and sensor condition (proper attachment of skin sensor) is highly recommended.

Poor oxygen control may cause hyperoxia or hypoxia. Excessive high oxygen concentration can lead to retrolental fibroplasia (formation of fibrous tissue behind the lens) in premature infants.

As the infant must stay inside the incubator around-the-clock, it is important to reduce the noise level inside the hood to protect the hearing of the infant. The main source of continuous noise is the motor and the blower. Most manufacturers are able to reduce the noise level to below 50 dB. However, using a nebulizer, opening and closing of access doors, et cetera can produce a temporary noise level as high as 100 dB.

The warm and moist environment inside the incubator and the water reservoir for humidification can become an incubator for bacteria. Care must be taken to clean and disinfect incubators after every use. Complete disinfection or sterilization should be done periodically.

FUNCTIONAL COMPONENTS AND COMMON FEATURES

Figure 29–2 shows the functional component diagram of an infant incubator. Common features of infant incubators are:

- Easy access–front, side, and rear access with cuffed ports to minimize temperature fluctuation
- Adjustable mattress elevator and tilt mechanism
- Skin or air temperature sensors for temperature control
- Proportional heating control to maintain temperature and minimize temperature fluctuation
- Oxygen sensor, regulator, and supply manifold to control oxygen level

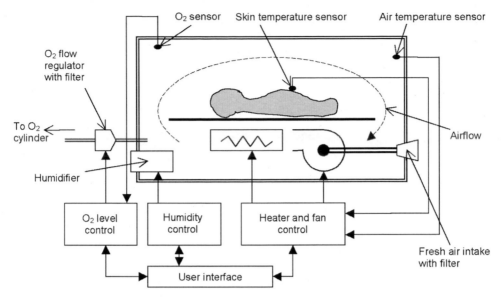

Figure 29–2. Functional Component Diagram of an Infant Incubator.

- Humidity sensor and water reservoir to maintain relative humidity inside incubator
- Low airflow across infant to reduce heat loss and dehydration
- Low internal audible noise to minimize noise and prevent hearing damage to infant
- Alarms–including temperature, overheat, oxygen level, humidity, heater, and loss of airflow
- Independent maximum air temperature (41°C) sensor and alarm to prevent overtemperature
- Display–numerical display including temperature, oxygen level, humidity level, and heater power
- Data trending and alarm log
- Air and oxygen inlet filters
- Easy to clean and disinfect

PHOTOTHERAPY LIGHTS

A phototherapy light is used to break down bilirubin in the newborn. Jaundice occurs when the liver of the infant has not reached full detoxification capability, especially in premature infants. During the first week of life, infants have poor liver function to remove bilirubin. A bilirubin level of 1 to

5 mg per 100 ml of blood within the first 3 days of birth is considered normal. This level should decrease as the liver begins to mature. Visible light spectrum of wavelength from 400 to 500 nm (blue) has been shown to be effective in transforming bilirubin into a water-soluble substance that can then be removed by the gallbladder and kidneys. A spectral irradiance of 4 $\mu W/cm^2/nm$ at the skin surface is considered to be the minimum level to produce effective phototherapy.

A phototherapy light can be placed directly over an infant in a bassinet or placed over the hood of an incubator. Blue light sources are used to increase the efficacy of phototherapy. However, blue light can mask the skin tone and is hard on the eyes of the caregivers. As a compromise, some manufacturers may use a combination of white and blue light sources and have built-in features to switch off the blue lights during observation.

Ultraviolet radiation (<400 nm) emitted from most blue light sources is harmful to the infant. Infants receiving phototherapy are required to wear eye protectors to prevent damage to their retinas. A Plexiglas™ (used as an enclosure) placed between the light source and the infant can cut out most of the wavelength below 380 nm. Far-infrared radiation (heat) can create hyperthermia and cause dehydration to the infant. As a precaution, monitoring or periodically checking the skin temperature of an infant receiving phototherapy treatment is recommended.

Some common features of a phototherapy light are:

- A blue light source (e.g., special blue fluorescent tubes, tungsten halogen, etc.) with a high-intensity blue spectrum (e.g., 400–500 nm) or a combination of blue and white light sources is used.
- The output of phototherapy lights in the range of wavelength from 400 to 500 nm measured at skin level should be greater then 4 $\mu W/cm^2/nm$. Most devices on the market have output much greater than this minimum level (e.g., 15 $\mu W/cm^2$).
- Filters (Plexiglas™) to remove ultraviolet (280–400 nm) radiation to avoid damaging the infant's eyes and skin.
- Equipped with white light for observation (with blue light switched off during observation)
- Observation timer to automatically switch back to phototherapy after observation
- Light bulb operation timer to signal light bulb replacement
- Light source housing on height adjustable stand

Many manufacturers are using a number (e.g., eight) of 50 cm (20 inches) fluorescent tubes in a metal housing for phototherapy units. The lower surface of the housing is a piece of Plexiglas™ for mechanical barrier as well as serving as an UV filter. A typical unit is shown in Figure 29–3. The light source housing is either mounted on a height adjustable stand or placed

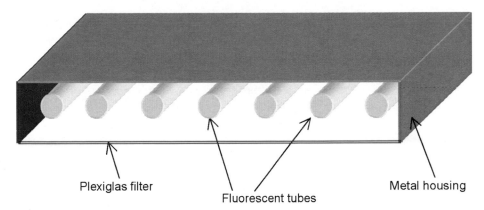

Figure 29–3. Cross-Sectional View of a Phototherapy Light.

directly on top of the hood of an infant incubator.

Experiments have shown that the spectral output of a fluorescent tube changes with the tube surface temperature as well as with time. An enclosed tube compartment as shown in Figure 29–3 can reach a temperature of 70°C after 2 to 3 hours of use. Figure 29–4 shows the typical characteristics of a phototherapy light output with respect to temperature inside the light source compartment. It shows that the light output will reach a peak value shortly after it is turned on and will drop to about 70% of its peak value after a few hours when it has risen to a steady temperature.

In addition, from manufacturers' specifications, the output of a fluorescent tube has a limited life span ranging from a few hundred hours to about

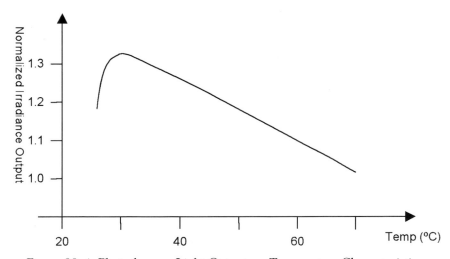

Figure 29–4. Phototherapy Light Output vs. Temperature Characteristics.

2,000 hours. The tube output decreases as it is being used (e.g., 10% drop after 300 hours). Blue fluorescent tubes generally have a shorter life span than ordinary white tubes. In order to ensure sufficient light output for phototherapy, some sites are measuring the output using a special light meter and replacing them when they are below a certain limit. Instead of performing periodic output measurements, some users implement a fixed schedule (e.g., monitoring the hours of operation) to replace these light sources.

Chapter 30

BODY TEMPERATURE MONITORS

OBJECTIVES

- Differentiate between core and peripheral temperature and list the sites for body temperature measurement.
- Differentiate between continuous and intermittent temperature monitoring.
- Describe the principles of operation of a typical bedside continuous temperature monitor.
- Analyze the transducer circuit diagram and the functional block diagram of a typical continuous temperature monitor.
- Describe the principles of operation of IR thermometry.
- Define the terms *emissivity* and *field of view*, and explain their significance in IR thermometry.
- Analyze the functional building blocks of a typical tympanic (ear) thermometer.
- State the sources of error in body temperature measurement using tympanic thermometers.

CHAPTER CONTENTS

457

7. Tympanic (Ear) Thermometers
8. Block Diagram of a Tympanic Thermometer
9. Potential Errors in Tympanic Thermometers

INTRODUCTION

The body temperature of a healthy person is regulated within a narrow range despite variation in environmental conditions and physical activity. Illness is often associated with disturbance of body temperature regulation leading to abnormal elevation of body temperature, or fever. Fever is such a sensitive and reliable indicator of the presence of disease that thermometry is probably the most common clinical procedure in use. Body temperature is also measured during many clinical procedures such as surgery, postanesthesia recovery, treatment of hyper/hypothermic conditions, et cetera.

A temperature monitor allows measurement and display of a patient's body temperature, sounds an alarm if it is above or below some preset limits, and tracks its variation over a period of time. Most monitors accept different sensors or probes to measure temperature at different body sites (e.g., oral, esophageal, rectal, etc.).

Temperature measurement can be continuous or intermittent. A continuous temperature monitor uses a sensor to acquire the temperature at the measurement site continuously. An example is skin temperature measurement of an infant in an infant incubator. A temperature sensor is placed on the infant's skin surface to continuously measure and display the infant's temperature and, using the measurand to control the heater inside the incubator, to achieve temperature regulation. An oral mercury-in-glass thermometer, which takes about 1 or 2 minutes to obtain a temperature reading between measurements, is an example of an intermittent temperature measurement device. This chapter describes two temperature measurement devices—a continuous temperature monitor that uses a contact temperature sensor; and a tympanic thermometer, which is a noncontact intermittent temperature monitor that senses the heat being radiated from the patient.

SITES OF BODY TEMPERATURE MEASUREMENT

Heat transfer within the body depends on conduction (heat transfer between adjacent organs) and convection (heat transfer through movement of body fluid). One can simply visualize the body as a central core at uniform temperature surrounded by an insulating shell. In body temperature measurement, it is often desirable to measure the core temperature as it reflects the true temperature of the internal parts of the body (skull, thorax, and abdomen). Peripheral or shell (skin and subcutaneous fat) temperature is often affected by the external environment.

It is not practical to define an exact upper level of normal body temperature because there are variations among normal persons as well as considerable fluctuations in a given individual. However, an oral temperature above 37.2°C in a person at rest is a reasonable indication of disease. Table 30–1 lists the range of temperature (in degree Celsius) measured from different sites on normal individuals of different age groups.

Body sites such as the tympanic membrane, rectum, esophagus, nasopharynx, bladder, and pulmonary artery are used for core temperature measurement. In a normothermic patient, these sites yield very similar temperature values. However, under hypothermic conditions, the rectal site can be cooler than the others by 1 to 2°C.

Table 30–1.
Normal Temperature Comparisons.

	Core	*Oral*	*Rectal*
Adult	36.5–37.6	36.0–37.2	36.3–37.6
Age 7–14 years	36.8–37.3	36.4–36.9	36.4–36.9
Age 3–6 years	37.3–37.6	36.9–37.2	36.9–37.2

CONTINUOUS TEMPERATURE MONITORS

Continuous temperature monitors are used in situations in which a patient's body temperature is required to be measured continuously. Examples of such situations are patients under general anesthesia, or receiving hypothermic or hyperthermic treatment. Many temperature transducers can be used in continuous temperature monitoring. However, the most common type of transducer for clinical application is a thermistor. The YSI series probes (patented by Yellow Spring Instruments) offer true interchangeability between probes and monitors from different manufacturers without the need for recalibration or adjustment. The temperature transducer element in a YSI 400 probe is a precision thermistor manufactured to achieve the resistance-temperature characteristics according to the YSI 400 specifications. The characteristics are shown in Table 30–2 with less than 0.1% resistance tolerance between 0 and 80°C.

Table 30–2.
YSI 400 Resistance/Temperature Characteristics.

Temp °C	Res. Ω	Temp °C	Res. Ω	Temp °C	Res. Ω	Temp °C	Res. Ω
–40	75.79 k	24	2,354	40	1,200	80	283.1
–35	54.66 k	25	2,253	41	1,153	85	241.3
–30	39.86 k	26	2,156	42	1,108	90	206.5
–25	29.38 k	27	2,065	43	1,065	95	177.5
–20	21.87 k	28	1,977	44	1,024	100	153.2
–15	16.43 k	29	1,894	45	984.2	105	132.7
–10	12.46 k	30	1,815	46	946.6	110	115.4
–5	9,534	31	1,740	47	910.6	115	100.6
0	7,355	32	1,668	48	876.2	120	88.1
5	5,720	33	1,599	49	843.2	125	77.4
10	4,483	34	1,534	50	811.7	130	68.2
15	3,539	35	1,471	55	672.9	135	60.2
20	2,814	36	1,412	60	560.7	140	53.4
21	2,690	37	1,355	65	469.4	145	47.4
22	2,572	38	1,301	70	394.9	150	42.3
23	2,460	39	1,249	75	333.5		

The normal output characteristics of a YSI 400 temperature probe is illustrated in Figure 30–1. It has a negative temperature coefficient and a highly nonlinear resistance-temperature relationship.

Often, it is desirable to have linear output characteristics. A YSI 700 series temperature probe is manufactured by combining two thermistor elements (Figure 30–2a) of different temperature characteristics to form a temperature transducer that can be wired to produce linear output characteris-

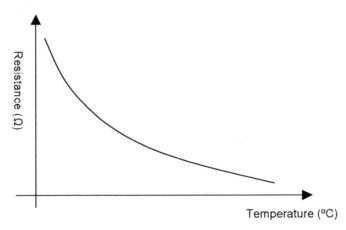

Figure 30–1. YSI 400 Series Temperature Probe Output Characteristics.

tics. The construction of a YSI 700 series thermistor and its application circuit is shown in Figure 30–2b. Figure 30–3 shows the equivalent resistance-temperature relationship of the circuit.

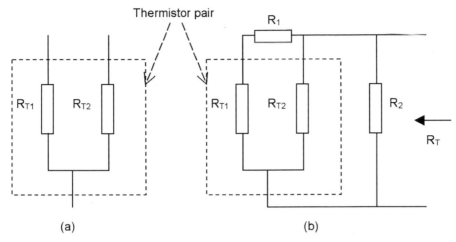

Figure 30–2. YSI 700 Series Thermistor (a) and Application (b).

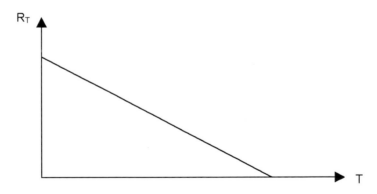

Figure 30–3. Linearized Characteristic of YSI 400 Series Thermistor Circuit.

Many continuous temperature monitors on the market can accept YSI 400 or YSI 700 temperature probes. As there are two lead wires for a YSI 400 series transducer, $1/4$ inch mono phono jacks are often used as connectors with YSI 400 probes. Whereas $1/4$ inch stereo phono jacks (3 wires) are used with YSI 700 probes.

A YSI 400 temperature probe can be connected to one arm of a Wheatstone bridge as shown in Figure 30–4. The output voltage V_0 will vary according to the change in resistance R_T of the probe. As the bridge output has a nonlinear relationship with the resistance R_T, the resistance values of R_a and R_b can be chosen such that the output voltage/temperature follows a piecewise-linear relationship.

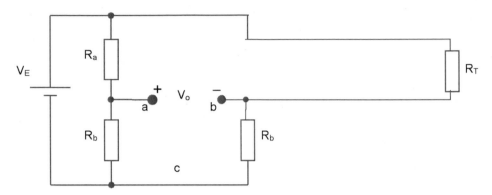

Figure 30–4. Wheatstone Bridge Temperature Monitor.

In a digital thermometer, the resistance-temperature relationship is stored in digital memory in a lookup table. Once the resistance of the probe is measured, the corresponding temperature is determined from the lookup table. No linearization circuit is required.

BLOCK DIAGRAM OF A CONTINUOUS TEMPERATURE MONITOR

Figure 30–5 shows a simple functional block diagram of a continuous temperature monitor. It consists of an excitation circuit to provide either a voltage or a current source to convert the change of resistance (due to change in temperature) to a voltage output. This output voltage is amplified, filtered, and sent to the processor and display modules. The purpose of signal isolation is for electrical safety.

INFRARED THERMOMETERS

Mercury-in-glass and electronic thermometers measure temperature by placing the probes under the tongue, in the rectum, or under the armpit. Temperature obtained from these sites may not reflect the true core temper-

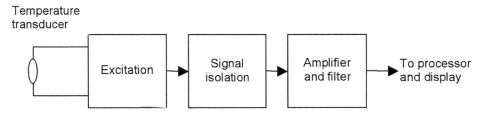

Figure 30–5. Frontend Block Diagram of Temperature Monitor.

ature as they are subject to thermal artifacts. Infrared (IR) ear thermometers, also known as ear thermometers or tympanic thermometers, allow users to measure temperature by inserting a probe into the patient's ear canal. These thermometers are quick and noninvasive. They can measure temperature without touching the mucous membrane and can be used on both conscious and unconscious patients. IR thermometers provide a convenient and fast alternative to other intermittent temperature measurement methods.

THEORY OF INFRARED THERMOMETRY

IR thermometry or pyrometry has long been used as a noncontact method to measure temperature in the industry. For example, in foundries, noncontact IR thermometers are used to measure the temperature of molten metals from a distance.

IR thermometry relies on the principle that radiation is emitted by all objects having a temperature greater than absolute zero (0 Kelvin) and that the emission increases as the object becomes hotter. The temperature of the object can be determined from the emission spectrum of the radiation in the infrared region. Devices based on IR thermometry are based on Planck's law and Wien's displacement law.

Planck's law states that if the intensity of the radiated energy is plotted as a function of wavelength (Figure 30–6), the area under the curve represents the total energy radiated at the associated temperature.

Wien's displacement law states that the wavelength λ_{max} corresponding to the maximum energy intensity in the radiated energy spectrum is given by the equation:

$$\lambda_{max} = \frac{2.89 \times 10^3}{T} \, \mu m,$$

where T is the object temperature in Kelvin.

For example, if the object is at temperature 37°C,

$$T = 37 + 273 = 310 \text{ K} \Rightarrow \lambda_{max} = 9.32 \text{ μm}.$$

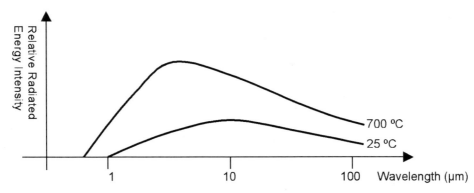

Figure 30–6. Radiated Energy Spectrum of an Object.

Another parameter important to IR thermometry is emissivity. Emissivity (ϵ) is defined as the ratio of the energy radiated by an object at a given temperature to the energy emitted by a perfect radiator, or a blackbody at the same temperature. Therefore, the emissivity of a blackbody is 1.0, whereas the emissivities for all "nonblack" objects lie between 0.0 and 1.0. The emissivity of body tissue is about 0.95. For most substances, the emissivity is wavelength-dependent except for a graybody. A graybody is defined as an object whose emissivity is the same for all wavelengths. As most objects are not close to being a blackbody, variation of emissivity without proper compensation will lead to error in IR measurement. Most IR thermometers restrict the sensing wavelength to a chosen narrow band so that near-graybody characteristics can be obtained.

In IR thermometry, a sensor is used to collect the radiant energy coming from the object. Therefore, it is important that the sensor's field of view (FOV) be aligned properly with the object to be measured. The FOV is the angle of vision at which the instrument operates. It is determined by the optics of the unit. The IR thermometer in Figure 30–7 will correctly read the temperature of Object A but will read a temperature lower than the temperature of Object B if the background is of a lower temperature than the object.

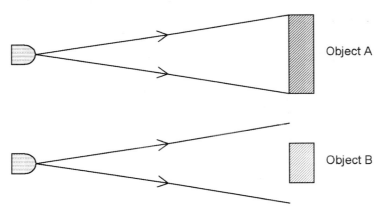

Figure 30–7. Field of View of Optical Sensor.

TYMPANIC (EAR) THERMOMETERS

A tympanic thermometer measures body temperature by measuring the IR energy emitting from the tympanic membrane in the ear. It is an intermittent temperature measurement device. The tympanic membrane is a good site to measure core temperature as it is vascularized by the carotid arteries, which also perfuse the hypothalamus. Since tympanic thermometers do not rely on thermal conduction, unlike most electronic thermometers, they take less time to reach temperature equilibrium. A typical tympanic thermometer takes less than 5 seconds to take a reading, and it is not subject to external thermal disturbances (such as air temperature fluctuation). Tympanic thermometers are recommended for temperature measurements on unsettled patients.

BLOCK DIAGRAM OF A TYMPANIC THERMOMETER

A functional block diagram of a tympanic thermometer is shown in Figure 30–8. In the diagram, the object is the tympanic membrane. The IR energy radiated from the membrane is collected by the optical lens and filter. The detector converts the radiated energy to an electrical signal. This electrical signal is processed to obtain the temperature. The following paragraphs provide a more detailed functional description of the building blocks.

The optical path consists of a lens, a filter, and an optical light pipe. The function of the lens and light pipe is to ensure that the FOV covers only the tympanic membrane instead of other tissue such as the wall of the ear canal. It also focuses the IR radiation to the detector. The filter allows only a cer-

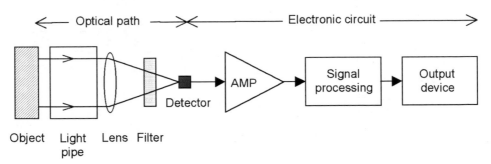

Figure 30–8. Functional Block Diagram of IR Thermometer.

tain bandwidth of wavelength to reach the detector. The wavelength of the IR spectrum lies between 0.7 and 20 μm. The bandwidth of a wideband IR thermometer is several microns wide (e.g., 8–14 μm), whereas a narrowband device allows only a single wavelength to reach the detector (e.g., 2.2 ± 0.5 μm). Instead of using a single band wavelength, a "two color" thermometer uses two narrowbands to reduce errors due to nonunity emissitivity and IR absorption in the optical path (e.g., due to water moisture in the atmosphere). Figure 30–9 shows the pass band(s) of a wideband, narrowband, and "two color" IR thermometer.

Several types of detectors can be used in IR thermometry. Common detectors are pyroelectric sensors and thermopiles.

In a pyroelectric sensor, conductive material is deposited on the opposite surfaces of a slice of a ferroelectric material. The ferroelectric material absorbs radiation and converts it to heat. The resulting rise in temperature changes the polarization of the material. The current flowing through the external resistor connected across the two conductive surfaces is proportional to the rate of change of temperature of the sensor. A shutter mechanism is often installed to provide a controlled period of exposure to the radiation.

A thermopile is made up of a number of thermocouples connected in series. Radiant energy landed on the hot junction area is first converted to heat, creating a differential temperature between the hot and cold junctions of the thermocouples. Each thermocouple generates a small voltage (on the order of μV) according to this temperature difference. The output of the thermopile is the summation of all the voltages from the thermocouples in the sensor. An IR thermometer using a thermopile sensor requires another temperature sensor, such as a thermistor, to measure the cold junction temperature. The construction of the thermopile in an IR sensor is shown in Figure 30–10.

To prevent sensing the ear canal temperature, some units use narrow FOV optics with multiple scanning to detect the highest temperature in the

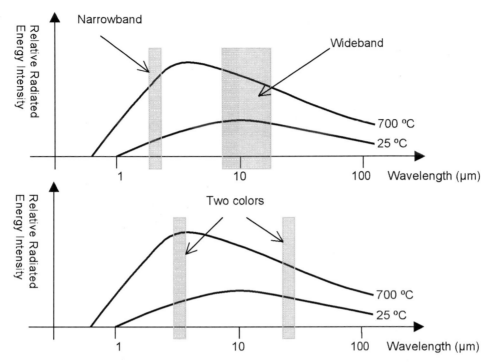

Figure 30–9. Detector Bandwidth of IR Thermometers.

ear canal. Within the ear canal, the hottest object is the tympanic membrane.

In most IR thermometers, the analog signal from the sensor is first digitized and sent to the signal processor. The main function of the processor is to determine the object temperature based on the signal from the sensor. Calibration curves or lookup tables are stored in the unit's memory for this purpose. Another function of the signal processor is to compensate for non-ideal conditions such as $\epsilon < 1.0$ and provide offset to estimate the oral, rectal, or core temperature from the tympanic reading.

POTENTIAL ERRORS IN TYMPANIC THERMOMETERS

Factors that affect accuracy unique to tympanic thermometers are:

- If the FOV of the sensor includes other tissue inside the ear canal, it will create a lower than normal temperature reading.
- Nonstraight ear canal can prevent direct line of view of the detector to the tympanic membrane. This situation often occurs in infants where the ear canal is narrow and curved.

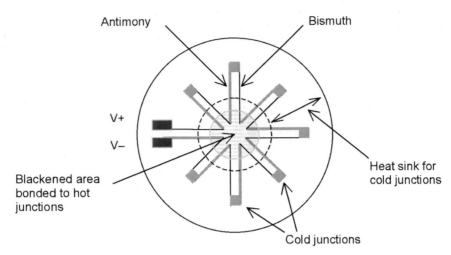

Figure 30–10. Construction of a Thermopile with Eight Thermocouples.

- Too much hair or ear wax in the ear canal will block the tympanic membrane from the detector.
- Finally, some units provide software compensation factors to the tympanic temperature reading in order to estimate the temperature of different body temperature measurement sites (e.g., rectal, oral, etc.). In these units, errors can be caused by incorrect selection of these compensation factors.

Chapter 31

PULSE OXIMETERS

OBJECTIVES

- State Lambert Beer's law.
- Define S_aO_2, S_pO_2, S_vO_2, fractional oxygen saturation, and functional oxygen saturation.
- State the clinical applications of pulse oximetry.
- Explain the principles of operation of pulse oximeters.
- Describe the construction of a typical pulse oximeter sensor.
- Sketch a typical block diagram of a pulse oximeter and explain the functions of each block.
- Discuss factors affecting signal quality and accuracy of pulse oximeters.
- Differentiate between the clinical application of oxygen analyzers and pulse oximeters.

CHAPTER CONTENTS

INTRODUCTION

One of the main functions of the cardiopulmonary system is to deliver oxygen and remove carbon dioxide to and from the cells. Hypoxia is a general term describing the condition of lack of oxygen in the system. Acute hypoxia produces impaired judgment and motor incoordination. When hypoxia is long-standing, the symptoms consist of fatigue, drowsiness, inattentiveness, and delayed reaction time. More severe hypoxia can affect brain function and lead to death.

Until the early 1980s, blood oxygen saturation levels were measured by drawing arterial blood samples from the patient and performing in vitro analysis using laboratory co-oximeters (a multiwavelength spectrophotometer). Pulse oximeters were developed in the early 1980s, providing a real-time, continuous, and noninvasive means to monitor the changing level of arterial blood oxygenation in patients; and allowing clinical intervention before the occurrence of significant hypoxia. In 1986, pulse oximeters were endorsed by the American Society of Anesthesiologists as a standard of care for use whenever anesthesia is performed. Since then, pulse oximeters have become the preferred method for measuring arterial oxygen saturation and are used in most areas of hospitals.

DEFINITION OF PERCENTAGE OXYGEN
SATURATION IN BLOOD

The primary function of red blood cells is to transport oxygen from lungs to tissue. This function is carried out by hemoglobin. When blood is circulated into the lungs, oxygen is attached to hemoglobin, forming oxygenated hemoglobin. Under normal conditions, hemoglobin in blood becomes almost fully saturated with oxygen before leaving the lungs. When blood is in the capillaries, oxygen is released from the oxyhemoglobin and delivered to the cells. The hemoglobin becomes deoxyhemoglobin. In studying oxygen transport in blood, the terms $\%S_aO_2$, $\%S_PO_2$, and $\%S_vO_2$ are commonly used. Here are their definitions:

- Percent oxygen saturation of hemoglobin in arterial blood ($\%S_aO_2$) is the percentage of hemoglobin in arterial blood that is bound with oxygen; it is determined by analyzing an arterial blood sample with a co-oximeter.
- Percent oxygen saturation of hemoglobin in venous blood ($\%S_vO_2$) is the percentage of hemoglobin in venous blood that is bound with oxygen; it is usually determined from a blood sample taken from or mea-

sured in the pulmonary artery.
- Percent oxygen saturation of hemoglobin in arterial blood (%SpO2) is determined by a pulse oximeter (instead of from a blood sample by a co-oximeter).

In addition to oxyhemoglobin and deoxyhemoglobin, there are two other forms of hemoglobin. Carboxyhemoglobin is hemoglobin bound with carbon monoxide. Methemoglobin is the oxidized form of hemoglobin. Methemoglobin is incapable of binding with oxygen. A high percentage of carboxyhemoglobin or methemoglobin compromises the oxygen-carrying capacity of blood as there is less hemoglobin available to bind with oxygen.

Table 31–1 shows the normal values of %SaO2 and %SpO2 with the corresponding blood gas values of normal adults and neonates.

Table 31–1.
Typical Values of Blood Oxygen Level

Adult	%SaO2	96–98%	PaO2	85–100 mmHg	PaCO2	38–42 mmHg
	%SvO2	70–75%	PvO2	35–40 mmHg	PvCO2	41–51 mmHg
Neonates	%SaO2	~94%	PaO2	63–87 mmHg	PaCO2	31–35 mmHg

PRINCIPLES OF OPERATION

The principle of pulse oximetry is based on Lambert Beer's law with differential light absorption of two wavelengths. The wavelengths of the most commonly used sources are red (660 nm) and the infrared (940 nm).

Lambert Beer's law states that for a substance of concentration C in a fluid, the absorbance (A) of light due to the substance in the fluid, which is defined as the natural logarithm of the ratio of incident light intensity (Io) to the transmitted intensity (I), is equal to the product of the absorptivity (a'), the substance's concentration (C) in the fluid and the distance of the optical path length (d). Figure 31–1 illustrates the concept.

For a mixture of two substances X and Y in the fluid, the total absorbance A is given by the sum of the absorbance due the substance X and the substance Y alone, or:

$$A = Ax + Ay.$$

Two equations are used by pulse oximeter device manufacturers to calculate oxygen saturation in blood. They are the fractional oxygen saturation and the functional oxygen saturation equations.

(i) Fractional oxygen saturation (% O2Hb) is equal to the ratio of the

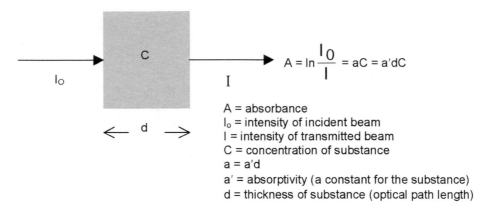

$$A = \ln\frac{I_0}{I} = aC = a'dC$$

A = absorbance
I_0 = intensity of incident beam
I = intensity of transmitted beam
C = concentration of substance
a = a'd
a' = absorptivity (a constant for the substance)
d = thickness of substance (optical path length)

Figure 31–1. Lambert Beer's Law.

concentration of oxyhemoglobin in blood to the sum of concentrations of all types of hemoglobin in blood.

$$\%O_2Hb = \frac{C_{O_2Hb}}{C_{HHb} + C_{O_2Hb} + C_{COHb} + C_{metHb}} \times 100\%, \qquad (1)$$

where:
C_{O_2Hb} = the concentration of oxygenated hemoglobin in arterial blood,
C_{HHb} = the concentration of deoxygenated hemoglobin in arterial blood,
C_{COHb} = the concentration of carboxyhemoglobin in arterial blood, and
C_{metHb} = the concentration of methemoglobin in arterial blood.

(ii) **Functional oxygen saturation** ($\%S_aO_2$) is equal to the ratio of the concentration of oxyhemoglobin in blood to the sum of the functional hemoglobin concentrations. That is, the concentrations of the oxyhemoglobin and the deoxyhemoglobin, which are responsible for the oxygen transport.

$$\%S_aO_2 = \frac{C_{O_2Hb}}{C_{HHb} + C_{O_2Hb}} \times 100\%. \qquad (2)$$

It is obvious from the preceding equations that the functional value is higher than the fractional value for the same blood sample. For most patients, the concentration of carboxyhemoglobin as well as that of the methemoglobin is negligible. In a healthy individual, the difference between $\%S_aO_2$ and $\%O_2Hb$ is less than 3%.

Figure 31–2 shows the absorption spectrum of oxyhemoglobin (O_2Hb) and deoxyhemoglobin (HHb). To measure the $\%S_aO_2$ (or $\%O_2Hb$) in a blood sample, two light sources of wavelengths $\lambda1$ and $\lambda2$ are used. In the blood sample, let:

C_o be the concentration of oxyhemoglobin (O_2Hb) in blood, and

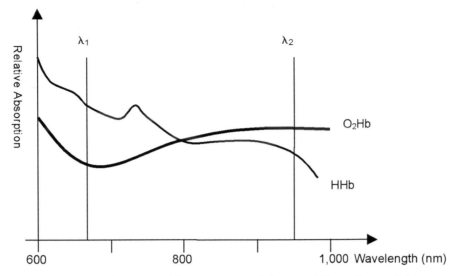

Figure 31–2. Absorption Characteristics of Oxy- and Deoxyhemoglobin.

C_d be the concentration of of deoxyhemoglobin (HHb).

At wavelength $\lambda 1$, using Lambert Beer's law:

$$A_1 = A_{1o} + A_{1d} = a_{1o}C_o + a_{1d}C_d, \qquad (3)$$

where A_1 = the total absorption due to wavelength $\lambda 1$
A_{1o} = the absorption of oxyhemoglobin due to wavelength $\lambda 1$
A_{1d} = the absorption of deoxyhemoglobin due to wavelength $\lambda 1$
a_{1o} = the product of the optical path length and the absorptivity of oxyhemoglobin due to wavelength $\lambda 1$, and
a_{1d} = the product of the optical path length and the absorptivity of deoxyhemoglobin due to wavelength $\lambda 1$

At wavelength $\lambda 2$, using Lambert Beer's law:

$$A_2 = A_{2o} + A_{2d} = a_{2o}C_o + a_{2d}C_d. \qquad (4)$$

One can solve equations (1) and (2) for C_o and C_d if A_1, A_2, a_{1o}, a_{1d}, a_{2o}, a_{2d} are known. Knowing C_o and C_d, the oxygen saturation can be computed. Using the functional oxygen saturation equation (Equation 2):

$$\%S_aO_2 = \frac{C_o}{C_o + C_d} \times 100\%$$

$$= \frac{1}{1 + \dfrac{C_d}{C_o}} \times 100\%.$$

In practice, the light beams travel through the tissue and are absorbed not only by the hemoglobin but also by other tissues (such as bone, muscle) in the light path. In addition, as the diameters of the capillaries are pulsating according to the blood pressure, the optical path length is not a constant. Therefore, a_{10}, a_{1d}, a_{20}, and a_{2d}, which are the product of the absorptivity and optical path length are not exactly constant values and hence C_o and C_d cannot be computed analytically.

Figure 31–3 shows the absorption waveform measured by the light sensor in a pulse oximeter probe. A red beam ($\lambda 1 = 660$ nm) and an infrared ($\lambda 2 = 940$ nm) beam are commonly used. The solid and dotted waveforms are results of the absorption characteristics of each of the beams.

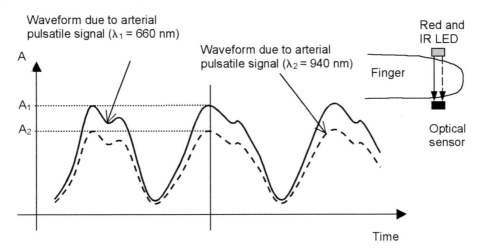

Figure 31–3. Absorption Signal from Pulse Oximeter Finger Probe.

Most pulse oximeter manufacturers derive the $\%SaO_2$ values from the optical intensity ratio (r) of the transmitted intensity of the red (I_{rd}) and infrared beam (I_{ir}) measured by the sensors in the probe.

$$r = \frac{I_{rd}}{I_{ir}}. \tag{5}$$

In most cases, an empirical equation or a lookup table between r and the $\%SaO_2$ values is established so the $\%SaO_2$ value can be determined from the measured I_{rd} and I_{ir}. This correlation between r and the $\%SaO_2$ is verified statistically by simultaneously reading the pulse oximeter output and drawing an arterial blood sample from the patient and analyzing the sample by a co-oximeter. Pulse oximeters are calibrated using arterial blood samples (blood oximeter) using either the $\%O_2Hb$ (fractional) or $\%SaO_2$ (functional) equations.

PULSE OXIMETER SENSOR PROBES

Many different types of sensor probes are used in pulse oximetry. A typical probe consists of two light-emitting diodes (LEDs), one emitting red light and the other emitting infrared. These LEDs are pulsed alternately to send a beam of light through the underlying tissues (see the top right figure in Figure 31–3). A photodetector in the probe on the other side of the tissue picks up the transmitted light signal and sends it to the processing circuits. Probes can be classified as reflectance or transmittance, disposable or reusable, or by their sensing locations. A disposable probe is one that will be discarded after being used on a single patient (however, some sites reuse some probes that are labeled "single use" for cost saving). The LEDs and the photodetector are mounted on each end of a flexible strip. The strip is applied on and often taped over the tissue (Figure 31–4). A reusable probe usually has a more robust and rigid cover to protect the LEDs and the detector. A transmitting probe has the LEDs on one side and the detector on the other side of the capillary bed. The light is transmitted through the capillary bed and tissues. On the other hand, in a reflecting probe, the detector is placed on the same side as the LEDs. As the light penetrates the tissue, some is absorbed and some is reflected back to the surface. The detector picks up the reflected signal and sends it to the processor. Pulse oximeter probes in theory can be placed over any part of the body with capillaries. However, common sites for transmitting probes are the index finger and the earlobe. For infants, probes are often taped to the big toe. Transmitting probes are usually placed on the forehead of the patient.

FUNCTIONAL BLOCK DIAGRAM

Figure 31–5 shows a typical functional block diagram of a pulse oximeter. It consists of:

- A probe consisting of a red LED, an infrared LED, and a photodetector.
- A timing control circuit to sequence the LEDs and synchronize them with the photodetector. There are three phases in one timing cycle: Red "on" and IR "off," Red "off" and IR "on," and both LEDs "off." The latter is to measure the dark signal to eliminate the effects of the ambient light.
- Analog and digital electronics to amplify and process the signal.
- A processor to compute the transmitted red and infrared light intensity ratio and match the $\%S_aO_2$ from the lookup table. It can also derive

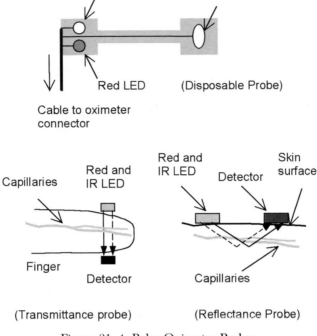

Figure 31–4. Pulse Oximeter Probes.

the heart rate from the pulsating waveform and compares the measured values (heart rate, $\%S_aO_2$) to the alarm settings.

• A display to show the $\%S_aO_2$ values, the alarm limits, and the heart rate. A plethysmograph showing the detected signal strength is often displayed to provide the user an idea of the signal to noise information of the measurement. A strong signal level indicates that the measured value is reliable. A plethysmograph can be a waveform similar to the absorption waveform shown in Figure 31–3 or simply a one-column bar graph proportional to the detected signal strength.

ERRORS IN PULSE OXIMETRY

Although we can empirically establish an accurate relationship under ideal situations between the optical intensity ratio (r) and $\%S_aO_2$, in the presence of patient motion or other interference, the optical densities will inevitably include noise components (N). Therefore, in the presence of noise, the measured beam intensity $I = S + N$ where S is the desired signal and N is the noise. The optical intensity ratio (equation 5) is now rewritten as

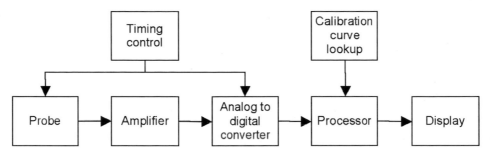

Figure 31–5. Block diagram of Pulse Oximeter.

$$r = \frac{S_{rd} + N_{rd}}{S_{ir} + N_{ir}} . \qquad (6)$$

A well-observed source of noise is the change in light absorption caused by patient motion. The movement changes the optical path length of blood vessels and tissues. In a poor signal to noise ratio situation, the noise level becomes significant in the optical intensity ratio. This will increase the error in the derived $\%S_aO_2$. If the noise (N) component is much larger than the signal (S), i.e. $N >> S$, the optical intensity ratio in equation (6) then becomes

$$r = \frac{N_{rd}}{N_{ir}} .$$

Under such conditions, if the noise level in the red and IR regions are similar (i.e., $N_{rd} \approx N_{ir}$), the optical intensity ratio r will approach unity.

For most systems with a good signal to noise ratio, $r = 1.0$ corresponds to a $\%S_aO_2$ of about 82%. For that reason, a pulse oximeter working under noisy conditions will tend to report a lower oxygen saturation reading. To maximize the signal to noise ratio, the transmitted beam intensity should be measured during the systolic region of the blood pressure cycle. There have been some reported successes by manufacturers using special digital signal processing techniques such as adaptive filtering or signal extraction to minimize the effect of noise in pulse oximetry.

In summary, errors in pulse oximetry measurement are due to the following causes:

- Poor perfusion–A patient suffering from poor perfusion usually has lower than normal blood pressure. A lack of blood in the capillaries will decrease the signal to noise ratio and therefore increase the error of the measurement.
- Excessive signal attenuation–Patients with dark skin pigment or too thick tissue (e.g., skin) at the measurement site will decrease the signal penetration (decrease the detector signal level) and increase measure-

ment error.

- External interference–EMI and ambient light can introduce errors in measurement. There were reported incidents that flashing light and fluorescent light sources were misinterpreted by machines as pulsating red or IR signals. To avoid external light interference, pulse oximeter probes are usually designed with a cover to block external light from reaching the sensor.
- Motion–Motion will cause changes in the optical path length, which will produce measurement errors.
- Substances in blood–Some substances in the bloodstream may affect the absorption of the light sources. A high level of dyshemoglobin in carbon monoxide poisoning, low hematocrit counts of an anemic patient, and artificial dyes in a patient's blood can all affect the accuracy of the measurement.

DIFFERENCES BETWEEN PULSE OXIMETERS AND OXYGEN ANALYZERS

Oxygen analyzers and pulse oximeters are the two devices commonly used today to monitor a patient's oxygen level in the clinical environment. An oxygen analyzer measures the percentage of oxygen gas in a gas mixture such as the inspired air of a patient. Oxygen analyzers are usually attached to the patient breathing circuit. A pulse oximeter measures the oxygen content in the patient's blood. Measuring oxygen saturation level in blood can detect hypoxia even before other signs such as cyanosis or hyperventilation are observed. Table 31–2 summarizes the main differences between the two devices.

Table 31–2.
Oxygen Analyzer and Pulse Oximeter Comparison.

	Oxygen Analyzer	*Pulse Oximeter*
Principle of operation	Electrochemical transducer	Lambert Beer's law
Parameter sensed	Partial pressure of O_2 in airway	Oxygen saturation in blood
Hypoxia detection	Detects oxygen deficiency in inhaled air	Detects insufficient oxygen in blood stream

Both devices are often used together to detect insufficient oxygen to the patient. They provide complementary protection against hypoxia. For example, in anesthesia, an oxygen analyzer is connected to the inspiratory limb of the patient breathing circuit to sound an alarm on low oxygen level in the patient's inspired gas. A pulse oximeter is connected to the patient (e.g., using a finger probe) to detect the actual level of oxygen in the patient's bloodstream.

Chapter 32

END-TIDAL CARBON DIOXIDE MONITORS

OBJECTIVES

- State the clinical applications of end-tidal CO_2 monitors.
- Sketch and explain the change in CO_2 concentration in expired air.
- Explain the principles of operation of end-tidal CO_2 monitors.
- Differentiate between mainstream and sidestream end-tidal CO_2 monitoring.
- Identify the functional components and the construction of a typical mainstream end-tidal CO_2 sensor.
- Sketch the functional block diagram of a typical sidestream CO_2 monitor.
- Discuss factors affecting the signal quality and accuracy of end-tidal CO_2 monitors.

CHAPTER CONTENTS

1. Introduction
2. Carbon Dioxide Concentration Waveform (Capnogram)
3. Principles of Operation
4. Mainstream Versus Sidestream Monitoring
5. Errors in Capnography

INTRODUCTION

Carbon dioxide is a by-product of cellular metabolism and is removed from the body through the circulatory and respiratory systems. The concentration of CO_2 in the exhaled air reflects the metabolic rate and indicates the status of the pulmonary and circulatory systems. Carbon dioxide is continuously produced in the body and transported to the alveoli. The two factors that determine the alveolar concentration of CO_2 are the rate of transport of CO_2 from the blood to the alveoli and the rate of removal of CO_2 from the alveoli by alveolar ventilation. The alveolar CO_2 concentration is directly proportional to the rate of CO_2 excretion and inversely proportional to the alveolar ventilation.

A CO_2 monitor can noninvasively measure the concentration of CO_2 in breathing air. It is primarily used in operating rooms to monitor patients' ventilation under general anesthesia. It can detect breathing circuit disconnection, airway leaks, and improper placement of an endotracheal tube. In intensive care units, it can be used together with other physiological monitoring parameters to evaluate a patient's cardiopulmonary function.

CARBON DIOXIDE CONCENTRATION WAVEFORM (CAPNOGRAM)

The expired air in a breathing cycle is a combination of the dead space air and alveolar air. Figure 32–1 shows the changes of CO_2 concentration in the expired air during the course of breathing. The expired air at the beginning of exhalation is dead space air, which is inspired air saturated with moisture. As expiration goes on, more and more alveolar air becomes mixed with the dead space air until the dead space air has been totally washed out. At the end of expiration, the expired air contains 100% alveolar air. For a normal adult breathing in atmospheric air, the partial pressure (or concentration) of the CO_2 in the inspired air (atmospheric air) is 0.3 mmHg (or 0.04%) and that of the alveolar air is about 40 mmHg (or 5.3%). At the beginning of expiration, the CO_2 concentration is 0.04% and it rapidly rises until reaching a plateau. At the end of the expiration, the CO_2 concentration is at its maximum (about 5%).

A normal capnogram includes a return to zero (0.04%) baseline, a sharp upstroke, and a relatively horizontal alveolar plateau. Significant deviations from this morphology suggest an abnormality in the patient or the gas delivery equipment.

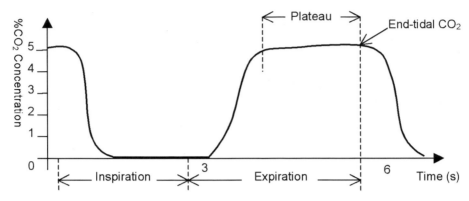

Figure 32–1. CO_2 Concentration in Breathing Air.

PRINCIPLES OF OPERATION

The principle of operation of an end-tidal CO_2 monitor is similar to that of a pulse oximeter. CO_2 monitors use infrared spectroscopy to measure the concentration of CO_2 in the exhaled gas. In normal exhaled gas, only CO_2 and water vapor contribute to the absorption of IR radiation. However, during anesthesia procedures, anesthetic gases such as N_2O may affect the IR absorption. Figure 32–2 shows the IR absorption spectrum of water vapor, carbon dioxide, and nitrous oxide. Based on Lambert Beer's law, the concentration of CO_2 in the gas is proportional to its absorption. Selecting the proper wavelength and correcting the effects of other absorptions allows the monitor to accurately determine the CO_2 concentration.

A typical setup to measure CO_2 concentration is shown in Figure 32–3. Infrared radiation passing through the gas mixture is absorbed by the CO_2 in the exhaled gas sample. The IR beam then passes through two filters; the first filter is within the IR frequency spectrum of CO_2 absorption and the second is outside. Behind each filter is an IR detector. The detector behind the first filter is for the data channel and the detector behind the second filter is for reference. The reference signal is to compensate for signal fluctuations such as variation of intensity of the light source.

MAINSTREAM VERSUS SIDESTREAM MONITORING

There are two types of capnographs, mainstream and sidestream, which are differentiated by the location of their CO_2 sensors. A mainstream capnograph has the sensor located right in the patient breathing circuit. Figure

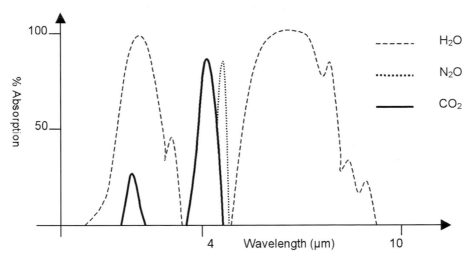

Figure 32–2. IR Absorption Spectra of H_2O, N_2O and CO_2.

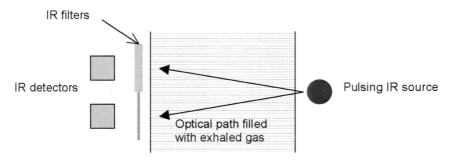

Figure 32–3. Functional Components of CO_2 Sensor.

32–4 shows a CO_2 sensor of a mainstream capnograph connected to the patient breathing circuit using a special airway adaptor. The windows on both sides of the airway adaptor allow IR from the light source to reach the detectors. As CO_2 gas mixture passes through the airway adaptor, the IR radiation of the pulsing source (e.g., 48 Hz) is partially absorbed by the CO_2 in the gas mixture. It then passes through the two optical filters before reaching the photodetectors. One filter is at the middle of the IR absorption spectrum (e.g., 4.2 µm) for carbon dioxide and the other is outside (e.g., 3.7 µm). To accurately measure the level of CO_2 in the gas mixture, the outputs of the detectors are sampled simultaneously and the level of CO_2 is determined from the ratio of the data and reference channels. The ratio is then compared to a lookup table in memory to determine the concentration of CO_2.

As the warm expired air is saturated with water vapor, water will condense on the cooler windows of the sensor, causing errors in the IR absorption measurement. To prevent condensation from forming on the window, a heater and a thermistor inside the sensor maintain a sensor temperature above the body temperature (e.g., 40°C).

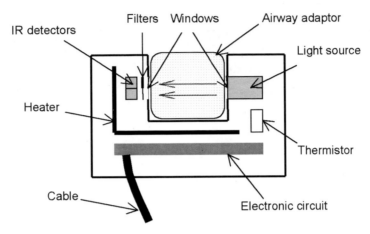

Figure 32–4. Internal View of a Mainstream CO_2 Sensor.

The sensor of a sidestream capnograph is inside the machine. The principle of CO_2 detection is similar to its mainstream counterpart. A small-diameter air sampling line connects the patient breathing circuit to the sensor inside the machine. During measurement, breathing gas sample is drawn into the sensor from the breathing circuit by an air pump. To prevent condensation, a water trap is located at the end of the air sampling line at the entrance of the machine. A heater is also used to raise the temperature of the sensor chamber to prevent water condensation. For both mainstream and sidestream monitors, the derived CO_2 concentration (or partial pressure) must be temperature and pressure corrected as it is measured at temperature and pressure different from those inside the patient's body. Figure 32–5 shows a functional block diagram of a sidestream CO_2 monitor.

ERRORS IN CAPNOGRAPHY

As discussed previously, moisture as well as its condensation absorb IR radiation. Water condensation is a major problem for sidestream monitors as it can block the small-bore air sampling tubing, causing a pressure and flow reduction in the circuit. Since the partial pressure of CO_2 is pressure-dependent, any pressure fluctuations will introduce errors in the measurements.

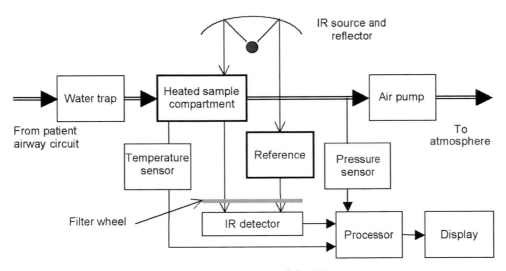

Figure 32–5. Sidestream CO_2 Monitor.

When a CO_2 monitor is used during anesthesia procedures, halogenated gases and nitrous oxide are present in the patient's exhaled gas. These gases absorb IR radiation and may cause measurement errors if they are not properly accounted for.

Although the presence of oxygen does not affect IR absorption, the collision of O_2 and CO_2 molecules will broaden the absorption peak and create a falsely low CO_2 concentration reading.

Capnographs may not be able to accurately measure the alveolar CO_2 concentration of neonates or patients with shallow breathing due to the relative large dead space volume. In addition, the gas sampling flow rate required in sidestream monitors may be too high (e.g., as high as the minute volume) for neonates.

Chapter 33

ANESTHESIA MACHINES

OBJECTIVES

- State the functions of an anesthesia machine.
- Name and explain the functional building blocks of an anesthesia machine.
- Sketch the gas circuit/piping diagram of a continuous-flow rebreathing anesthesia machine.
- Trace the oxygen, nitrous oxide, and anesthetic gas flow in a typical anesthesia machine and its patient breathing circuit.
- List potential hazards associated with the use of an anesthesia machine and the built-in features in anesthesia systems to minimize such risks.

CHAPTER CONTENTS

1. Introduction
2. Principles of Operation
3. Gas Supply and Control Subsystem
4. Breathing and Ventilation Subsystem
5. Scavenging Subsystem
6. Major Causes of Injury and Preventive Measures

INTRODUCTION

Since Dr. Crawford Long of Jefferson, Georgia, administered the first ether anesthetic in 1842 for the painless removal of a neck tumor, anesthesiology has evolved into a branch of medicine that is concerned with the administration of medication or anesthetic agents to relieve pain and support physiological functions during a surgical procedure. In a surgical procedure, an analgesic or anesthetic agent is administered to the patient for pain relief. For a major or long surgical procedure, the patient may undergo general anesthesia. General anesthesia is a reversible state of unconsciousness produced by anesthetic agents in which motor, sensory, mental, and reflex functions are lost. While depressing the cerebral cortex to achieve anesthesia, the anesthetic agents may cause respiratory depression or even respiratory arrest. An anesthesia machine is a collection of medical instrumentations to assist the anesthetist to induce and maintain anesthesia. It serves three major functions:

1. Dispense a controlled mixture of gases consisting of anesthetic agents (such as halothane, enflurane, nitrous oxide, etc.) and oxygen to anesthetize the patient during surgery.
2. Assist patient's respiration (ventilation) when normal breathing is compromised due to the anesthetic effect.
3. Monitor the patient's condition, such as vital signs and depth of anesthesia, during the surgical procedure.

Physiological parameter monitors with alarm functions are often integrated into the anesthesia machine. Automatic record keeping of vital signs and ventilation parameters, networking capabilities, and data management functions are available in modern anesthesia systems.

This chapter introduces the backbone of a typical anesthesia machine, which includes the gas supply and control, breathing and ventilation, and scavenging subsystems. Technology and instrumentation in physiological monitoring is discussed in other parts of this book.

PRINCIPLES OF OPERATION

A basic anesthesia machine consists of three main subsystems:

1. Gas supply and control
2. Breathing and ventilation
3. Scavenging

Patient monitoring equipment may be considered as the fourth subsystem (which is not discussed in this chapter). The most commonly used anesthesia machine is the continuous-flow rebreathing anesthesia machine. In this type of machine, the exhaled gas from the patient is supplied back to the patient after it is processed and mixed with a proportion of fresh anesthetic gas. Figure 33–1 shows a simple functional block diagram of such a machine. The gas supply and control block takes oxygen and nitrous oxide from the wall outlet and combines them with an anesthetic agent to produce a mixture of anesthetic gas. This gas mixture, being regulated to an appropriate level of flow and pressure, is supplied to the breathing and ventilation circuit. The function of the breathing and ventilation circuit is to deliver the gas mixture to the patient as well as to remove the expired gas from the patient. The scavenging block is to prevent the exhaled or released anesthetic gas from polluting the operating room environment. The scavenging system captures the waste anesthetic gas and discharges it safely outside the operating room.

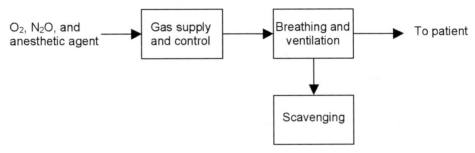

Figure 33–1. Functional Block Diagram of a Basic Anesthesia Machine.

Figure 33–2 shows a basic anesthesia machine. The following sections describe the principles of operation of each of the three subsystems.

GAS SUPPLY AND CONTROL SUBSYSTEM

Figure 33–3 illustrates a gas piping diagram showing the major components of the gas supply and control subsystem of an anesthesia machine.

Under normal operation, oxygen and nitrous oxide gases are supplied from the wall piped gas outlets to the oxygen and nitrous oxide gas inlets of the machine. The pressure of the gases at the wall outlets is about 50 psi. Oxygen flow through a check valve (one-way valve) is reduced to about 16 psi by the second-stage oxygen regulator before it reaches the flow control valve of the oxygen flowmeter. Nitrous oxide gas from the wall outlet passes through the pressure-sensing shutoff valve and reaches the nitrous oxide flow control valve of the nitrous oxide flowmeter. The shutoff valve is held open by the oxygen pressure, which is normally at 50 psi. If the oxygen pressure drops to below 25 psi, the valve will shut off the nitrous oxide supply to the

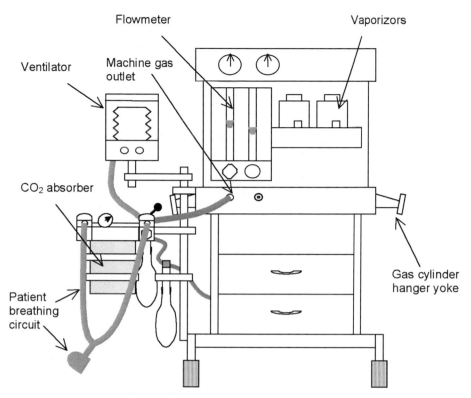

Figure 33–2. Basic Anesthesia Machine.

machine. In addition, the shutoff valve will discharge the oxygen stored in the alarm cylinder through a whistle to alert the anesthetist to the failing oxygen supply. This shutoff and alarm mechanism will protect the patient from unknowingly breathing in a low oxygen level gas mixture in case of supply oxygen failure.

By adjusting the flow control valves, the anesthetist can achieve a suitable mix and flow of oxygen and nitrous oxide gas mixture. The gas mixture then flows through a calibrated vaporizer, where it picks up a selected amount of an anesthetic agent before it is delivered to the patient via the breathing and ventilation circuit. An oxygen flush valve is available to flush the patient circuit during setup.

Under rare circumstances in which piped-in wall gases are not available, oxygen and nitrous oxide supplies are automatically switched to gas cylinders mounted on the machine. There are usually two cylinders of oxygen and two cylinders of nitrous oxide mounted on the hanger yokes on the sides or the rear of the anesthesia machine. One cylinder of each gas is on standby (turned on) and the other one serves as backup in case the first cylinder is depleted. As the maximum pressure of oxygen and nitrous oxide from

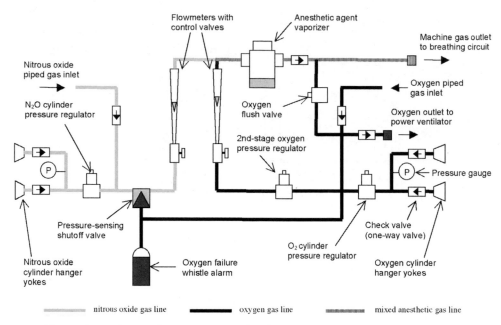

Figure 33–3. Major Components of the Gas Supply and Control Subsystem.

their cylinders are 2,200 psi and 750 psi, respectively, cylinder pressure regulators are installed to reduce the pressure of these gases to about 50 psi. Pressure gauges at hanger yokes provide an indication of whether the cylinders are full or empty. As oxygen in the gas cylinder is in gaseous state, the level of gas in the cylinder is proportional to the pressure in the cylinder. However, it is not possible to tell the amount of nitrous oxide left in the cylinder by reading the cylinder pressure. Since nitrous oxide is in liquid form inside the cylinder, the cylinder pressure will start to drop only when it is almost empty (no more liquid N_2O in the cylinder).

A vaporizer is used in the gas supply and control circuit to introduce a selected concentration of the anesthetic agent into the oxygen and nitrous oxide mixture to form the anesthetic gas. Two types of vaporizers are found on anesthesia machines: the conventional variable-bypass vaporizers and the electronically controlled vaporizers. Variable-bypass vaporizers are used to deliver liquid anesthetic agents such as halothane, enflurane, isoflurane, and servoflurane. Anesthetic agents (such as desflurane) that are in gaseous form under room temperature require the electronically controlled vaporizer. There is usually more than one vaporizer (with a different agent in each) mounted on the output manifold of the anesthesia machine. However, only one vaporizer can be active at one time.

Figure 33–4a shows the simplified construction of a variable-bypass vaporizer. The oxygen and nitrous oxide gas mixture enters the vaporizer from the inlet. It is then split into two flow paths, one into the vaporizing chamber and the other through a bypass into a mixing chamber. The percentage of the total flow into the vaporizing chamber is determined by the position of the agent concentration control valve. The gas mixture flowing into the vaporizing chamber flows over a reservoir of liquid anesthetic agent, picks up the vaporized agent, and exits the vaporizing chamber. The gas then meets and mixes with the bypassed gas and flows to the vaporizer outlet. The concentration of anesthetic agent in the final gas mixture is higher when a larger volume of gas is allowed to flow into the vaporizing chamber. Temperature-sensing flow control devices are necessary to compensate for temperature variations during the procedure.

In an electronically controlled vaporizer, the anesthetic agent is pressurized into its liquid state and heated inside the agent chamber. The pressurized vapor of the anesthetic agent is released through a regulating valve into the mixing chamber. The concentration of the agent in the gas mixture is adjusted by the control valve. To maintain a constant agent concentration, the electronic controller of the regulating valve determines the valve's position from a number of factors: the selected agent concentration, the gas flow rate, the pressure and temperature inside the vaporizer chamber, as well as the pressure and temperature of the inlet gas mixture.

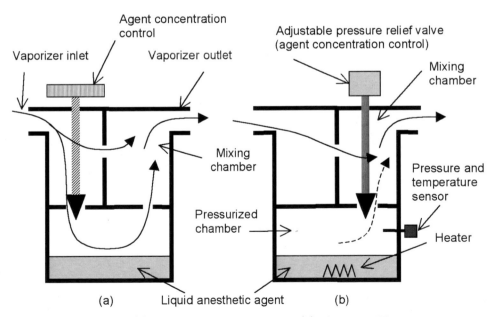

Figure 33–4. (a) Variable-Bypass Vaporizer, (b) Electronic Vaporizer.

BREATHING AND VENTILATION SUBSYSTEM

The function of the breathing and ventilation subsystem of an anesthesia machine is to deliver the anesthetic gas mixture (which is a mixture of oxygen, nitrous oxide, and an anesthetic agent) to the patient. During a procedure when the patient's respiration function is suppressed, a mechanical ventilator in controlled ventilation mode is used to ventilate the patient. Most anesthesia machines deliver a continuous flow of anesthetic gas and oxygen mixture to the patient. Two types of breathing circuits are used: the circle system and the T-piece system. Both types allow a certain level of rebreathing to conserve moisture and heat as well as anesthetic agents.

Figure 33–5 shows the circle breathing/ventilation subsystem of an anesthesia machine under ventilator mode. The ventilator valve is used to select between manual breathing mode using the breathing (or reservoir) bag and automatic ventilation mode using the built-in mechanical ventilator. The

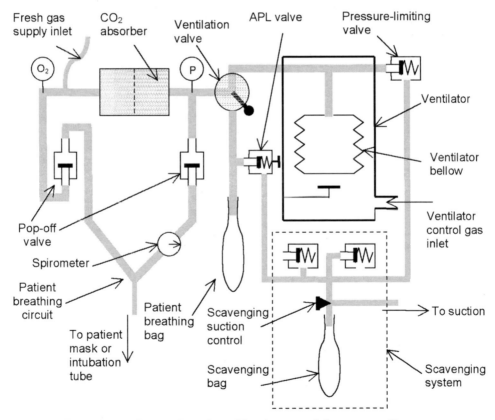

Figure 33–5. Patient Breathing/Ventilation and Scavenging Systems.

scavenging subsystem for waste anesthetic gas removal is also shown in the diagram.

Figure 33–6 shows the machine in manual breathing mode. The Y-connection of the patient breathing circuit is connected to a face mask covering the patient's mouth and nose or to an endotracheal tube inserted into the trachea of the patient. During patient inhalation, fresh gas from the anesthesia machine enters the inspiratory limb of the breathing circuit into the lungs of the patient (flow direction in solid arrows). During exhalation (flow direction in dotted arrows), expired gas from the lungs goes through the expiratory limb of the breathing circuit into the breathing bag. A pair of check valves is used to prevent reverse gas flow in the inspiratory and expiratory limbs of the breathing circuit. These check valves are also referred to as pop-off valves due to their construction (they consist of a circular disk sitting on top of a circular opening of the breathing circuit). When positive pressure is created in the circuit by manually squeezing the breathing bag, the gas collected in the bag is driven through a CO_2 absorption canister, through the inspiratory limb of the breathing circuit, and back to the patient. The canister contains a CO_2 absorber (such as soda lime) to remove CO_2 from the rebreathed

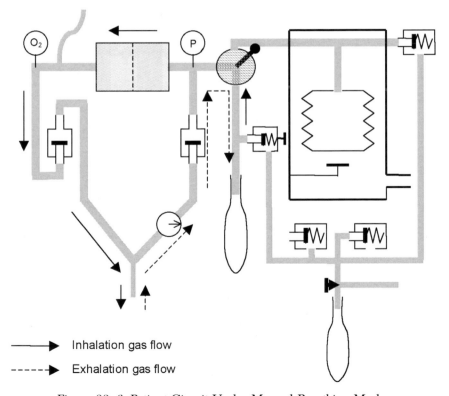

Figure 33–6. Patient Circuit Under Manual Breathing Mode.

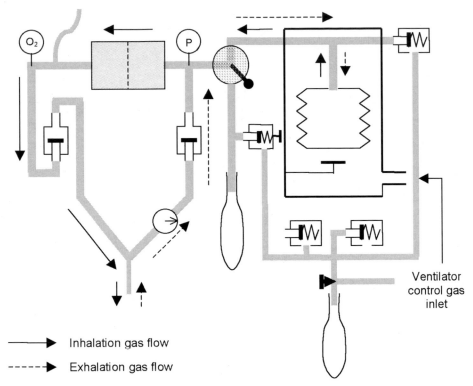

Inhalation gas flow

Exhalation gas flow

Figure 33–7. Patient Circuit under Ventilator Mode.

gas. The maximum pressure in the breathing circuit is limited by the adjustable pressure-limiting (APL) valve located near the patient bag. The APL valve is adjusted by the anesthetist during the procedure to maintain a slightly inflated breathing bag.

When the machine is in ventilator mode (Figure 33–7), expired gas flows into the bellow of the ventilator instead of into the patient breathing bag. During inhalation, the positive pressure of the control gas compresses the bellow in the ventilator, forcing the accumulated gas in the bellow to flow through the CO_2 absorber, and then through the inspiratory limb of the breathing circuit to the patient. The maximum pressure in the breathing circuit is limited by the pressure-limiting valve of the ventilator. In the controlled mode, the ventilator is cycled to deliver a fixed volume of gas to the patient at a fixed time interval. The volume and frequency of ventilation are set by the anesthetist.

No CO_2 absorber is used in the T-piece design (Figure 33–8). Fresh gas is mixed with rebreathed gas before entering the patient's lungs. The percentage of rebreathing is controlled by the flow rate of fresh gas from the gas supply and control system. The exhaled anesthetic mixture leaves the circuit

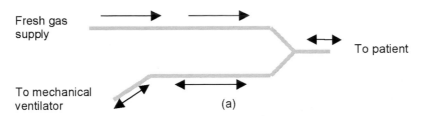

Figure 33–8. Rebreathing Circuit Using T-Piece Design.

through an APL valve. The rate of elimination of exhaled CO_2 in the rebreathed air mixture is proportional to the flow rate of the fresh gas. This design is often used in pediatric anesthesia.

SCAVENGING SUBSYSTEM

Prolonged personal exposure to anesthetic agents, including nitrous oxide, has been shown to be related to some illnesses such as liver disease and premature infant birth. Exposure to anesthetic agents is classified as an occupational hazard for operating room personnel. The scavenging subsystem is designed to capture and remove waste anesthetic gases from the operating room to reduce such health hazards. Instead of being released into the operating room, waste anesthetic gases are collected from the exhausts of the APL valve and pressure-limiting valve of the breathing/ventilation circuit (Figure 33–9). Scavenging systems remove gas by connecting to either a vacuum or a passive exhaust. A vacuum scavenging system uses the wall suction in the operating room, whereas the passive exhaust scavenging system connects to the exhaust of the room air ventilation system. System pressure adjustment is critical to ensure that the scavenging system is of just enough negative pressure to prevent waste anesthetic gases from being released into the operating room but not so much as to remove too much of the patient breathing gases. A scavenging bag is attached to act as a reservoir to absorb fluctuations. As a safety measure, a pair of pressure-limiting valves are placed near the scavenging bag to limit the pressure to within ±0.5 cmH_2O of the atmospheric pressure. When the gas flow and APL valve are properly adjusted, no anesthetic gas should be released to the atmosphere from these valves.

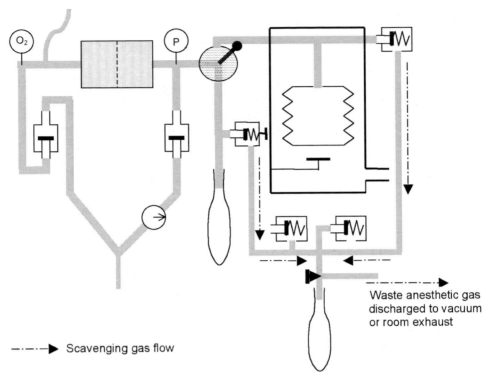

Figure 33–9. Scavenging Subsystem.

MAJOR CAUSES OF INJURY AND PREVENTIVE MEASURES

A patient under general anesthesia is unconscious and cannot react or signal for help. Patients under general anesthesia are vulnerable to operating errors or malfunctions of instrumentation. A list of potential safety hazards to patients under general anesthesia follows.

- Insufficient oxygen supply to patient
- Insufficient carbon dioxide removal from the rebreathing gas
- Excessive or wrong anesthetic agents being delivered to the patient
- Excessive breathing circuit pressure leading to trauma to the lung
- Introduction of foreign particles into the airway

Insufficient oxygen supply to the patient will lead to hypoxia. An oxygen analyzer is used to monitor the oxygen level of the inspired gas. To detect hypoxia in the patient, a pulse oximeter probe is connected to the patient to measure the oxygen saturation level in the arterial blood. An oxygen ratio monitor on the flow regulators of the anesthesia machine prevents the oxygen level in the gas mixture from being set below 30%. Touch-coded oxygen and nitrous oxide control knobs prevent the anesthetist from mistaking the nitrous oxide control for the oxygen control. Backup cylinders of oxygen and nitrous oxide are in place to ensure an uninterrupted supply of oxygen and nitrous oxide during a procedure. Color-coded gas cylinders and hoses (oxygen–white in Canada or green in the U.S., nitrous oxide–blue) are used to prevent reversed connection of the gases. Different sizes of hose are used to prevent misconnection of gas lines (breathing circuit–22 mm, fresh gas supply and patient Y–15 mm, scavenging hose–19 mm). A diameter-indexed safety system (DISS) using different diameters of connectors prevents an oxygen cylinder from being connected to nitrous oxide pipelines. A pin-indexed safety system prevents the wrong gas cylinder from being connected to a cylinder yoke of another gas. Vital sign monitors are used to assess the patient's physiological condition.

Failure to remove carbon dioxide from the patient can lead to hypercapnia. An end-tidal CO_2 monitor can detect an abnormal level of carbon dioxide in the patient's exhaled gas. A low oxygen saturation level in arterial blood (by a pulse oximeter) may also be an indication of excessive carbon dioxide in the patient's system. Carbon dioxide absorbers are used to remove CO_2 from the exhaled gas.

Delivery of a wrong anesthetic agent can be fatal. The filling spout of a vaporizer is keyed to accept only the bottle of the correct agent. Vaporizers on an anesthesia machine are interlocked to allow only one vaporizer to be turned on at one time. To ensure a correct mixture of anesthetic gases being supplied to the patient, agent monitors are built into anesthesia machines to monitor the concentration of the anesthetic agent during the procedure. Bispectral (BIS) index monitoring, a special EEG measurement, may be used to assess the depth of anesthesia (level of consciousness) of the patient.

Overpressure in the airway will create injury to the patient. Pressure monitors and overpressure alarms are installed on all machines. The APL valve and pressure-limiting valves limit the maximum pressure in the patient air circuit. Filters and traps are used to prevent patient injury from foreign particles.

Table 33–1 summarizes the preceding discussion. Daily functional verifications of anesthesia machines as well as their accessories are performed by the operating room staff, whereas performance inspection is done by biomedical engineering personnel during scheduled inspections.

Table 33–1.
Summary of Hazards and Mitigation Related to Anesthesia Machines

Potential Hazards	Methods to Minimize Hazards
Insufficient oxygen supply to the patient	• Oxygen analyzer • Pulse oximeter • Oxygen ratio monitor • Backup oxygen supply • Color-coded gas cylinders and hose • Touch-coded oxygen and nitrous oxide control knobs • DISS and pin-indexed safety system • Different diameters of hoses used • Vital sign monitoring
Insufficient carbon dioxide removal from the patient	• End-tidal carbon dioxide monitor • Pulse oximeter • Carbon dioxide absorber with color indicator
Excessive or wrong anesthetic agent delivered to the patient	• Agent specific keyed filling spouts on the vaporizers with color coding • Interlock to prevent turning on more than one anesthetic agent • Agent concentration monitors • BIS index monitor
Trauma to the lung caused by excessive pressure	• Pressure monitors • APL (adjustable pressure-limiting) valve • Pressure-limiting valve
Foreign matters injuring the airway	• Particle filters and traps • Dust-free carbon dioxide absorber
General	• Regular service by qualified personnel (daily functional check and regular quality assurance inspection and maintenance)

Chapter 34

DIALYSIS EQUIPMENT

OBJECTIVES

- List the basic kidney functions and the functions of a hemodialyzer.
- Describe the principles of diffusion, osmosis, and ultrafiltration.
- Define ion/molecular clearance in a hemodialyzer.
- Describe methods of vascular access and their advantages and disadvantages.
- Analyze the construction of the artificial kidney (AK).
- State the properties of the membrane in an AK and evaluate the mechanisms of molecular and fluid transport across the membrane.
- Explain different methods of dialysate preparation and delivery in hemodialysis.
- Sketch line diagrams and identify the basic functional components in the extracorporeal blood and dialysate delivery circuits.
- Differentiate between peritoneal dialysis and hemodialysis.
- Explain the needs and describe methods of water treatment in dialysis.
- Compare different cleaning and disinfection methods for dialysis equipment.

CHAPTER CONTENTS

INTRODUCTION

A healthy kidney maintains the level of body fluid, electrolytes, and acid/base balance, and removes some of the metabolic wastes. For patients with impaired renal function, renal dialysis supplements or replaces some of these functions to restore a reasonable state of health to the patient and minimize damage to other organs and physiological systems. The two most commonly used renal dialysis methods are hemodialysis and peritoneal dialysis.

The artificial kidney (AK) or dialyzer is a device that supplements or replaces some of the many functions of the human kidney (e.g., water and electrolyte balance, elimination of waste products, etc.). A very simplified representation of the AK kinetics is shown in Figure 34–1. It consists of a blood compartment and an electrolyte (or dialysate) compartment separated by a semipermeable membrane.

Movement of substances, including water molecules across the membrane, occurs in such an arrangement due to:

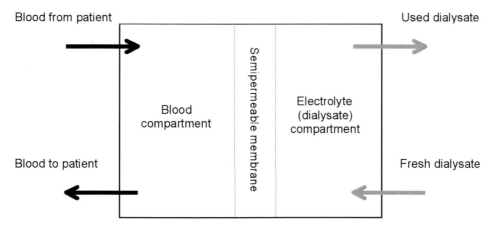

Figure 34–1. Artificial Kidney (Dialyzer).

- Differences in concentrations of various substances in the two compartments
- Particle sizes of these substances with respect to the membrane pores
- Pressure difference between the two compartments

These phenomena are the result of diffusion and osmosis (or ultrafiltration). The procedure to use these physical principles in a controlled fashion for medical purposes is known as hemodialysis.

BASIC PHYSICAL PRINCIPLES

Diffusion

Diffusion is the movement of molecules and ions in a solution as a result of repeated intermolecular collisions. When two regions of a system have different concentrations, a concentration gradient is said to exist between the regions. The rate of diffusion is proportional to the product of the concentration gradient and the cross-sectional area separating the two regions.

In hemodialysis, the factors governing diffusion are complex because of the presence of the membrane. The diffusion of substances (molecules) in a solution through the membrane is substance-dependent as well as membrane-dependent. The membrane may be characterized for a particular substance i by the permeability P_i of the membrane on the substance. The mass diffusion rate J_i of the substance i of the membrane is given by:

$$J_i = P_i \times \frac{C}{l},$$

where C = the difference in concentration of the substance across the membrane, and
l = the membrane thickness.

Note: Not all molecules can go through the membrane.

Osmosis

Osmosis takes place when a concentration gradient exists across a semipermeable membrane. A true semipermeable membrane is a membrane through which only water molecules can pass. In dialysis, the membrane has pores that allow certain sizes of molecules to go through. It is therefore not a true semipermeable membrane.

The net movement of water across a membrane against a solute concentration gradient is called osmosis. By means of osmosis, the system tends to achieve a situation of uniform concentration. This tendency for water to move in response to a solute concentration gradient develops a force called osmotic pressure. Osmotic pressure may also be defined as the hydrostatic pressure that must be exerted on a solution to prevent the movement of water through the semipermeable membrane. Osmotic pressure is a function of the absolute temperature and the concentration gradient of substances in the solution.

Ultrafiltration

If the opposing pressure to prevent movement of water through the membrane is increased to a level above the osmotic pressure of the solution, water is forced to flow from the solution against the osmotic pressure. This event is called ultrafiltration. In hemodialysis, this can be used to remove excess water from the patient. The mass of water transfer per unit time is proportional to the pressure across the membrane.

KIDNEY FUNCTIONS REVIEW

Figure 34–2 shows the daily water transport of an average adult. About 2 liters of water is ingested per day; 200 ml of those is excreted from the bowel and the rest is absorbed into the body. About 350 ml is lost to the atmosphere during respiration in the form of water vapor in the expired air. About 1,000 ml is excreted as urine through the urinary tract and 450 ml is evaporated from the surface of the body. There are three water compartments in the body: blood, intracellular (within the cells) fluid, and interstitial (outside the cells) fluid.

An average person (70 kg) has about 40 liters of water (or about 40% by weight) in the body. The percentage of water in a newborn is about 75%, much higher than that of an adult. Of the 40 liters of water, 25 liters is within the cells and 15 liters is in the interstitial fluid. There is about 5 liters of blood in the body, of which 3 liters is plasma and 2 liters is red blood cells. With a cardiac output of 5 liters per minute, about 1.2 l/min flows into the renal arteries. The capillaries in the kidneys create about 2.2 m^2 of membrane contact surface area to process and filter the blood. On an average day, 180 liters of fluid passes through the membrane inside the kidney but almost all of it is reabsorbed, leaving only about 1 liter of fluid excreted as urine.

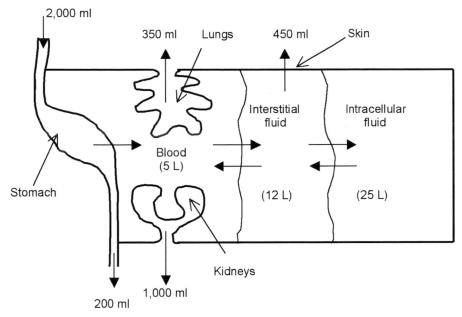

Figure 34-2. Body Fluid Transport.

Kidney Functions

The functions of a normal kidney include:

1. Removal of waste products from body fluid (blood and body water)
2. Regulation of blood volume
3. Regulation of extracellular fluid volume and composition
4. Maintenance of acid-base balance (pH)
5. Control of specific concentration of ions (e.g. Na, K balance)
6. Regulation of externally overtaken products such as glucose
7. Control of volume and composition of urine
8. Regulation of endocrine and metabolic functions

An artificial kidney (AK) replaces or supplements, to varying degrees, many of these processes (except the last two functions).

One of the main functions of the kidney is the removal of waste products from the blood. The parameter to measure the performance of the kidney in terms of product removal is called plasma clearance. Similar parameters called clearances are also used to evaluate a dialyzer's performance to remove substances from the blood or bodily fluid.

Plasma clearance is substance-dependent. CL_x (ml/min) of a substance x is given by:

$$CL_x = Q_u \times \frac{C_{ux}}{C_{px}},$$

where Q_u = rate of urine production (ml/min),
C_{ux} = concentration of substance x in urine, and
C_{px} = concentration of substance x in plasma.

Renal deficiency refers to underperformance of the renal system. Some of the possible causes of renal deficiency are:

- Kidney overload
- Kidney disease or damaged kidneys
- Inadequate renal blood flow

Some of the effects of renal deficiency include:

- Uremia (increase in urea and other nonprotein nitrogen)
- Water retention and edema
- Acidosis in renal failure
- Elevated K concentration in uremia
- Uremic coma
- Reduced availability of calcium to bones (osteomalacia)

Symptoms of renal failure include:

- Loss of appetite, increased blood pressure, nausea, decreased urine output, edema, itching, fatigue, and neurological disturbances. If left untreated, will lead to convulsion, coma, and death.
- One of the best means to assess renal failure is to measure concentrations of the nitrogenous nonprotein substances (e.g., urea).

Treatment of renal problems includes:

- Vigorous control of the intake of different materials into the body (diet control)
- Avoidance of excessive supply of water, cations, and nonessential nitrogenous material
- Hemodialysis treatment using an artificial kidney
- Peritoneal dialysis: the use of the peritoneal membrane in the peritoneal cavity as the interface between blood and dialysis
- Kidney transplantation

MECHANISM OF DIALYSIS

The dialyzer, also known as the artificial kidney (AK), is the main component of the hemodialysis system in which blood solutes (metabolic wastes) are removed from the blood and dialysate solutes (electrolytes) are added to the blood. During the process of dialysis, blood and dialysate are simultaneously circulated through the dialyzer, separated only by the semipermeable membrane. Substances (including water) to be added to and removed from the blood are exchanged across the membrane by the principles of diffusion and ultrafiltration. The process usually continues for 4 to 5 hours per treatment and consists of two to three treatments a week. The principles applicable to dialysis are explained next.

Diffusion

Within a dialyzer, as the semipermeable membrane separating the blood and dialysate is not an ideal membrane, ions (solutes) are selectively exchanged across the membrane according to their molecular weight. Water and waste products in the blood (e.g., urea, creatinine, uric acid), which have relatively low molecular weights, can diffuse easily and rapidly through the membrane into the dialysate; higher molecular weight substances, such as glucose and proteins, cannot easily pass through the membrane and are not significantly exchanged. Since the rate of diffusion depends on the concentration gradients of the solutes, it is necessary to maintain a fresh supply of blood and dialysate to facilitate these two-way transports.

Ultrafiltration

Ultrafiltration is the primary method to remove water from the blood using the semipermeable membrane. In ultrafiltration, water is forced through the membrane by applying a hydrostatic pressure across the membrane. The physician may require intermittent adjustment of the ultrafiltration rate based on the observation and the long-term trend of the patient.

HEMODIALYSIS SYSTEM

Figure 34–3 shows a simplified functional block diagram of a hemodialysis system. It consists of a vascular access serving as the interface between the machine and the blood vessels of the patient. The blood circuit takes the blood from the patient to the dialyzer and returns it to the patient. The blood and dialysate are separated by the semipermeable membrane in the dialyzer where the substance and water exchange between the blood and dialysate take place. The dialysate circuit takes the dialysate from the supply, feeds it to the dialyzer and removes it from the dialyzer, and disposes it to the drain.

Table 34–1 lists the functions described above plus other monitoring and control tasks of each of the functional blocks.

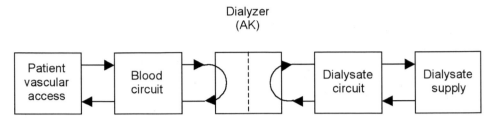

Figure 34–3. Hemodialysis System.

Table 34–1.
Functions of a Hemodialysis System

Vascular Access	Blood Circuit	Dialyzer	Dialysate Circuit	Dialysate Supply
Remove blood from patient	Introduce and remove blood to dialyzer	Provide blood/dialysate interface	Introduce and remove dialysate to dialyzer	Prepare and control dialysate composition
Reintroduce blood to patient	Control/monitor blood flow rate	Remove waste from blood	Control/monitor dialysate flow rate	Remove air from dialysate
	Control/monitor blood output pressure	Remove water from blood	Control/monitor dialysate pressure	Control/monitor dialysate temperature
	Control/monitor blood input pressure	Introduce solute to blood	Detect blood leak into dialysate	
	Trap air bubbles and produce alarm		Monitor dialysate pH	
	Prevent blood clot		Monitor dialysate conductivity	

DIALYZER (OR ARTIFICIAL KIDNEY)

The dialyzer (or AK) is the heart of the hemodialysis system where the exchange of substances and removal of water between blood and dialysate take place. The membrane within the AK allows such exchange to occur.

A membrane that permits substances to pass through is said to be permeable to those substances. A true or ideal semipermeable membrane is permeable to water but impermeable to all other substances. Most membranes pass only molecules of certain sizes. Hence they are called selective membranes. Membrane permeability may be passive or active. Active permeability transports molecules against the concentration gradient. Passive permeability depends on the concentration gradient as the driving force. The ability of a particle to pass through a membrane passively is dependent on the molecular size, ionic charge, and the degree of ionic hydration (e.g., OH⁻ is smaller and passes through the membrane easier than Ca^{++}).

The basic properties of a dialyzer depend on:

- Type of membrane used (porosity, size of pores, clearances, etc.)
- Effective membrane surface area
- Membrane's ability to withstand hydrostatic pressure
- Transmembrane pressure
- Blood flow rate
- Dialysate flow rate

Performance Parameters

As discussed in the previous section, the parameter to measure the performance of the kidney in terms of product removal is called plasma clearance. A similar parameter known as clearance Cl_x is also used to evaluate an AK's performance to remove a substance x from the blood or bodily fluid.

In hemodialysis, CL_x is redefined as:

$$CL_x = Q_B \times \frac{(C_{ax} - C_{vx})}{C_{ax}},$$

where Q_B = blood flow (ml/min),
C_{ax} = arterial concentration of substance x, and
C_{vx} = venous concentration of substance x.

Another performance parameter of a hemodialysis system is the ultrafiltration coefficient (KUf). KUf is a concept used to evaluate an AK's performance to remove water. KUf is defined as the volume (ml) of fluid that will be transferred per unit time (hour) across the membrane per unit pressure (mmHg) difference across the membrane of the dialyzer. Typical value of KUf is 2 to 6 ml/hr/mmHg. However, it can be as high as 50 ml/hr/mmHg for a high permeability dialyzer. Dialyzers with KUf greater than 8 ml/hr/mmHg are generally referred to as high flux dialyzers.

Example

In a 4-hour dialysis treatment, it is necessary to remove 2 liters of water from the patient. A dialyzer with KUf = 2.0 ml/hr/mmHg is used. It is estimated that during the treatment, 100 ml of fluid will be ingested by the patient. At the end of the treatment, 300 ml of water will be used to rinse the dialyzer free of blood (back into the patient). What is the pressure setting in the dialysate compartment if the blood compartment has a position pressure of 50 mmHg?

Solution

The total water removal taking into account fluid ingestion and dialyzer rinsing is

$$(2,000 + 100 + 300) \text{ ml} = 2,400 \text{ ml}.$$

Let X be the pressure setting in the dialysate compartment. The transmembrane pressure P is therefore equal to

$$(50 - x) \text{ mmHg}.$$

Using the definition of KUf: Volume of water removal = KUf $\times$ time $\times$ P, and substituting the values into the equation:

$$2,400 = 2 \times 4 \times (50 - x) \Rightarrow X = -250 \text{ mmHg}$$

to obtain a total transmembrane pressure of 300 mmHg.

Types of Dialyzers

Several types of AK with different physical constructions are available. The more common types are coil, parallel plate, and hollow fiber. These AKs are named according to the construction of the semipermeable membrane. A coiled construction AK consists of a circular cross section tube made of semipermeable membrane material wound into a coil. During dialysis, blood flows inside the tube and the coil is immersed in a container filled with dialysate. A parallel plate AK consists of multiple layers of semipermeable membrane in parallel. Blood is circulated between alternate pairs of plates and dialysate is circulated between the other plates. A hollow fiber AK consists of a large number (10,000 to 15,000) of hollow fibers connected in parallel inside a container (Figure 34–4). Each fiber has an internal diameter of about 0.2 mm and a length of about 150 mm. Blood flows inside the lumens of the fibers with dialysate surrounding them. Although the lumen is small, the diameter of an erythrocyte is 8 μm, a monocyte is 14 to 19 μm, and a thombocyte is 2 to 4 μm. Hollow fiber AKs are the most popular type used today. Common membrane materials are cellulose acetate, cuprophane, nephrophane, and visking. The total surface area of the membrane ranges from 0.6 to 2 m² and supports a blood flow rate from 100 to 300 ml/min. A typical dialysate flow rate is between 400 and 600 mL/min. Ultrafiltration can be achieved by creating a positive pressure on the blood side or a negative pressure on the dialysate side.

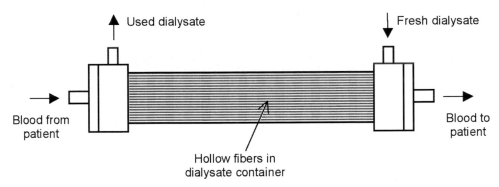

Figure 34–4. Hollow Fiber Artificial Kidney.

Table 34–2 lists the construction and performance specifications of a hollow fiber artificial kidney for hemodialysis.

Table 34–2a.
Physical Specifications of AK.

Housing Construction	Rigid transparent plastic
Tube Sheets Material	Medical-grade silicon rubber
Dimensions	21 cm long × 7.0 cm diameter
Weight	650 g (filled)
Blood Volume	135 ml
Dialysate Volume	100 ml
Fiber Material	Regenerated cellulose
Number of Fibers	11,000
Effective Length per Fiber	13.5 cm
Fiber Lumen	225 μm
Fiber Wall Thickness	30 μm
Effective Membrane Area	1.0 m^2

Dialyzers are evaluated by comparing:

- Clearances for different substances (e.g., urea, creatinine, phosphate, vitamin B12, uric acid, blood serum phosphate, glucose, NaCl)
- Ultrafiltration rate (KUf)
- Priming volumes

Table 34–2b.
Performance Specifications of AK.

Blood Compartment Flow Resistance		At blood flow rate of 200 ml/min	15 to 55 mmHg
Dialysate Compartment Flow Resistance		At dialysate flow rate of 500 ml/min with negative pressure of 400 mmHg	< 50 ml/mm
Average Ultrafiltration Rate		At 500 ml/min dialysate flow and 300 mmHg negative pressure	300 ml/hour
Typical Clearances	Urea Creatinine Phosphate	At 200 ml/min blood flow and 500 ml/min dialysate flow	135 ml/min 105 ml/min 85 ml/min

- Cost (taking into account single or multiple use)
- Clotting properties

PATIENT INTERFACE

As hemodialysis is often done three times a week, a semipermanent interface between the dialysis unit and the patient's circulatory system to allow repeated dialysis is required. This interface is called the vascular access. Several common methods to access the bloodstream are described in the following sections.

A-V Shunt

An A-V shunt is a pair of cannulae of polytetrafluoroethylene (PTFE) inserted through the skin into an artery and a vein near the inner surface of the forearm or the lower leg. Between dialysis treatments the two cannulae, which are permanently implanted, are joined by a short length of Silastic™ tubing to allow blood circulation. During dialysis, the Silastic™ tubing is removed and replaced by two plastic tubings that direct the blood to and from the dialyzer. These A-V connections can provide natural blood pressure differential to circulate blood through the dialyzer. However, due to the low differential pressure, it requires a low flow resistance dialyzer; otherwise a pumping mechanism is necessary to provide enough blood flow. A-V shunts are used in acute as well as chronic therapies.

A-V Fistula

In this method, an internal shunt is developed by joining an artery and a vein within the limb by a short length of fibrin tubing. Blood is obtained by venous puncture using either one or two large-bore needles. A blood pump is necessary to create enough blood flow.

In the double-needle technique, blood is continuously and simultaneously withdrawn from one needle and reinfused through the other. The single-needle technique requires a Y-connection and a controller to alternately withdraw and infuse blood to and from the patient. A special pump or a pair of synchronized pumps is required for this technique. To provide continuous blood transfer, a special double-lumen needle/catheter can be used.

A-V fistula is the most commonly used method for vascular access as it requires no permanent open site, which minimizes infection problems encountered with a normal A-V shunt. It has a 3-year 70% average site survival rate.

A-V Graft

Similar to an A-V fistula, this vascular access method surgically puts in a graft (a section of autogenous saphenous vein or PTFE Teflon™) to connect an artery to a vein (e.g., graft between the radial artery and basilic vein). It has a 3-year 30% average site survival rate.

Percutaneous Venous Cannula

This method is only for acute cases. To create the vascular access, a cannula can be inserted into the subclavian, femoral, or internal jugular vein. A percutaneous venous cannula can be single or double lumen.

DIALYSATE

Dialysate is a solution to effect diffusion and ultrafiltration. It is also used to carry away waste products and neutralize excess body acid by transferring either acetate or bicarbonate from the dialysis solution. There are two basic types of dialysate: acetate base and bicarbonate base. Dialysate is prepared in batch before dialysis or on demand during dialysis. Batch processing is done only in large dialysis centers where the dialysate is prepared and stored in large holding tanks. In a smaller center or when prescription dialysis is required, the dialysate is prepared by blending dialysate concentrate in proportion with treated water during the dialysis process. The concentration must be continuously monitored using thermally compensated conductivity meter. The mechanism for dialysate blending, monitoring, and control is often an integral part of the dialysis machine. Examples of dialysate compositions are listed in Table 34–3. The unit of concentration is mEq/l.

Table 34–3.
Dialysate Compositions.

	Na	*K*	*Ca*	*Mg*	*Cl*	*Acetate*	*Dextrose*
Standard	134	2.6	2.5	1.5	104.0	36.6	2.5
K Free	134	0	2.5	1.5	101.0	37.0	2.5
Low Ca	134	2.6	1.0	1.5	102.5	36.6	2.5
Low Na	130	2.0	3.0	1.0	101.0	35.0	2.0

In any case, the following processes are necessary before the dialysate is introduced into the AK or during dialysis:

- Treat water before it is used to prepare the dialysate (water treatment is discussed in the latter part of this chapter)
- Warm the dialysate to body temperature (37°C) before entry into the dialyzer
- Deaerate the dialysate to prevent gas evolution at body temperature and subatmospheric pressure (for AK using negative pressure ultrafiltration) and to prevent supersaturation of blood with nitrogen at body temperature
- Monitor dialysate pressure at entry to and exit from the dialyzer to ensure that the blood pressure is always greater than that of the dialysate
- Detect blood leaks across the membrane using photoelectric or ultrasound detector

In modern day dialysis, the dialysate is continuously fed into and removed from the AK. The used dialysate is disposed of during dialysis. This is referred to as a single-pass dialysate system. In earlier day dialysis, in order to conserve chemicals (and cost), dialysate was reused on the same patient. Many methods to reuse dialysate have been employed. For example, sorbent materials are used to remove some chemicals from the dialysate so that it can be regenerated and reintroduced into the AK (sorbent regenerative system). In another method, the used dialysate may be mixed with a certain proportion of fresh dialysate and reintroduced into the AK (single-pass recirculation system). In the extreme case, the used dialysate is recirculated back into the

AK until the performance of dialysis has decreased to such a level that the old dialysate must be replaced with a fresh batch (total recirculating system).

BASIC COMPONENTS OF A
TYPICAL HEMODIALYSIS MACHINE

Figure 34–5 shows the basic components and fluid flow diagram of a typical hemodialysis machine. Blood enters the machine from the vascular access via the arterial blood line, through the artificial kidney (dialyzer), and returns to the patient via the venous blood line. Dialysate is prepared and fed into the AK, where water and substance exchange take place. After passing through the AK, the dialysate is dumped into the drain. The blood circuit is separated from the dialysate circuit. Blood is separated from the dialysate as long as the membrane in the AK remains intact. The basic components in the extracorporeal blood and dialysate delivery circuits are described in the following sections.

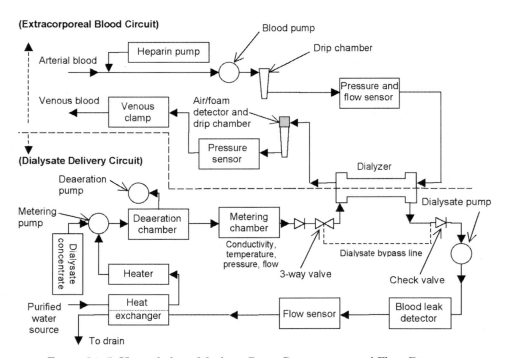

Figure 34–5. Hemodialysis Machine Basic Components and Flow Diagram.

Extracorporeal Blood Circuit

Heparin is administered intermittently or continuously (e.g., at a rate of 1.5 ml/hr) to the incoming blood from the venous access. Blood clots decrease the efficiency of the AK and are hazardous if they are reintroduced into the patient. Regional heparinization is used in some clinical conditions (e.g., to avoid worsening of existing bleeding sites). During regional heparinization, careful neutralization of heparin is achieved by injecting coagulants (such as protamine) into blood returning to the patient.

A roller pump in the dialysis machine controls the blood flow rate and creates a positive pressure in the blood compartment of the AK. The blood flow rate is controlled by varying the speed of the pump. The pressure in the blood line is regulated by the roller pump and the venous clamp located at the end of the blood circuit in the machine. The positive pressure in the blood circuit also prevents ingress of air and dialysate fluid into the blood circuit.

An arterial drip chamber provides a visual indication of the blood flow in the circuit. The pressure and flow rate of blood before entering the AK are monitored. As the blood exits the AK, it passes through another drip chamber. As the pressure becomes less, foaming occurs as air exits the blood. To prevent excessive air from getting into the bloodstream of the patient via the returning blood, an air/foam detector is located at the drip chamber. A pressure sensor monitors the blood pressure at the exit of the AK. Together with the upstream pressure sensor, the sensors monitor the blood average compartment pressure in the AK for ultrafiltration control as well as measuring the resistance of the AK. If the hollow fibers are blocked by blood clots, a large pressure drop will develop across the AK in the blood circuit.

Dialysate Delivery Circuit

Water from the purified water source enters the dialysate circuit of the dialysis machine. It is first heated when passing through the heat exchanger and the heater compartment. A metering pump accurately introduces concentrated dialysate into the water path to produce the right concentration of dialysate to the patient. Gas in the dialysate is removed by passing the dialysate through the deaeration chamber, where a reduced pressure is created by the deaeration pump. Excessive gas in the dialysate can diffuse across the membrane into the patient's blood.

Temperature, pressure, flow rate, pH, and conductivity of the dialysate are measured in the metering chamber. To prevent cooling or heating the patient's blood, the temperature sensor ensures that the dialysate is at body temperature before entering the AK. Correct flow rate and pressure are required to ensure removal of substances and water from the patient. The dialysate pH and conductivity are indications of the dialysate composition and concentration.

After passing through the metering chamber, the dialysate is introduced via a check valve (one-way valve) into the AK. A dialysate pump maintains the flow rate and produces a negative pressure in the dialysate chamber of the AK. The positive pressure in the blood circuit and the negative pressure in the dialysate circuit create the transmembrane pressure that controls the ultrafiltration rate, whereas the blood flow and dialysate flow rates control the substance removal rate (clearances) of dialysis. Before going through the heat exchanger and being dumped into the drain, the dialysate passes through a blood leak detector. If blood is detected in the dialysate, which indicates rupture of the membrane in the AK, the machine will sound an alarm and have to be shut down. The dialysate bypass line can be used to facilitate replacement of the AK.

Table 34–4 shows the typical range of control and monitoring parameters of a hemodialysis machine.

Table 34–4.
Range of Control and Monitoring Parameters.

Parameters	Typical Range
Dialysate flow rate	200–1,000 ml/min
Dialysate temperature	35–39°C
Conductivity	7–17 mS/cm
Blood flow rate	50–650 ml/min
Heparin flow rate	0.0–5.5 ml/hr
Venous/arterial pressure display	–300 to +600 mmHg
Transmembrane pressure	–100 to +500 mmHg
Blood leak detector sensitivity	0.35–0.45 ml/min
Air detector sensitivity	Air bubble size > 5–25 µl in blood line
Ultrafiltration rate	0–4 l/hr

PERITONEAL DIALYSIS

Hemodialysis requires removing blood from the patient and processing the blood in the AK external to the patient's body. Another form of dialysis can be performed using a natural membrane inside the human body to achieve substance and water exchange. As the peritoneal cavity is lined with blood vessels and capillaries, peritoneal dialysis uses the peritoneal membrane as the blood–dialysate interface instead of a membrane in an external dialyzer. A peritoneal dialysis setup is much simpler than a hemodialysis system. It uses gravity feed and drain instead of blood and dialysate pumps. The dialysate stays in the peritoneal cavity instead of being circulated through the external AK. Figure 34–6 shows a setup for continuous cycler-assisted peritoneal dialysis (CCPD).

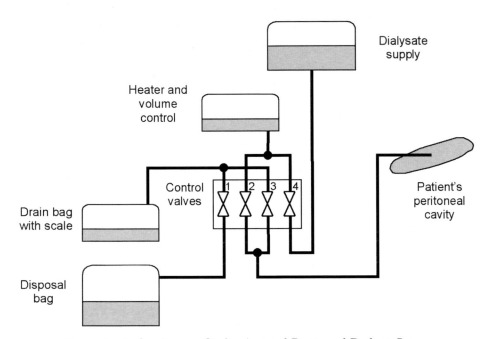

Figure 34–6. Continuous Cycler-Assisted Peritoneal Dialysis Setup.

At the start of a dialysis cycle, valve number 4 opens (all others remain shut) to allow a selected volume of dialysate to flow from the supply reservoir to the volume control and heater compartment. The dialysate stays in the compartment until it is warmed to body temperature. Valve number 2 is then opened so that the dialysate flows by gravity to the patient's peritoneal cavity through an indwelling catheter. The dialysate stays inside the peritoneal cavity for a period of time (e.g., 45 minutes) to allow substances and water exchange between the blood in the capillaries and the dialysate. After the preset time, valve number 3 opens to drain the used dialysate (together with the additional water from osmosis) from the peritoneal cavity to the first drain bag. The scale measures the weight of the dialysate to monitor the fluid removed from the patient. After the measurement, valve number 1 is opened to allow the dialysate to flow into the disposal bag to complete the cycle.

Although peritoneal dialysis takes more time due to slower transport, the rate and process have more resemblance to those of natural kidneys and therefore reduce the possibility of shock to the patient. Peritoneal dialysis is often performed at home due to its relatively simple operation and less sophisticated equipment setup. However, because of the high risk of developing peritonitis (due to careless handling of indwelling catheters by patients or home caregivers), patients are often forced to switch to hemodialysis due to repeated peritonitis. Continuous ambulatory peritoneal dialysis (CAPD) and continuous cycler-assisted peritoneal dialysis (CCPD) are the two commonly performed types of peritoneal dialysis.

Continuous Ambulatory Peritoneal Dialysis (CAPD)

In CAPD, the dialysate is constantly present in the abdomen but is changed three to five times daily with a per-fill-volume from 1.5 to 3.0 liters (typically 2 liters). Dextrose (1.5, 2.5, or 4.25%) in the dialysate is used to create osmosis for water removal. Drainage and replenishment of dialysate are performed using gravity.

Continuous Cycler-Assisted Peritoneal Dialysis (CCPD)

CCPD is performed at bedtime using an automated cycler to change dialysate four to five times during the night. The dialysate used is similar to that used in CAPD.

OTHER MEDICAL USES OF DIALYSIS TREATMENT

Other than treating patients with renal problems, dialysis may be used to eliminate toxic materials in the blood, to perfuse isolated organs, to reduce abnormally high ammonia concentration found in the blood following liver malfunction, or to supplement renal function during and after major surgery.

WATER TREATMENT

Normal tap water contains traces of metal ions (e.g., copper, lead) and chemicals (e.g., chlorine or chloramines). During a 4-hour dialysis treatment using a dialysate flow of 500 ml/min., 120 liters of dialysate interface with the patient's blood. Under repeated dialysis, if untreated water is used to prepare the dialysate, these ions and chemicals, which normally are not harmful under usual consumption, can quickly accumulate in a patient's body. Therefore, it is necessary to remove ions (e.g., Cu^{++}) and other molecules (suspended particles) in the water used for dialysate preparation.

Raw water usually goes through a pretreatment process that consists of:

1. Cartridge filter to remove particles greater than 0.05 µm (but cannot remove dissolved toxin or endotoxin)
2. Water softener to remove ions such as Ca^{++} or Mg^{++}
3. Activated carbon to remove chlorine or chloramines

A second-stage water treatment process is carried out to remove smaller particles and remaining chemicals in the water. Reverse osmosis (RO) is the most commonly used method. Distillation can also be used. RO (using the same principle as ultrafiltration) is achieved by applying pressure, forcing water to pass through a true semipermeable membrane while leaving impurities behind. RO removes over 90% of impurities and is acceptable in most cases.

To further purify the water, ion exchange resins can be used to remove all charged ions from the water. Activated charcoal is used to remove non-toxic contaminants. Heat or ultraviolet radiation can be used for sterilization. However, in most cases, there is no need for water sterilization since the membrane in RO or distillation can remove the majority of bacteria and endotoxins. For dialysis applications, water with a bacteria count below 200 colonies per ml is acceptable.

CLEANING AND DISINFECTION

As dialysis is an invasive procedure, care must be taken to reduce the chance of infection. Dialysis machines are required to be flushed and disinfected between patients. Heat disinfection (e.g., heat fluid to 85°C for 15 min) can eliminate waterborne bacteria such as Pseudomonas cepacia (a gram-negative bacterium). Although heat disinfection is convenient, it is ineffective to kill spore-forming bacteria such as Bacillus varieties. Chemical disinfection (e.g., using formaldehyde) can be used instead of heat treatment. Disinfection treatment using heat or chemicals is usually done daily on every machine and after each patient's treatment.

In addition to daily disinfection, sodium hypochorite (bleach) is used to disinfect the machine weekly. It is important to rinse the machine thoroughly after chemical or bleach disinfection to remove all chemical residuals before the machine is used on patients.

A dialysis center must set up standard operation procedures to take regular bacteria cultures in order to monitor the effectiveness of disinfection and detect possible contamination.

The blood and dialysate lines are single use disposable items. Although all dialyzers are labeled single-use, many centers reuse a dialyzer on the same patient. Studies have shown that following proper cleaning and disinfection procedures, reusing a dialyzer on the same patient is easier on the patient (i.e., it has less chance to cause adverse reactions). Some centers have shown that after taking into account the time and materials for processing, reusing dialyzers can achieve cost saving.

Chapter 35

MEDICAL LASERS

OBJECTIVES

- Describe the characteristics of lasers and their applications.
- Explain the effect of lasers on tissue.
- Describe the physics of laser action.
- List different surgical lasers and their applications.
- Explain the two common methods of laser delivery.
- Identify the benefits and limitations of laser surgery over conventional surgical methods.
- List the hazards associated with the use of lasers and the methods to mitigate the risks.
- State the maintenance requirements and handling precautions of laser systems.

CHAPTER CONTENTS

INTRODUCTION

Laser is the acronym for **L**ight **A**mplification by **S**timulated **E**mission of **R**adiation. Albert Einstein in 1917 described the absorption, spontaneous emission, and stimulated emission of light, which eventually lead to the development of lasers in 1940 in the former Soviet Union.

An electron, at its resting or ground state, when struck by a photon, can absorb the energy of the photon, become excited, and move to a higher energy level. On spontaneous return to its ground energy level, the electron emits a photon of energy equal to the difference between the two energy levels. This emitted photon can interact with an atom with an excited electron to produce another photon with the same frequency and phase traveling in the same direction. When there are many excited atoms in the medium (known as having a high degree of population inversion), this mechanism will set up a chain reaction of stimulated emission. Stimulated emission under the right conditions creates light amplification.

The first laser used in surgery was a ruby laser for treatment of retinal hemorrhages in the United States in the 1960s. It was not until 1972, when Gezo Jako adapted a CO_2 laser to an operating microscope, that laser became a viable surgical instrument in operating rooms. This chapter discusses some of the applications of lasers in medicine.

CHARACTERISTICS OF LASERS

Although both are electromagnetic waves, a laser is different from a normal light source. Lasers have the following characteristics:

• Monochromatic—Lasers have one or a few discrete wavelengths due to the fixed energy band gaps of the atoms, whereas normal light consists of a relatively wide spectrum of wavelengths. However, in practice, a laser has a finite (but narrow) width of wavelength (Figure 35–1a).

• Coherent—Due to stimulated emission, the waves or photons coming from the laser are all in phase, whereas those from normal lights have different phase angles (Figure 35–1b).

• Collimated—Due to the repeated reflection between the parallel mirrors (generation of laser is discussed in the latter part of this chapter), all the waves of the laser beam are parallel along the longitudinal axis of the mirrors. Compared to normal light, the trajectory of the laser beam coming from the lasing medium has minimal divergence or convergence (Figure 35–1c).

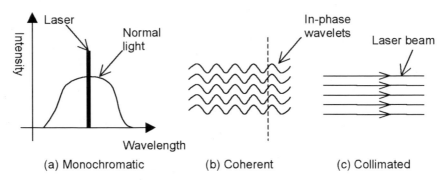

Figure 35–1. Laser Characteristics.

LASER ACTION

Although there are many types of lasers, they all have three basic components:

1. A lasing medium, which can be gas, liquid, or solid
2. An external excitation source that pumps energy into the lasing medium
3. A resonator or optical cavity with two parallel mirrors housing the lasing medium. One mirror is totally reflective and the other is partially reflective

Using a ruby laser as an example, it consists of a flash lamp (excitation source), a ruby crystal (lasing medium), and two mirrors as shown in Figure 35–2. The flash lamp ignites and pumps energy into the ruby atoms. Light energy is absorbed by the atoms in the ruby crystal to excite electrons to higher energy levels. Some of the excited electrons return to their ground state and emit photons. The photons traveling in the direction perpendicular to the mirrors are bounced back and forth between the two mirrors. As they travel inside the crystals, they stimulate more photon emissions from the excited atoms. The beam intensity therefore increases as it undergoes multiple reflections along the longitudinal axis between the mirrors. A portion of the beam is allowed to leave the laser through the partially reflective mirror.

APPLICATIONS OF LASERS

Lasers are used in a wide range of products and technologies. Applications of lasers can be separated into three categories.

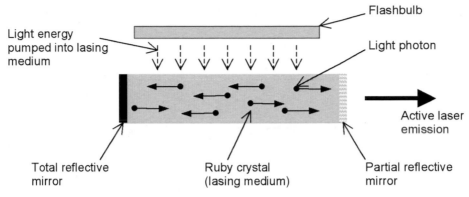

Figure 35–2. Laser Action.

Thermal Effect

When a laser is absorbed by a target, it converts to heat energy. A lens system or a light pipe can be used to focus and redirect a laser. This property is used in the industry in cutting materials such as metal or burning a compact disc. In the military, its heating effect is used in laser guns to destroy military targets. In medicine, lasers are used in surgery and physiotherapy.

Straight Collimated Beam

The collimated property of a laser beam produces a parallel beam of light that has little convergence and divergence. That is, the beam diameter of an ideal laser will stay constant irrespective of the distance. Due to this property, a laser beam can travel a long distance without losing its intensity (except from absorption in the optical path). Lasers are widely used in industry such as in land survey and in precision alignment. In the military, laser beams are used in guidance systems such as laser-guided missiles. In medicine, this property is used in position alignment such as beam alignment of linear accelerators in cancer treatment.

Photostimulation Effect

As a laser produces a monochromatic beam of high-intensity light, it can be used as a stimulant. In medical applications, a laser beam can be used to stimulate blood circulation and in cell healing in physiotherapy. In addition, it can be used in conjunction with a photodynamic drug to selectively activate the drug by a laser beam.

TISSUE EFFECTS AND SURGICAL APPLICATIONS

The surgical effect of a laser is primarily due to its thermal effect on tissues. Laser tissue effect depends on:

1. Type of tissue
2. Type of laser
3. Power density at the lasing site
4. Exposure time (continuous/pulsed)

The general tissue effect inflicted by a surgical laser is shown in Figure 35–3. In essence, when the laser beam hits the tissue, the laser energy is absorbed by the tissue to create three zones of injury. Due to the intense heat, the cell membranes rupture and vaporize at the center of the laser beam (zone 1). Next to the vaporized zone is a zone of cell necrosis where the tissues undergo irreversible heat damage (zone 2). Beyond the necrosis zone is a layer of cells that were injured due to the elevated temperature (zone 3). Tissues in zone 3 are able to repair and recover.

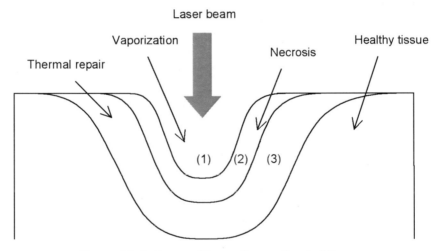

Figure 35–3. Zones of Injury from a Surgical Laser.

The rise in temperature and temperature distribution in the tissue during laser irradiation depends on the energy absorbed and the thermal parameter of the tissue. For short irradiation (less than a few seconds), tissue heated to less than 60°C undergoes little or no permanent damage. Denaturation of protein will result when the tissue temperature is above 60°C. Coagulation of blood occurs when the blood temperature is above 82°C. Tissue charring and vaporization starts to occur above 90°C. The heat absorption effect of tissue when hit by a laser depends on the type of tissue and the type of laser. For examples, an argon laser is highly absorbed by hemoglobin but not by water. Using this property, an argon laser can be used as a photocoagulator to stop bleeding at the back of the eye. In the procedure, the laser beam passes through the cornea with very little or no absorption and delivers its energy to the blood vessels on the retina. On the other hand, a CO_2 laser is highly absorbed by water, which makes it a general surgical laser as all soft tissues contain a high percentage of water.

The power density or intensity of a laser beam striking an object is equal to the power divided by the beam area on the object. A laser, like light, can be reflected by a mirror or focused by a lens. A laser beam can be focused to a tiny spot to produce a very high intensity beam. Figure 35–4 shows the tissue effects of different focal spot size of the same laser. In general, the higher the beam intensity, the deeper the vaporization zone.

For a continuous laser, the longer the exposure time, the more energy the tissue will absorb; in terms of a surgical laser, the deeper and wider the zone of injury will be. A laser can be pulsed to increase its peak power, creating intense heat in short durations. A pulsed laser creates a deep zone of vaporization but allows periods of cooling between pulses. Such cooling periods slow heat conduction to adjacent tissues. A pulsed laser will provide a deeper vaporization with less surrounding tissue damage than continuous laser at the same power output. By manipulating these parameters, different surgical effects can be created.

When an intense beam of laser slides across the surface of a soft tissue, it produces a zone of vaporization along the path of the laser. This action pro-

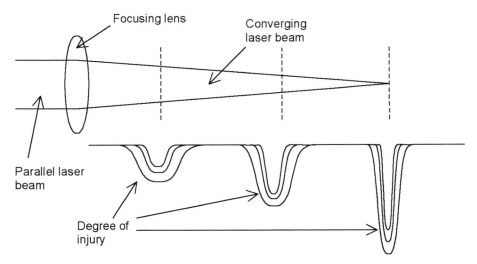

Figure 35–4. Tissue Effect on Power Density (or Focal Spot Size).

duces a sharp, clean cut. Abrasion effect (removal of a thin layer of surface tissue) is created by moving a defocused beam of laser with sufficient intensity over the tissue. Laser energy absorbed by the tissue may create destruction and charring effects on the tissue. Absorption of laser energy by blood produces coagulation effect. Retina reattachment, vision correction, vascular surgery, and microsurgery are some of the many examples of laser surgical applications.

CHARACTERISTICS OF MEDICAL LASERS

There are many types of lasers. Lasers are often classified by their lasing media. A solid laser has lasing material in solid crystal form such as a ruby crystal. In gas lasers, the lasing media are gas mixtures. Examples of gas lasers are helium neon (HeNe) and carbon dioxide (CO_2) lasers. The name *excimer laser* is derived from "excited and dimmers." A reactive gas mixture is electrically stimulated to form a pseudomolecule (dimer) and when excited produces a cool laser. A dye laser uses a fluorescent liquid dye as the lasing medium. When exposed to an intense laser such as an argon beam, it absorbs the laser energy and fluoresces over a broad spectrum. A tunable prism can be used to adjust the wavelength. A semiconductor diode can be manufactured to emit laser. However, the output power of a semiconductor laser is usually too low for surgical applications. Table 35–1 lists the characteristics and applications of common surgical lasers.

Transverse electromagnetic modes (TEM) of the laser beam are due to the oscillatory behavior of the electric and magnetic fields at the boundary of the laser resonator. The shape of the transverse mode is shown by the shape of the output beam. Figure 35–5 shows the shapes of selected transverse laser modes. These modes can be visualized by the burn mark on a wooden tongue blade by irradiating the laser beam vertically on the tongue blade. The fundamental mode of TEM$_{00}$ with a Gaussian beam intensity profile is the best mode structure to maximize the energy density propagation.

FUNCTIONAL COMPONENTS OF A SURGICAL LASER

Figure 35–6 shows the functional components of a surgical laser. A low power helium neon (HeNe) laser producing red light is often used as the "aiming beam." An alignment optical system is used to align the HeNe beam with the main laser beam. Most surgical lasers require high power output and

Table 35–1.
Laser Characteristics and Applications.

Laser	Wavelength	Color	Lasing Medium	Applications
CO_2	10.6 μm	Far-infrared	Mixture of carbon dioxide, nitrogen, and helium gas	Absorbed by water. For vaporization and cutting tissue.
Holmium: YAG	2.1 μm	Mid-infrared	Crystal of holmium, thulium, and chromium	Absorbed by tissue containing water. Precise cutting and less generalized heating of tissue
ND: YAG	1.064 μm	Near-infrared	Crystal of neodymium, yttrium, aluminum, and garnet	Poorly absorbed by hemoglobin and water, but absorbed by protein. For denaturation of protein and shrinkage of tissue and coagulation
Ruby	694 nm	Red	Ruby crystal	Not absorbed by blood vessels and transparent tissues. High energy pulses selectively vaporize tissue, use in dermatology and plastic surgery such as port-wine stain removal
HeNe	630 nm	Red	Helium neon gas	Use as aiming beam of medical lasers
KTP/532	532 nm	Green	Crystal of potassium titanyl phosphate	Highly absorbed by red or dark tissue. Use for coagulation and precision work
Argon	514 nm	Green	Argon gas	Passes through water and clear fluid but highly absorbed by red-brown pigments. Use in coagulation, ophthalmology, dermatology, and plastic surgery
	488 nm	Blue		
Excimer	193 nm	Ultraviolet	Argon fluoride gas	Precision cutting and coagulation with little thermal damage to surrounding tissue. Use in ophthalmology, angioplasty, orthopedics, and neurosurgery
	308 nm		Xenon chloride gas	
	351 nm		Xenon fluoride gas	
Dye-tunable	400–900 nm	Entire visible spectrum	Fluorescent liquid dyes	Use in photodynamic therapy, dermatology, and plastic surgery

therefore a cooling system must be in place to take away the heat generated from the laser production. The laser will then be coupled to the surgical site via a system of delivery device (or transport medium).

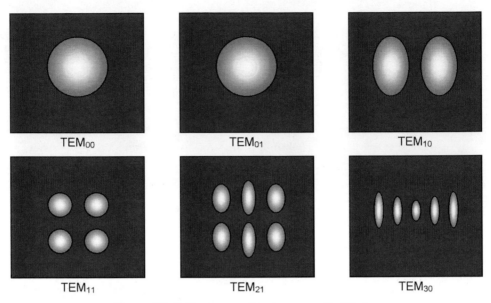

Figure 35–5. Transverse Electromagnetic Modes.

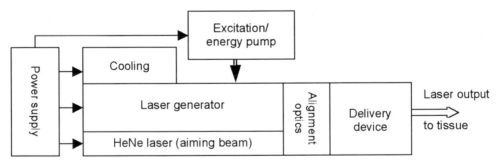

Figure 35–6. Functional Components of a Surgical Laser.

LASER DELIVERY SYSTEM

A laser procedure may be contact or noncontact. In noncontact procedures, the surgical delivery of the laser to the surgical site can be via a system of mirrors or through an optical fiber. Some lasers (such as Nd:YAG, Argon) can be delivered using optical fibers while others (far-infrared lasers such as CO_2) can be delivered only through a system of mirrors. Figure 35–7a shows an articulation arm system for CO_2 laser delivery. The laser travels inside a hollow rigid tube and is reflected to another tube segment by a first surface mirror located at the junction of the two tube segments. After

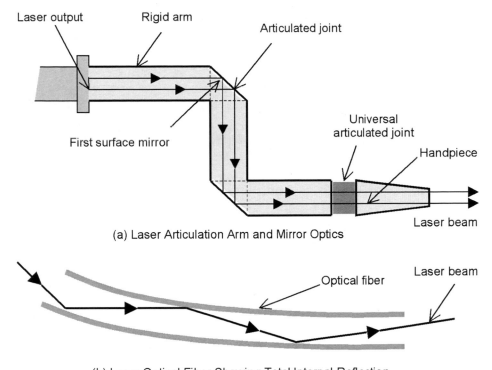

Laser output Rigid arm Articulated joint

First surface mirror

Universal articulated joint

Handpiece

Laser beam

(a) Laser Articulation Arm and Mirror Optics

Optical fiber Laser beam

(b) Laser Optical Fiber Showing Total Internal Reflection

Figure 35–7. Laser Delivery Systems.

several reflections, the laser will reach the handpiece and can be directed at the surgical site.

Instead of using mirrors, the laser may travel inside a flexible optical fiber by total internal reflection (Figure 35–7b). The laser travels inside the optical fiber until it has reached the other end of the fiber. Due to its small diameter and flexibility, optical fiber can easily move around the surgical sites. Silica fibers are good for ultraviolet and visible lasers and glass fibers are good for visible lasers. Special fibers are required for near- and mid-infrared lasers.

Contact laser probes offer a completely different method of delivering laser energy to tissue. Instead of laser directly transferring its energy to the tissue, the laser first heats the contact probe, and the heat of the probe in contact with the tissue is used to create the surgical effect. Similar to noncontact lasers, contact laser probes will cut, coagulate, vaporize, and ablate. These probes can be attached to a variety of handles for use in open surgical procedures or can be affixed to a standard optical fiber and passed through any rigid or flexible endoscope. Contact laser probes can be manufactured to any shape and are made of synthetic sapphire crystals with great mechanical strength, low thermal conductivity, and high melting temperature. The tip of a probe can be heated to 2,000°C.

ADVANTAGES AND DISADVANTAGES OF LASER SURGERY

Lasers are selectively absorbed by different tissues to produce different surgical effects. Lasers offer many advantages over other surgical techniques.

- The laser beam can be precisely focused for localized destruction of tissue. The depth of penetration can also be regulated by the power density, duty cycle, duration, and focus.
- Using fiber optics, a laser can access areas that are inaccessible to other surgical instruments.
- The laser beam simultaneously cuts and coagulates blood vessels and seals lymphatic vessels.
- Less tissue trauma due to no pressure and no traction applied on tissue.
- Quick healing with minimal postoperative edema, little pain, and little scarring.
- Noncontact procedure reduces risk of contamination and infection.

Some of the disadvantages of laser surgery are:

- Safety risks to patient and staff in terms of potential eye injuries, burns, and fire hazards.
- Higher cost per procedure due to expensive equipment and setup.
- Need for special facility support, supplies, and staff training.

SAFETY HAZARDS AND RISK MITIGATION

Surgical lasers present hazards to patients and to clinicians. Their use must comply with regulations, standards, manufacturers' recommendations, and professional practices. Lasers must be operated only by trained users, in designated areas, and adhering to institutional policies and procedures. To ensure laser safety in a surgical procedure, all users must be familiar with the specific laser to be used, its accessories, modes of operations, tissue effects, and potential risks.

Eye Protection

In addition to hazards common to all electromedical devices, a high-energy laser beam (with its collimated property) can cause damage at a distance far from its source. Inadvertent firing of a laser may cause burns on patient or staff, ignite a fire, or even cause an explosion in an oxygen-enriched environment. Many lasers are in the infrared or ultraviolet range in the electromagnetic spectrum, which are invisible to the human eye. An operator may not be aware of the laser path until damage is done. When a laser beam is directed to the eye, the collimated beam of a laser will be focused by the lens to a small dot of high-energy density on the back of the eye. This high-intensity beam will create irreversible damage to the eye. Even a low-energy laser beam, which normally will not create tissue burns, will have enough power density to inflict ocular injuries after being focused by the lens of the eyes. An acute exposure to laser can cause a scotoma (permanent damage of a small area of the retina), resulting in a blind spot in the field of vision. Long-term exposure to low-energy laser may lead to slow degenerative changes due to thermal or photochemical injuries. Examples of such injures are slow cataract formation in damaged lens and chronic reduction of color-contrast sensitivity from a damaged retina.

Laser Classifications

Based on these potential hazards, lasers are classified according to their risks, especially in ocular exposure. According to these classifications, safety measures and special precautions are required during laser procedures. The following classifications are taken from the Standards "CAN/CSA-Z386-92–Laser Safety in Health Care Facilities." Similar definitions are found in "ANSI Z136.3-1988–Standards for the Safe Use of Lasers in Health Care Facilities." The Standards also stipulate responsibilities of health care facilities; composition and responsibilities of laser safety committee and the laser safety officer; safety control measures; risk management and quality assurance guidelines; training, education, and credentialing of laser users.

Class I.   Laser equipment emitting radiation that is not considered hazardous. These lasers do not require hazard-warning labeling.

Class IIa.   Laser equipment emitting radiation that is not considered hazardous when viewed for up to 1,000 seconds. However, frequent viewing may cause degenerative changes in the eye.

Class II.   Laser equipment emitting radiation (usually low-power visible lasers) that presents a hazard when viewed directly for periods of time longer than 0.25 second.

Class IIIa. Laser equipment emitting radiation considered harmful with direct viewing, especially when viewed with optical instruments.

Class IIIb. Laser equipment emitting radiation considered hazardous with direct exposure to the skin and eyes.

Class IV.   Laser equipment emitting radiation considered hazardous to the skin and eyes from direct and scattered radiation.

The 0.25-second time interval is the average human reflex time for eye closure when a visible beam of light hits the eye. For high-power lasers, even the beam reflected from a shiny surface or scattered from a dull surface can cause injuries. In medicine, most lasers are Class III and Class IV. The helium-neon (HeNe) lasers used in the aiming beam for invisible lasers are usually Class II lasers.

To prevent eye damage, all personnel inside the operating room during laser surgery must wear appropriate protective eyewear (eyeglasses or goggles). Protective eyewear must be certified for the type of laser and of a specific optical density. The lens of the protective eyewear must attenuate the laser beam to an acceptably safe level. It must be free from scratch and shield the wearer's eyes from all directions of the visual field.

Skin Protection

Skin burns (patient or operating room personnel) can occur from exposure to direct or reflected laser energy. Overexposure to ultraviolet lasers may create skin sensitivity. To reduce the power density of the reflected laser beam, metallic instruments with a polished surface should not be used during laser procedures. The area surrounding the surgical site should be covered with fire-retardant materials.

Laser Plume

The smoke or laser plume arising from vaporization and charring of tissue may become airborne from the surgical site into the surrounding atmosphere. Sample analysis has revealed that it contains water, carbonized particles, DNA, and intact cells. The plume has a distinct odor and may include toxic substances, viruses, and carcinogens and therefore should not be inhaled. The plume can scatter and attenuate the laser beam and obscure the surgical site. Removal of laser plume enhances the visibility of the target site for the surgeon. Smoke evacuation from the laser site and face masks can prevent personnel from inhaling this plume. Laser smoke evacuators are high-efficiency vacuum machines with submicron filters (to remove bacteria and viruses) and active charcoal filters (to remove odor).

Fire Hazards

Since a high-energy laser beam is used in laser surgery, operating room personnel should be aware of and prepared for fire hazards. Flammable prep solution should not be used. Fire-resistant drapes and gowns should be used. A basin of sterile water should be available at the sterile site. A halon fire extinguisher must be available in the operating room. Oxygen concentration in the room should be as low as possible. Instruments used near the surgical site must be nonreflective and noninflammable.

Access Control

During a laser procedure, only properly trained personnel with proper eye protection should be allowed to enter and stay in the operating room. Others must be aware of the hazards. To maintain a safety zone, the laser operating location must be enclosed with access control. See-through windows should be covered to prevent the laser beam from passing outside the operating room (except for CO_2 laser as it is absorbed by glass). Warning signs should be posted on the doors outside the operating room when lasers are being used. The wording and symbols on these signs should be specific for the type of laser in use. An example of a laser warning sign is shown in Figure 35–8. Walls and ceilings should have nonreflective surfaces. Reflective surfaces (glass on windows, mirrors, X-ray view boxes, etc.) should be covered with nonreflective materials to prevent reflection of the laser beam.

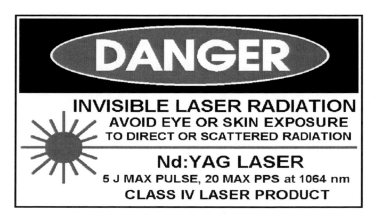

Figure 35–8. Laser Warning Sign.

Laser Safety Program

The CAN/CSA Z386 and ANSI Z136.3 Standards recommend laser safety programs to be set up in workplaces using Class IIIB or Class IV lasers. The program should include the following components: administrative (develop laser policy, establish laser safety committee, etc.), engineering control (install and maintain exhaust ventilation, window covers, etc.), and personal protection (provide eye protections, appropriate training, etc.).

The Standards also recommend the appointment of a laser safety officer (LSO) whose duty is to ensure the safe use of lasers in the workplace. Duties of the LSO include:

- Determine laser classifications
- Ensure that laser equipment is properly installed and maintained.
- Limit access to laser areas.
- Arrange training for workers in safe use of lasers.
- Recommend and ensure appropriate personal protection such as eyewear and protective clothing

MAINTENANCE REQUIREMENTS AND HANDLING PRECAUTIONS

In addition to knowledgeable and trained staff, the performance and safety of lasers rely on an effective preventive maintenance program. Performance inspection of medical lasers and their accessories should be carried out periodically to ensure that they conform to the manufacturers' specifications as well as current performance and safety standards. Output characteristics, including laser power output, pulsing sequence, and timing accuracy, are measured by calibrated laser power meters. The gas mixture of a gas laser must be replaced or recharged after being used for a period of time. Failure to replace the gas will result in reduced laser power output. The lenses and mirrors in the laser delivery system are fragile; they are easily scratched and damaged. Shock and motion from rough handling and even from normal use will cause misalignment of the optical path in the handpieces and laser arms. A misalignment in the delivery system of a laser will result in little or no laser output. Optical alignment of the system should be performed according to manufacturers' procedures. The transverse electromagnetic mode (should be close to a TEM_{00}) of the laser beam should be verified after every optical alignment. Dirt on the first surface mirror will eventually lead to heat damage of the mirror from absorbing the laser energy. Glass or silicon optical fibers are brittle and therefore cannot be bent too much. Care must be taken to inspect the tips of bare fibers or the tips of contact laser probes for signs of cracks and heat damage.

Chapter 36

ENDOSCOPIC VIDEO SYSTEMS

OBJECTIVES

- Describe clinical applications of endoscopic video systems.
- Analyze the construction and function of rigid and flexible endoscopes.
- Evaluate essential features of an endoscopic video system.
- Differentiate between fiberscopes and videoscopes.
- State the advantages and disadvantages between a three-chip and single-chip color CCD camera in endoscopy.
- List common types of light sources for surgical video illumination.

CHAPTER CONTENTS

INTRODUCTION

An endoscopic video system allows the physician to look inside the patient's body by inserting a light pipe with viewing optics (an endoscope) into the body through a natural lumen or a small surgical puncture. The first endoscopic instrument was developed in 1876 by Maximilian Nitze in Austria. Endoscopic inspection of the abdominal cavity was introduced in 1902 and has since been refined and become widely used in many diagnostic and therapeutic procedures. Endoscopy such as laparoscopic cholecystectomy (removal of gallbladder using a surgical video system) or arthroscopy has replaced many open surgical procedures. Endoscopic procedures are less traumatic to patients, cause less discomfort, and enable shorter recovery time. Surgical procedures using endoscopy instead of open surgery are often called minimally invasive surgeries (MIS).

APPLICATIONS

Laparoscopy refers to the minimally invasive treatment and examination of organs and tissues in the peritoneal cavity using an endoscope and other special instruments. In a multipuncture laparoscopic procedure, a small incision is made to allow the insertion of a trocar or cannula. A viewing laparoscope is inserted through the cannula. Another incision is made for the insertion of the surgical instrument. Procedures such as cholecystectomy and appendectomy can be performed by viewing the surgical site and inserting the surgical instrument through the laparoscope without opening the abdominal cavity. An external light source is required to illuminate the surgical site. An insufflator helps to maintain a pneumoperitoneum to enlarge the working space for the surgical instruments and increase the field of view of the surgeon within the peritoneal cavity. Similar to laparoscopy, arthroscopy allows the diagnosis and treatment of some joint injuries and diseases without open arthrotomy. In gastrointestinal and bronchial endoscopy, flexible endoscopes are inserted through the rectum, esophagus, or trachea to allow the diagnosis and treatment of diseases in the gastrointestinal and respiratory tracts.

SYSTEM COMPONENTS

A typical endoscopic video system consists of the following components:

- An endoscope
- A light source
- A video camera
- An image processor
- One or two video display monitors
- An image management system

Depending on the procedure, some of the following instruments and devices may be used in endoscopic procedures:

- Trocars/cannulae
- Gas insufflators–CO_2 or N_2O
- Air, water, and suction pumps
- Laser, ESU, U/S, cutters, forceps, scissors, biopsy snares, etc.

The following sections describe the basic components of a typical system.

ENDOSCOPES

An endoscope or viewing scope is used by the surgeon to view anatomical structures and perform therapy to the interior of the body. The diameter of an endoscope varies from the 1.7-mm needle fetoscope to the 5-mm arthroscope to the 22-mm colonoscope. The length of the endoscope must be appropriate to reach the desired structure. Endoscopes can be rigid or flexible.

Rigid Endoscope

Rigid scopes (Figure 36–1) are either hollow sheaths that allow straight viewing (such as laryngoscopes) or a sheath with an eyepiece and lens system that allows viewing in a variety of directions (such as cystoscopes). The sheaths of most rigid scopes are made of stainless steel, although plastic-sheathed scopes (mostly disposable) are available.

A laparoscope is an example of a rigid endoscope. A viewing laparoscope employs a series of rod lenses to convey high-resolution, wide field of view images to the eyepiece. Objects seen through a laparoscope may be magnified or reduced depending on the distance between the object and the tip of the scope. Optical fibers surrounding the rod lenses transmit illumination to the object from an external light source connected to the laparoscope

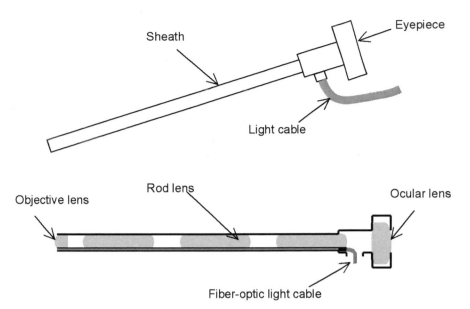

Figure 36–1. External and Cross-Sectional View of a Rigid Endoscope.

via a fiber-optic light cable. An insufflator is connected to the laparoscope or the trocar via an air hose. Through an air channel in the shaft of the laparoscope (or the trocar), N_2O or CO_2 gas is injected into the abdominal cavity. The external diameter of a typical viewing laparoscope ranges from 5 to 10 mm. In an operating laparoscope, the eyepiece is offset from the shaft (by a set of prisms) to allow insertion of the instrument through a separate instrument channel in the shaft. The external diameter of a typical operating laparoscope ranges from 8 to 12 mm. During a procedure, the object can be viewed directly through the eyepiece. In practice, the eyepiece is often coupled to a video camera and the images are displayed on a video monitor.

Flexible Endoscope

Instead of a rigid shaft, a flexible fiberscope has a long flexible insertion tube connected to a proximal housing (Figure 36–2). Flexible endoscopes can be inserted into curved orifices of organs such as colon, lung, and stomach. To facilitate scope insertion and viewing, wires running from the control head to the distal tip enable the user to angulate the distal end of the insertion tube.

A flexible endoscope consists of the following sections:

• Insertion tube
• Control head

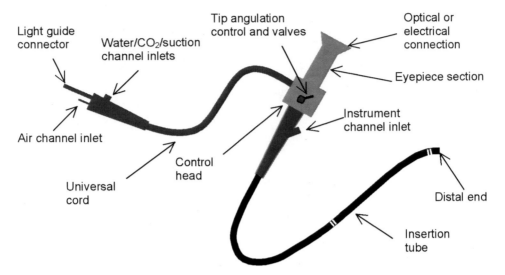

Figure 36–2. Flexible Endoscope.

- Light guide connector
- Universal cord (or light guide tube)

In a typical fiberscope, the insertion tube contains two bundles of optical fibers, one for the illumination and the other for the image. A water channel, an air channel, and an instrument channel are also included in the insertion tube. Figure 36–3 shows the viewing and illumination optical pathway. Figure 36–4 shows the cross-sectional view of the insertion tube. In a videoscope, the viewing optical fiber bundle is replaced by a video camera chip mounted at the tip of the insertion tube to pick up the image and convert it to electrical signal directly. A videoscope generally has a larger diameter than a fiberscope due to the larger size of the camera chip. To facilitate insertion and viewing, the distal tip can be bent or angulated by moving a control mechanism on the control head. The external diameter of the insertion tube of a bronchoscope ranges from 0.5 to 6.4 mm with a working length from 550 to 600 mm, whereas it can be up to 14 mm in diameter and 2,000 mm working length for a colonoscope.

During an endoscopic procedure, the physician holds the control head to manipulate the insertion tube, introducing water or air to flush the site. The control head houses the up/down and left/right angulation control knobs to move the distal tip of the insertion tube as well as the air/water and suction control valves. The opening of the instrument channel is also located on the control head.

The light guide tube is a flexible tube containing the fiber-optic bundle for the light source. It also has separate air, water, suction, and CO_2 channels

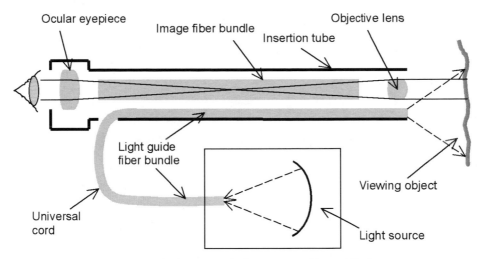

Figure 36–3. Image and Illumination Optical Path.

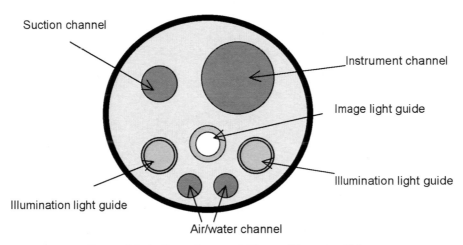

Figure 36–4. Cross-Sectional View of Insertion Tube.

connected to those in the insertion tube via valves on the control head. The light guide connector houses the adaptor for the fiber-optic bundle to the light source. The connectors for air, water, suction, and CO_2 (as well as the electrical connector for videoscope) are also located on the light guide connector. Figure 36–5 shows the water, air, suction, and CO_2 channels of a typical gastrointestinal endoscope.

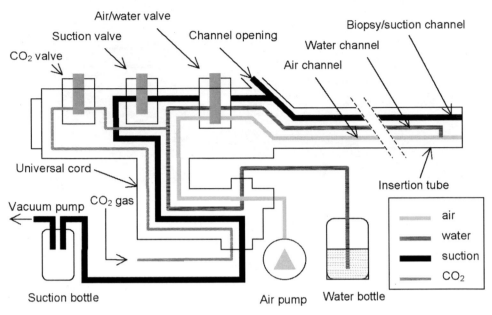

Figure 36–5. Air, Water, Suction, and CO_2 Channels of an Endoscope.

LIGHT SOURCES

A light source is connected to the illumination light guide of the rigid or flexible endoscope to provide illumination for viewing the surgical fields or body cavities. Light sources are intended to provide the physician a sufficient level of visible light for diagnostic observations and surgical procedures. A light source usually emits a wide spectrum covering the visible, infrared, and sometimes ultraviolet radiation. Infrared filters are installed in the light source to prevent infrared radiation from entering the body, which otherwise can cause thermal burn or even fire. A surgical light source can use a variety of lamps, including xenon, quartz halogen, metal halide, and mercury vapor. Xenon (color temperature from 5,600 to 6,600 K) and quartz halogen (from 3,200 to 5,500 K) are popular lamps for endoscopic procedures due to their high intensity and near-daylight spectrum (5,000 to 6,000 K). The output intensity of a light source can be adjusted either by an adjustable aperture or by changing the brightness of the lamp. Changing the brightness of the source by changing its supply voltage or current may be more energy efficient, but doing so may alter the color temperature of the light. In systems that have automatic brightness control, the light source is connected to the video processor to automatically maintain the level of illumination throughout the procedure. The output intensity and color temperature of light sources usually decrease with time. A typical xenon lamp has an approximate useful life span of 500 operating hours. Most lamps require forced cooling to maintain a safe operating temperature.

CAMERA, PROCESSOR AND DISPLAY

With traditional rigid endoscopes and fiberscopes, an endoscopic camera head is attached to the eyepiece (through an adapter) of the rigid scope or the proximal end of the flexible endoscope. The most commonly used single-chip mosaic color filter CCD (charge-coupled device) camera consists of a single CCD chip with red, green, and blue colored filters overlaying each CCD pixel. The light reflected from the object is filtered by each of the color filters and incident on the underlying CCD elements. Each group of red, green, and blue filters and CCD element combination forms one color image pixel. The intensity of this filtered light is measured. After each exposure, the mosaic signal from the CCD pixels is sent to the image processor. The three signals (RGB) from each group of pixel are combined and reverted to the color and intensity of the original light source. Another single-chip design uses a rotating color wheel containing the red, blue, and green filters. In essence, each CCD element is time-shared by the filters to measure the intensity of the color components of the incident light. In a three-CCD-chip system, the incoming light is split into red, green, and blue beams and each beam is directed to one of the three dedicated CCDs. A three-CCD-chip system provides a higher resolution image than the mosaic filter system and a higher refreshing rate than the rotating color wheel system.

In a videoscope, the CCD chip is integrated into the tip of the scope to provide a high-quality picture free from image distortion and degradation from optical misalignment and deterioration of the optical fibers and lens system. However, this may increase the size or diameter of the endoscope.

The image or video processor is responsible for white balance, brightness, contrast, color control, focus, and shutter control. Some video processors can support automatic gain control (AGC), multiformatting, and character generation.

During a minimally invasive surgical procedure, video or still images are displayed on one or more color monitors. Typical medical-grade video monitors have low leakage current with high brightness and high contrast, allow gamma curve calibration, and can support resolution better than 800 lines per frame. Both cathode ray tube (CRT) monitors and liquid crystal displays (LCD) are used in endoscopic systems.

IMAGE MANAGEMENT SYSTEM

Some surgical video systems are integrated with a computerized information management system. The basic functions of such a system include organization of patient data; image storage, retrieval, and transfer; and production of hard copies. More sophisticated systems can be networked with the hospital information system (HIS) to download patient information and upload test results and images.

INSUFFLATORS

An insufflator helps to maintain a pneumoperitoneum to enlarge the working space for the surgical instruments and increase the field of view of the surgeon within the peritoneal cavity. Nitrous oxide (N_2O) or carbon dioxide (CO_2) gas is introduced into the peritoneal cavity to distend the abdomen during the procedure. The device acts as a pressure-controlled flow regulator converting the high-pressure gas source (either from a cylinder or from a gas wall outlet) to about 10 to 15 mmHg before delivering it to the patient. An insufflator automatically regulates the flow to maintain a user-selected pressure throughout the procedure. High and low flow as well as high and low pressure alarms are built in to ensure patient safety.

ADVANCED DEVELOPMENT

The field of endoscopy is evolving very rapidly. New applications and procedures are being developed along with new instruments and devices. A few new applications and features of endoscopic video systems are:

- Three-dimensional endoscopy–Using two image sensors at slight distance apart to produce stereo images to improve visualization.
- Cancer detection–use special light spectrum or dye to detect malignant tissues in endoscopic procedures.
- Wireless endoscopic camera capsules–A miniature wireless camera with signal transmitter is enclosed in a capsule. The capsule is swallowed by the patient. As the capsule travels through the digestive tract, video image is captured and transmitted to an external receiver.

COMMON PROBLEMS

Two major complications of endoscopy are:

1. Perforation–Perforation is a major cause of concern when rigid scopes are used. The risk of perforation for flexible scopes is lower but it remains a potential complication.
2. Bleeding–Excessive bleeding can occur from a biopsy site, removal of a polyp, or areas where tissue has been cut.

Patients may also suffer from burn injuries when electrosurgery is used with endoscopy.

Apart from mechanical wear and tear and electronic component failures, problems associated with endoscopic system can be separated into three categories:

1. Cleaning, disinfection, and sterilization
2. Water leakage
3. Optics

All parts of endoscopes and accessories must be thoroughly cleaned, disinfected, or sterilized after every use. The primary causes of infection transmission in endoscopic procedures are inadequate cleaning and disinfection or sterilization of the endoscopic equipment. It is important to clean all parts of the endoscope as soon as possible after use while organic debris is still moist. Tissue, mucus, blood, feces, and protein residue can become trapped in the channels and are difficult to remove when dried. Nonresidual liquid detergent are used with small brushes to clean the inside lumen of all channels. Special ultrasonic cleaners may be used. If the scope can be sterilized with ethylene oxide, it must be thoroughly cleaned and dried before sterilization. Scopes that cannot be sterilized are disinfected by soaking them in activated glutaraldehyde, acetic acid, or formaldehyde solution. Care must be taken to fill all the lumens with the disinfectant. Endoscope processors are available to clean and disinfect flexible scopes. An automatic endoscope processor cycles through wash, disinfect, rinse, and dry to clean and disinfect the scope once it is set up properly in the washer.

An insertion tube of a flexible endoscope is covered with a waterproof plastic sheath. If this waterproof sheath has a leak, water or bodily fluid will enter the internal part of the scope. Water leak will cause deterioration of internal components (e.g., rusting of the angulation cables) and prevent effective disinfection or sterilization. Moisture will fog up and damage optical components. Leak tests on flexible endoscopes should be done on a regular basis.

Optical fibers in the light guide or image bundles may break, causing lower light illumination or black spots on the image. Poor handling of the scopes may damage the lens or cause misalignment. Moisture inside the sheath may decrease transmission and damage the optical components.

The heat from the intense light source may cause patient burn. Although infrared filters in the light source are used to remove IR radiation, care must be taken not to shine the light onto the same position for a prolonged period of time. Radio frequency (RF) leakage current may cause a secondary site burn in a patient undergoing an endoscopic electrosurgical procedure. Electrical leakage and insulation tests are performed periodically on endoscopes to detect potential current leakage problems.

As most injuries are internal, they may not be observable immediately after the procedure. Moreover, extreme care must be taken to observe the patient after an endoscopic procedure. Ambulatory outpatients must not leave the facility until vital signs are stable and the surgical side effects have passed.

Appendix A–1

A PRIMER ON FOURIER ANALYSIS

Consider a symmetrical square waveform with amplitude of ±1 V and a period of 1 sec. (Figure 1)

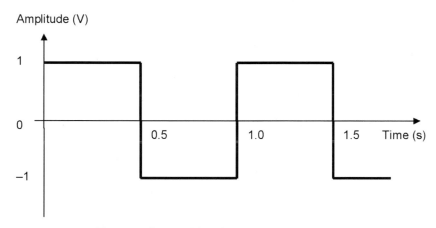

Figure 1. Square Waveform in Time Domain.

This signal can be expressed by the following summation of sinusoidal signals, known as the Fourier series:

$$V(t) = 4V/\pi \ (\sin 2\pi t + 0.33\sin 6\pi t + 0.20\sin 10\pi t + 0.14\sin 14\pi t + \ldots).$$

The sinusoidal components in the Fourier series constitute the frequency spectrum of the square wave signal. Such a spectrum can be graphically represented in Figure 2, where the horizontal axis represents the frequency in Hz. The lowest nonzero frequency f_0 of the spectrum, in this case equal to 1 Hz, is called the fundamental frequency and the others, which are in multiples of f_0, are called the harmonics. In the case of this square wave signal, the frequency spectrum contains the fundamental frequency and only the odd harmonics (i.e., 3rd, 5th, 7th, etc.).

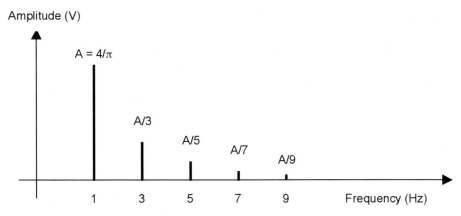

Figure 2. Square Wave (Fig. 1) in Frequency Domain.

Note that the amplitude of the higher harmonics decreases with increasing frequency. In general, harmonics of very low amplitude are insignificant and can be ignored (which means that the signal is considered to have a finite bandwidth).

Figure 3a shows three sinusoidal waveforms of frequencies 1Hz, 3Hz, and 5Hz with amplitudes equal to 1.0, 0.333, and 0.20 V, respectively. The three waveforms can be represented in mathematical form as:

$$V_1 = 1.0\sin(2\pi t)$$
$$V_3 = 0.33\sin(3\pi t)$$
$$V_5 = 0.20\sin(10\pi t)$$

Figure 3b shows the sum of the waveforms $V_1 + V_2$ and Figure 3c shows $V_1 + V_2 + V_3$.

We note that as more waveforms are added together, the more it will resemble a square wave. As it turns out, if we keep adding the higher harmonics, we will eventually get back a perfect square wave like we have seen in Figure 1. This simple example illustrates that a signal in the time domain can be fully represented by its frequency and phase spectrum in the frequency domain (note that we have not discussed the effect of phase shifts of the harmonics).

We have shown that the frequency spectrum for a periodic square wave is composed of discrete frequency components. These frequency components are at multiple frequencies of the fundamental frequency. Other than

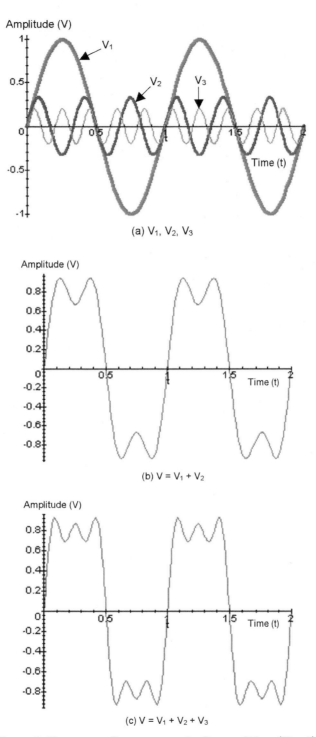

(a) V_1, V_2, V_3

(b) $V = V_1 + V_2$

(c) $V = V_1 + V_2 + V_3$

Figure 3. Frequency Component of a Square Wave (Fig. 1).

periodic signals, Fourier transform may be applied to a nonperiodic function of time. A nonperiodic signal produces a continuous frequency spectrum (instead of a discrete spectrum). That is, unlike the spectrum of a periodic function of time, the frequency spectrum of a nonperiodic waveform spreads over the entire bandwidth, as shown in Figure 4.

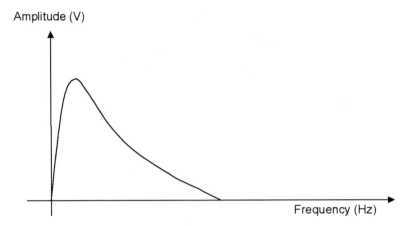

Figure 4. Frequency Spectrum of a Nonperiodic Waveform.

Figure 5 shows a time domain signal of a blood pressure waveform and its frequency spectrum. (Note that the signal has no significant frequency components above 9 Hz and it has a positive amplitude at zero frequency due to a nonzero average pressure in the time domain.)

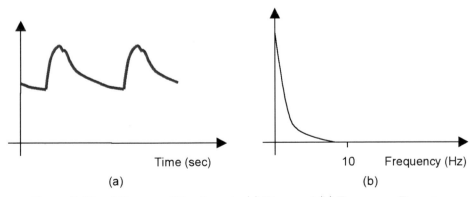

Figure 5. Blood Pressure Waveform in (a) Time and (b) Frequency Domains.

Appendix A–2

OVERVIEW OF MEDICAL
TELEMETRY DEVELOPMENT

1. INTRODUCTION

Purpose

Medical telemetry is defined (by the AHA's Spectrum Selection Workgroup) as

> The wireless transfer of information associated with the measurement, control, and/or recording of physiological parameters and other patient related information between points separated by a distance, usually within the healthcare institution.

Note that the modulated signal can also be transmitted via hard wires such as a telephone network. The most common patient vital sign transmitted in patient monitoring systems is the ECG waveform. Telemetry has substantially reduced the risk to patients who may otherwise require continuous monitoring.

Typically, a telemetry ECG transmitter would be used on a patient who has been released from ICU and is now in a step-down inpatient ward. It is critical for the patient's recovery that they become ambulatory. In the past, without telemetry, this was not possible due to the monitoring requirements.

Advantages in use of telemetry

- Mobility of subject under study or monitor
- Minimal disturbance of routine
- Centralization of expensive equipment (e.g., automatic arrhythmia monitors)

Examples of biomedical applications

- ECG, EEG, Temp., Resp., EMG, pH transmission
- Position localization
- Stimulation via telemetry
- Pacemaker programming and information download
- Transmission of image information over long distances (e.g., teleradiography)

2. PROBLEMS WITH TELEMETRY

Problems with telemetry are primarily related to data rate and reliability. Some factors are:

- Bandwidth requirements
- Channel overcrowding
- EM interference and immunity
- Transmission range
- Power requirement for mobile units (MU)
- CRTC/FCC licensing
- Primary (registered users who have the right to use the bandwidth) versus secondary (users who do not have the exclusive right to use the bandwidth) users

3. DEVELOPMENT AND TREND IN MEDICAL TELEMETRY

Development

Started in the VHF band (174–216 MHz) Using Analog Modulation Techniques

- Migrate to UHF (460–470 MHz) using digital modulation.
- New wireless medical telemetry system (WMTS) bands: 608–614 MHz in 2000, 1,395–1,400 MHz in 2006.
- The 2.4 GHz Industrial, Scientific and Medical (ISM) band limits transmission power and requires users to use spread-spectrum technology. Users are all sharing the bandwidth with equal rights.
- Currently, some manufacturers use the ISM bands; others choose to use the WMTS band.

Medical Telemetry Using General VHF Band

- 174–216 MHz
- Nonprimary user
- Sharing frequencies with other nonmedical users (e.g., TV Channels 7–13)
- Unidirectional
- No voice or video
- Obsolete

Medical Telemetry Using General UHF Band

- 460–470 MHz
- Nonprimary user
- Sharing frequencies with other no-medical users
- Unidirectional
- No voice or video
- Will be phased out

Medical Telemetry using WMTS Band

- 608–614 MHz, 6 MHz bandwidth, and 1,395–1,400 MHz (will expand to include 1,429–1,432 MHz)
- Dedicated band for medical telemetry
- Unidirectional
- No voice or video
- Primary user protected against intentional interference but not out-of-band interference (e.g., EMI sources from other medical or nonmedical devices such as foot massagers)

Medical Telemetry Using ISM Band

- 2.4000–2.4835 GHz, 83.5 MHz bandwidth
- Allow voice and video data (e.g., can use VoIP)
- All users must use spread-spectrum technology
- Wireless Ethernet: IEEE802.11 (a wireless extension of Ethernet: IEEE802.3)
  - 802.11: 2.4 GHz, 1 and 2 Mb/s using DSSS or FHSS
  - 802.11b: 2.4 GHz, 11 Mb/s using DSSS
  - 802.11a: 5.7 GHz, 54 Mb/s using OFDMSS
- WLAN connects to LAN via an access point (AP)

4. SPREAD SPECTRUM TECHNOLOGY

The characteristics of spread-spectrum technology are:

- Use packet (short burst of data) transmission

- Bandwidth of transmitted signal is spread over a much greater bandwidth than the original signal
- 79 channels available in North America (79 × 1 MHz wide channels from 2.402 to 2.480 GHz)
- A two-step modulation process—one modulation step to spread the data and the second step to modulate the spread signal (e.g., the second step uses frequency modulation)
- Increased processing gain
- Robust—high resistance to noise and interference
- Bidirectional—allow data retransmission in case of interference (receive acknowledge). May reduce throughput but ensure data integrity.
- Allow two-way communications
- Low spectral power density: average energy in a specific frequency band is very low; less chance of signals interfering with other systems
- Three methods: direct sequence spread spectrum (DSSS), frequency hopping spread spectrum (FHSS), orthogonal frequency division multiplexing spread spectrum (OFDMSS)

Appendix A–3

MEDICAL GAS SUPPLY SYSTEMS

In a typical acute care hospital, medical gases are available through piped-in wall outlets. A typical operating room is equipped with oxygen, nitrous oxide, medical air, nitrogen gas, and suction outlets on the wall or on the ceiling column. At the bedside of a typical patient ward, oxygen, medical air, and suction are available. Cylinder gases are used to supply some less common gases and also used as backup in case the central supply is interrupted. The pressure for piped-in gas supply is usually about 50 to 55 psig. The absolute pressure of wall suction is usually about 200 mmHg.

Figure 1 shows a typical cryogenic bulk central supply system. During normal operation, gas is drawn from the primary operating supply reservoir. A secondary operating supply reservoir is used when the primary is depleted. The primary reservoir is filled soon after the supply has been switched to the secondary reservoir. To ensure uninterrupted supply, a number of gas cylinders are connected to the central supply line as reserve supply. These cylinders are checked regularly but will not normally be used to supply the system.

Four sizes of gas cylinders are available. The dimensions are tabulated in Table 1.

Table 1.
Gas Cylinder Dimensions

Cylinder Size	Height w/Cap (in.)	Outside Diameter (in.)
D	20	4
E	29	4
M	49	7
H	57	9

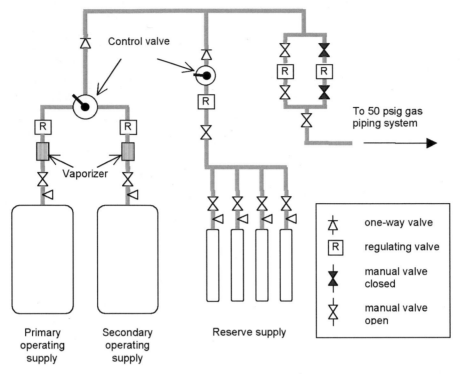

Figure 1. Medical Gas Central Supply System.

Table 2 shows the characteristics of common medical gas cylinders. The pressure at room temperature, capacity (H-cylinder), color coding, and the state of the gas inside the cylinder of the gases are listed.

In order to prevent a wrong medical gas cylinder from being connected to the gas line or the inlet of a device, a pin-indexed safety system (PISS) is used. In this safety system, the stem of a gas cylinder can be allowed to connect only to the cylinder yoke of the same gas. A pin-indexed safety system

Table 2.
Cylinder Data of Common Medical Gases

Gas	Pressure (psig)	Capacity (liters)	State	Color Code
Oxygen	2,217	7,000	Gas	White
Nitrous oxide	745	15,540	Liquid	Blue
Medical air	2,217	6,500	Gas	Black and white
Helium	2,217	8,200	Gas	Brown
Carbon dioxide	838	12,360	Liquid	Gray
Nitrogen	2,217	6,400	Gas	Black

uses a set of pins on the yoke and a set of holes on the stem to encode the medical gases. The cylinder can connect to the yoke only when the pins are at the same matching location as the holes. For the same gas, the location of the pins on the yoke aligns with the locations of the holes on the stem.

A diameter-indexed safety system (DISS) is designed to prevent a wrong hose from being connected to the piped-in outlets. In this system, the diameter of the connector on the flexible hose is encoded together with the connector of the wall outlet for the medical gas. Only the hose connector of the gas can be connected to the piped-in wall gas outlet of the same gas. The flexible hoses are color-coded according to the gases to further minimize connection errors.

INDEX